EVERYDAY LIFE IN THE COVID-19 PANDEMIC

The Mass-Observation Critical Series

The Mass-Observation Critical Series pairs innovative interdisciplinary scholarship with rich archival materials from the original Mass-Observation movement and the current Mass Observation Project. Launched in 1937, the Mass-Observation movement aimed to study the everyday life of ordinary Britons. The Mass Observation Project continues to document and archive the everyday lives, thoughts and attitudes of ordinary Britons to this day. Mass-Observation, as a whole, is an innovative research organization, a social movement, and an archival project that spans much of the 20th and early 21st centuries.

The series makes Mass-Observation's rich primary sources accessible to a wide range of academics and students across multiple disciplines, as well as to the general reading public. Books in the series include re-issues of important original Mass-Observation publications, edited and introduced by leading scholars in the field, and thematically-oriented anthologies of Mass-Observation material. The series also facilitates cutting-edge research by established and new scholars using Mass-Observation resources to present fresh perspectives on everyday life, popular culture and politics, visual culture, emotions, and other relevant topics.

Series Editors:

Jennifer J. Purcell is Professor of History at Saint Michael's College in Vermont, USA. Using Mass-Observation diaries and directives, her first book, *Domestic Soldiers* (2010), seeks to understand the day-to-day lives of six women on the home front during the Second World War. She is also the author of *Mother of the BBC: Mabel Constanduros and the Development of Light Entertainment on the BBC, 1925-1957* (Bloomsbury, 2020).

Benjamin Jones is Lecturer in Modern British History at the University of East Anglia in Norwich, UK. He is the author of *The Working Class in Mid-Twentieth-Century England* (2012), which was positively reviewed in *Sociology, American Historical Review, Journal of Modern History, Journal of British Studies, The Historical Journal, Economic History Review, Contemporary British History, Twentieth Century British History* and *Planning Perspectives*.

Lucy Curzon is Associate Professor of Contemporary and Modern Art History, University of Alabama, USA.

Editorial Board:

Fiona Courage, Head of Special Collections, University of Sussex in Brighton, UK
Claire Langhamer, Director of the Institute of Historical Research, School of Advanced Study, University of London
Jeremy MacClancy, Professor of Anthropology, Oxford Brookes University, UK
Kimberly Mair, Associate Professor of Sociology, University of Lethbridge, Canada
Rebecca Searle, Lecturer in the Humanities, University of Brighton, UK
Matthew Taunton, Lecturer in the School of Literature, Drama and Creative Writing, University of East Anglia, UK

Published Titles:

The Biopolitics of Care in Second World War Britain, Kimberly Mair (2022)
Mass Observers Making Meaning, James Hinton (2022)
Mass-Observation, edited by Jennifer J. Purcell (2023)
Reflections on British Royalty, edited by Edited by Jennifer J. Purcell and Fiona Courage (2024)

EVERYDAY LIFE IN THE COVID-19 PANDEMIC

MASS OBSERVATION'S 12TH MAY DIARIES

Edited by Nick Clarke

BLOOMSBURY ACADEMIC
LONDON • NEW YORK • OXFORD • NEW DELHI • SYDNEY

BLOOMSBURY ACADEMIC
Bloomsbury Publishing Plc
50 Bedford Square, London, WC1B 3DP, UK
1385 Broadway, New York, NY 10018, USA
29 Earlsfort Terrace, Dublin 2, Ireland

BLOOMSBURY, BLOOMSBURY ACADEMIC and the Diana logo are trademarks
of Bloomsbury Publishing Plc

First published in Great Britain 2024

A catalogue record for this book is available from the British Library.

A catalog record for this book is available from the Library of Congress.

ISBN: HB: 978-1-3504-3470-7
PB: 978-1-3504-3469-1
ePDF: 978-1-3504-3471-4
eBook: 978-1-3504-3472-1

Typeset by Deanta Global Publishing Services, Chennai, India
Printed and bound in Great Britain

To find out more about our authors and books visit www.bloomsbury.com and sign up
for our newsletters.

Dedicated to the memory of Clive Barnett (1968–2021)

Diarist 26 (male, 40s, South East England, journalist)

Today marks nearly two months my family and I have spent in 'lockdown' because of the covid-19 pandemic. That means it's been a lot like the last 60 days!

Diarist 602 (female, 50s, Wales, university tutor)

Feed the cat and prepare supper and listen to the news – the death rate has risen again.

Diarist 858 (female, 40s, East Midlands, communications worker)

It's funny how a day can have such a lot in it and yet never leave the confines of the house.

Diarist 1005 (female, 19, West Midlands, student)

History is happening [. . .] all around us as I write this, and as far as crises go it's all so . . . *mundane.*

Diarist 1580 (female, 50s, Yorkshire and Humber, administrative assistant)

We are now in week 8 of 'lockdown', a word which is the 'norm' along with 'pandemic', 'testing' and 'death'. The coronavirus or Covid 19 is the reason.

Diarist 2164 (male, 40s, London, student)

It's strange sometimes, the contrast between everyday normality inside and the knowledge that in houses and flats – even in the same streets – dramas of life and death are being played out.

CONTENTS

Contents

FIGURES

ACKNOWLEDGEMENTS

The idea for this book emerged from research funded by the British Academy Special Research Grants Covid-19 Scheme (grant number COV19\200422: 'Learning to Live with Risk and Responsibility: Understanding Popular Responses to COVID-19'). I was the principal investigator. The co-investigator was Clive Barnett. Clive was a friend, mentor, inspiration and early supporter of the idea behind this book. He died suddenly from a heart attack in December 2021. I've missed him intensely while writing the book, which is dedicated to his memory.

Much of the book is comprised of extracts from diaries collected by the Mass Observation Archive. I'm grateful to the trustees of the MOA, who granted permission to reproduce these extracts (© The Mass Observation Archive). I'm grateful to the archivists, especially Jessica Scantlebury and Kirsty Pattrick, whose expertise and generosity I've now been depending on and benefiting from, on various projects, for almost a decade. I'm also grateful to the diarists themselves. As many scholars of Mass Observation have pointed out, those who write for the archive, whether for the 12th May project or the Mass Observation Project, are not simply 'respondents' or providers of 'data'. They are *correspondents* who shape the archive. They are frontline analysts of their own everyday lives. To my editor, they are the true authors of this book.

My ideas on how to edit the book were developed through a series of engagements during 2020–23. These included: participation in a seminar series on 'Using Mass Observation's COVID-19 collections', which I co-organized with Clive, Jessica and Kirsty; participation in Mass Observation's 85th Anniversary Seminar Series; participation in a session of the RGS-IBG Annual International Conference on 'Governing the COVID-19 pandemic', which I co-organized with Clive; participation in the School of Geography and Environmental Science Seminar Series at the University of Southampton; publication of a special section of *History of the Human Sciences* on 'Archiving the COVID-19 pandemic in Mass Observation and Middletown', which I co-edited with Clive under the expert guidance of Felicity Callard and Rhodri Hayward, two of the journal's editors, and in response to helpful comments from reviewers; and publication of an article on 'Good citizenship during the COVID-19 pandemic' in *Transactions of the Institute of British Geographers*, again under expert editorial guidance (from Matt Sparke) and in response to helpful comments from reviewers.

I discussed early ideas for the book project with Ben Highmore and Nigel Thrift, who kindly provided encouragement and advice. I shared early drafts of material with Ben, Annebella Pollen and James Hinton. The suggestions and questions I received in response helped to shape later drafts, which I think are improvements on earlier drafts, though probably still don't do justice to the comments received from these generous, insightful, critical readers.

After the proposal was submitted to Bloomsbury's Mass-Observation Critical Series, I received further helpful comments, advice and encouragement from the publisher, Rhodri Mogford, the series editors, Jennifer Purcell and Benjamin Jones, and three anonymous reviewers.

I'm very grateful to all these people. And I'm especially grateful to Kath Burton. It helps to live with an experienced publishing professional when preparing a book manuscript for submission! Moreover, during the pandemic, amid the anxiety, cancellations, fear, funerals, grief and guilt – and especially when Clive died – it helped to stay home with someone so attuned to the birdsong. This was my luck during the Covid-19 pandemic.

INTRODUCTION
REMEMBERING THE COVID-19 PANDEMIC

Towards a humanizing and democratic account

How will the Covid-19 pandemic be remembered in the UK? One account is provided by the health sciences, the social sciences and evidence provided to House of Commons committees during 2021.[1] They describe a sequence of events. On 30 December 2019, the Medical Administration of Wuhan Municipal Health Committee posted an alert on ProMED, the Programme for Monitoring Emerging Diseases of the International Society for Infectious Diseases, of 'undiagnosed pneumonia'. Genetic sequencing identified a new coronavirus: SARS-CoV-2 or Covid-19. On 30 January, the World Health Organization announced a Public Health Emergency of International Concern. On 31 January, the first cases in the UK were described. On 11 March, the WHO declared a pandemic.

The UK responded slowly to these events. The government's scientific advisors were cautious, having been accused of overreacting to H1N1 (swine flu) in 2009. Some advocated a strategy of herd immunity by infection – managing the spread, flattening the curve – which may have been appropriate for influenza, but not for Covid-19. Some worried about the UK's capacity for an alternative strategy of test-trace-isolate after a decade of austerity. Some worried about whether such an alternative strategy could work in the UK, given its high degree of international connectivity and supposedly liberal political culture. Leadership from Prime Minister Boris Johnson, who missed numerous key meetings during early 2020, was lacking. The UK eventually went into national lockdown on 23 March, days after most neighbouring countries (when days mattered because cases were doubling every few days). Support and compliance from citizens were high – at least initially, until late May when the messaging changed (from 'stay home' to 'stay alert') and reports emerged that Dominic Cummings, the prime minister's chief advisor, had broken lockdown rules (yet retained Johnson's support and would continue in post).

In the first months of the pandemic, the UK's performance was comparatively poor. In May 2020, as the first lockdown was lifted, the UK had 180 excess deaths per 100,000 people – one of the worst performances in the world, suggesting that many of these deaths were avoidable. There were particularly bad outcomes for certain groups: people in care homes, to which patients were discharged from hospitals without adequate testing and isolation; ethnic minorities, for whom mortality rates were higher than expected; women, who shouldered more of the additional caring responsibilities generated by the pandemic; and young people, who lost education and employment opportunities during this period. As the pandemic proceeded, however, the UK at least performed well in developing and delivering treatments and vaccines. In December 2020, the UK became the first Western country to approve a vaccine.

This account will be expanded and firmed up by the UK Covid-19 Inquiry, an independent public inquiry launched in June 2022, with public hearings scheduled for June 2023 to summer 2026, aiming to provide a 'factual narrative account' of the pandemic in the UK covering preparations, response, impact and lessons. Perhaps one outcome of that inquiry will be an official national memorial to those who lost their lives due to Covid-19. There is no such memorial at the time of writing. There are numerous local memorials, though, and there is an unofficial national memorial (the National Covid Memorial Wall) alongside St Thomas's Hospital, across the Thames from the Palace of Westminster. On this Memorial Wall, established by Covid-19 Bereaved Families for Justice with support from campaigners Led by Donkeys, each hand-painted heart is meant to represent one death.

The future of this Memorial Wall is uncertain, much like the outcome of the public inquiry. What can be said now is that we need ways of remembering the pandemic in the UK that fall between the 'factual narrative account' of a public inquiry and the (potentially powerful, but necessarily limited) representation of a memorial. Such a need has been articulated by Richard Horton, editor-in-chief of *The Lancet*. In 2020, reflecting on how the pandemic was described and reported, he wrote:[2]

> This was a pandemic that was described and reported in terms of statistics – numbers of infections, numbers of patients in critical care and numbers of deaths. Lives were transformed into mathematical summaries. Graphs of the epidemic were drawn. And countries were compared for their rates of mortality.
>
> But those who died cannot and should not be summarised. They must not become lines on squared paper. They must not become mere rates used to argue differences between nations. Every death counts. A person who died in Wuhan is as important as one who died in New York. Our way of describing the impact of the pandemic erased the biographies of the dead. The science and politics of COVID-19 became exercises in radical dehumanisation.

Later in the same book, *The COVID-19 Catastrophe*, Horton asks:[3]

> So what must we say about the politics of COVID-19? We must say, I think, that it is our task to uncover the biographies of those who have lived and died with COVID-19. It is our task to resist the biologicalisation of this disease and instead to insist on a social and political critique. It is our task to understand what this disease means to the lives of those it has afflicted and to use that understanding not only to change our perspective on the world but also to change the world itself.

These words carry particular weight because of their author's central position in the health sciences – the world of biology, epidemiology and statistics. Horton's call – for 'biographies of those who had lived and died with COVID-19' and a better understanding of 'what this disease means to the lives of those it has afflicted' – cannot be answered fully by inquiries or memorials. Hopefully, though, it can be answered by books like the present one, at least in part.

The purpose of this book is to provide an alternative account of the Covid-19 pandemic as it was experienced in the UK, as a supplement to the statistics, mathematical summaries, graphs and comparisons between countries available elsewhere. It is to provide a *humanizing* account, concerned with understanding what the pandemic meant to those living (and dying) through it. The purpose of this book is also to provide a *democratic* account of the pandemic, concerned with capturing the multiple perspectives and voices of people across the UK – with capturing everyday life in the pandemic, described by ordinary people in their own terms. Such an account is made possible by Mass Observation's Covid-19 collections and especially the 5,000 day-diaries MO collected on, or soon after, 12 May 2020.

Mass Observation's 12th May projects

The original M-O (with a hyphen) existed in the 1930s and 1940s. It was founded in 1937 as part of a world of early social investigation, survey research and market research (think: Booth, Rowntree, the New Fabien Research Bureau, the Pilgrim Trust, Political and Economic Planning, Gallup's British Institute of Public Opinion).[4] Its three main founders gave M-O a distinctive character: the anthropologist Tom Harrisson; the journalist, poet and surrealist Charles Madge; and Madge's fellow surrealist, the artist and film-maker Humphrey Jennings. All three were interested in mass culture, which they researched using volunteer observers, initially via Harrisson's Worktown Project (focused on Bolton, where a team of observers reported on what they saw of everyday life in the town) and Madge's National Panel (managed from London, but involving panellists spread across the UK, who kept diaries and answered occasional sets of questions – known as 'directives' – about themselves, their lives and those close to them). Later, during the Second World War, M-O took commissions from the Ministry of Information. This is what the original M-O is probably best known for today: research on morale for the Home Intelligence Division during the Second World War.

The original M-O fizzled out in the late 1940s. Its papers are archived at the University of Sussex, Brighton. Since being founded in 1975, this Mass Observation Archive (MOA) has evolved from an archive focused on the original M-O to a research organization with its own active research projects.[5] One project of this contemporary MO is the Mass Observation Project (MOP), established in 1981 and still going strong, inspired by Madge's National Panel and involving hundreds of volunteer writers across the UK responding to directives every four months or so. This MOP is the longest-running and best-known project of the contemporary MO, and it overlaps with other projects in so far as members of the panel (the contemporary Mass Observers) often contribute writing to other projects too. However, the basis for the present book is another project of the contemporary MO: the 12th May project. This was established in 2010 and

involves the collection of day-diaries annually on 12 May from people across the UK –
Mass Observers who write regularly for the MOP, but also anyone who hears about the
project from news or social media in the days and weeks before 12 May each year. This
particular research project was inspired by *May the Twelfth*, one of the first publications
of the original M-O.[6]

May the Twelfth was focused on 12 May 1937, the day of the Coronation of George
VI. Madge organized observers to report on the ceremony, procession and speeches –
and associated broadcasts – and their reception by ordinary people. The idea was to
produce a street-level view of the day, a contrast to the official record of the day that
would puncture the official rhetoric of national unity.[7] Jennings edited the observers'
reports using techniques from surrealist film: montage, collage, juxtaposition, close-ups
and long shots, detail and ensemble. The effect is that no single clear image or narrative
whole is presented.[8] Instead, we get fragments, partial perspectives, different points of
focus and different voices allowed to speak for themselves. For anthropologist David
Pocock, a director of the MOA, 'The very lack of analytic commentary has the effect
of putting the reader there, as though he or she were watching from the top of a slow-
moving bus, sitting in the corner of the public bar, strolling through the street.'[9] For
cultural theorist Ben Highmore, a trustee of the MOA, the effect of so many perspectives
and voices, presented with so little mediation, is a portrait of society as multiple, diverse,
complex, contradictory, eccentric:[10]

> Day-surveys took the basis of commonality (everyone experienced the same day,
> the same coronation) to emphasise the diversity of the lives being lived. It is the
> mixture of diversity and commonality (diversity as commonality) that I think is
> particularly important to Mass-Observation, and crucial to its understanding of
> everyday life. What continually needs asserting is the historical context of these
> experiments – crucially, their critically dialogic response to the image of society
> where diversity was being brutally and systematically eradicated (Nazi Germany),
> in comparison to their political support for the Popular Front and the possibilities
> of a consensus of radically different political positions against a common enemy.
> How Mass-Observation translates this is in the practice of promoting a 'totality
> of fragments', of a society 'united' by a heterogeneous everyday, a commonality of
> diversity. What remained was how to find a form for producing such an image of
> society.

May the Twelfth was M-O's attempt to find a form for producing this image of society as a
totality of fragments. It was a 'collective poem', 'a giant cubist account of a historical event
– history not just seen from "below" but seen from every conceivable (and inconceivable)
angle'.[11] It was M-O's attempt to confront myths of 'the people', elite representations of
the masses in Parliament and the new mass media, with the 'heterogeneous actuality' of
people.[12]

When the contemporary MO established its own 12th May project in 2010, a
similarly populist historical context was just around the corner. In the following years,

however, the project received only a small number of day-diaries (in the low hundreds) in response to annual calls made via news and social media. Then 12 May 2020 came around and something changed. With many people confined at home due to the Covid-19 pandemic, with time on their hands and sensing they were living through events of historical significance (perhaps in the same way the original Mass Observers had lived through the Second World War), the MOA received 5,000 diaries in response to its call. These diaries form the basis for the rest of this book, which is itself inspired by the original *May the Twelfth* book and the project behind it.

Introducing the diarists and diaries

So who are these diarists and what can their day-diaries tell us about the Covid-19 pandemic? Like any contributors to MO, whether the original M-O or the contemporary MO, they are a particular group of people by definition. They are volunteers. Beyond this basic starting point, however, we can say that among the 5,000 diarists who responded on 12 May 2020 can be found a wide range of positions, experiences and voices. Roughly a third are of working age, with a third of retirement age (including the odd diarist in their nineties) and a third of school age (including some diarists of primary school age). All genders, regions and occupational classifications are covered. To ensure I captured this wide range, and because of the sheer volume of material in the archive, I sampled 10 per cent of the diaries (500 of the 5,000) for this project. This allowed me to fill quotas for age, gender, region and occupation, as well as include recommendations from the archivists of diarists who seemed particularly interesting, reflective, articulate or notable in some other way. Of course, it also means this book presents only a small part of MO's vast Covid-19 collections.

One thing I was unable to do was to fill quotas for race or ethnicity. MO did not start collecting information about ethnicity – or sexuality, disability and religion – until 2021. There are complex reasons for this, but it fits the history of MO, which has long been characterized by whiteness.[13] In their founding pamphlet, Madge and Harrisson described the original M-O as 'the anthropology of whites',[14] by whom they appear to have meant people in Britain, assumed to be white and assumed to be different in this respect from the usual subjects of anthropology at the time. These assumptions carried through into the kinds of questions asked of Mass Observers; for example, questions about racialized others – especially Jewish people (a topic of particular interest in the late 1930s in the context of rising Fascism and anti-Semitism in Europe).[15]

My sampling exercise, then, did not leave me with a set of diarists formally representative of the UK population. We can assume that white people are over-represented – since attempts by MO in recent decades to diversify its correspondents have met with only partial success[16] – though we can't be sure, and some of the diaries do appear to be from people of colour. From the metadata collected by MO, we can be sure that certain other groups are slightly over-represented: women; teenagers and people in their fifties and sixties; people from South East England; and people with professional and associate professional and technical occupations. We can also be sure that certain groups are slightly under-represented: men; people in their twenties; people from the West Midlands; process, plant and machine operatives; and people with elementary occupations. Nevertheless, the sampling exercise did generate a wide range of diarists in at least some respects. The diarists quoted in this book include the usual suspects: those more likely to be aware of and interested in MO (archivists, academics, students, teachers) and those with time to volunteer (especially retirees). However, they also include many other people, positions and voices: bereavement services managers, cabin crew members, carers, chaplains, church ministers, cleaners, company directors, customs officers, delivery drivers, diplomats, doctors, electricians, engineers, farmers, finance managers, funeral celebrants, garage forecourt workers, hairdressers, midwives, nurses, online retail workers, painters and decorators, publicans, priests, sales assistants, sex workers, vicars.

It should also be noted that demographic characteristics only tell us so much about people's lived experiences during the pandemic anyway. Rather than describing diarists by their occupation, for example, often it makes more sense to describe them in other ways: as the daughter with a mother whose dementia has been getting worse during the period of lockdown; or the child whose mother has been in intensive care for three weeks with Covid-19; or the recently self-employed person who fell through the cracks of the various government support schemes (eligible for neither furlough nor self-employed income support); or the person living apart from their partner, who last saw them physically more than two months ago; or the woman who took a risk and moved into her new partner's one-bedroom flat just a couple of days before lockdown began; or the child whose father is not currently living at home because he is a consultant cardiologist fearful of bringing the virus home from work. These are all positions – with associated experiences and voices – included in the sample.

It should also be noted that many diarists, in the tradition of MO, wrote about not only their own day (and its context) but also the days of others they observed – on the street, at the supermarket or via news and social media. Also in the tradition of MO, which guarantees contributors anonymity while granting them space and time to express themselves (and encourages them to do so), many diarists wrote in particularly thoughtful and frank ways. Therefore, instead of thinking of MO materials as less helpful in understanding experiences of the pandemic than survey, focus group or social media data – because of concerns about representativeness – we might think of MO materials as being *more* helpful because of their *quality*. In the 12th May diaries, we see evidence of serious interpretive work: 'I have spent time reflecting on this and I think I feel this way because [. . .]' (Diarist 479). And we see evidence of serious expressive work: 'I feel quite detached from this description as I'm writing, as it doesn't fully convey the fear, dread and horror I've been experiencing the last two months' (2957). Diarists often took care to reflect and interpret, and to capture reflections and interpretations in their writing.

Also in the diaries, we see what appears to be frankness, honesty and full disclosure by many diarists. They tell us their secrets: 'I practised the piano in secret for a few minutes [. . .] Starting again at the piano makes me confront one of several failed careers, and a lot of bad memories. I don't want my parents to hear me' (2627). They tell us things they would not have the courage to say in other settings: 'My friend has taken to chanting "PPE, PPE" [Personal Protective Equipment] during the Thursday Night Clap, and I wish I were brave enough to do the same' (2394); 'I daren't admit to liking lockdown in any public arena [. . .] as it feels so wrong when people are dying in their thousands' (1122). They tell us things they have not told their closest loved ones: 'Today makes it 58 days since I've seen the face I love in front of me [. . .] He doesn't even know I love him; well I think he does. But we've never said it out loud' (200); 'My children are adamant that I should not go out at all, anywhere [. . .] I do not tell them about my shopping trips' (3210). And some diarists lay themselves bare for us: 'I found myself in a moment yesterday where I didn't even know how to feel anymore. I sat in the bath and cried so hard I couldn't breathe' (14); 'Writing this now, I am flooding with tears' (2205); 'So now I'm [. . .] crying over the keyboard' (1289).

These are all lines that appear in diary extracts included later in the book, where fuller contexts for these lines can be found. They suggest that MO diaries might open a unique and valuable window into everyday life during the pandemic. They may not be as representative or numerous as poll results or social media posts, which others may choose to analyse. But the representativeness of MO diaries should not be underestimated, just as that of polling or social media should not be overestimated. And the unique value of MO diaries should be recognized. They allow correspondents time, space and anonymity, which in turn encourage thoughtfulness, interpretation and apparent honesty – including regarding polling results and social media posts encountered during the pandemic (on which, see Anxiety, Lockdown projects, Stay alert, Stay apart, Stay home and, of course, WhatsApp).

What of the fact that such diaries were kept on one particular day (12 May 2020 – the focus of this book) in one particular place (the UK – when a pandemic, by definition, is global or at least multinational)? We have seen how the UK's experience of the pandemic was particular. It responded slowly to events in early 2020. It was not a country that prioritized test-trace-isolate. It locked down relatively late compared to neighbouring countries. The UK's response to the pandemic was quite different from those Asian countries with recent experience of SARS and MERS.[17] We have also seen how the UK's experience of the pandemic developed over time. Its performance, measured by excess deaths, was relatively poor in the early stages of the pandemic (including the period around 12 May 2020). Later, during much of 2021, its performance was better – exemplary even – if measured by development and delivery of vaccines and treatments.

So the diaries capture life in a particular place (the UK) on a particular day (a Tuesday towards the end of the UK's first national lockdown). But they capture so much more than that. They capture much that was shared among people across the world during the early stages of the pandemic: uncertainty over what was happening and how to respond; fear of the virus and its potential consequences; policy responses including elements of quarantine, test-trace-isolate, lockdown and PPE. And many of the diaries look forward beyond 12 May 2020, describing plans, hopes and fears for the future, and back over previous days, weeks and months (the road to 12 May 2020). In these respects, the diaries capture much of everyday life in the pandemic for millions of people in the UK and beyond: the activities, events and rituals of pandemic life (birdsong, cancellations, clap for carers, deliveries, funerals, home schooling, lockdown projects, PE or physical education, (dog) walking, working from home); the sites or stages on which everyday life played out during the pandemic (homes, shops, WhatsApp, Zoom); the roles or subject positions offered by the pandemic (furloughed workers, key workers, shielding or vulnerable people); the frames in which the pandemic was viewed (luck, the new normal); and the moods of the pandemic (anxiety, fear, gratitude, grief, guilt, hope). The rest of this book contains chapters on each of these items. It is worth noting that other items were included in earlier drafts, which far exceeded the publisher's word limit: baking, boredom, facemasks, gardens, grandchildren, hair (and teeth), hugging, neighbours, war.

In the tradition of MO, which has been interested in dreams ever since the original M-O was influenced by Surrealism and psychoanalysis, the diaries capture both conscious and unconscious responses to the pandemic (not least in reports of dreams). Overall, the diaries capture responses of people to the pandemic, to news of the pandemic, to new government regulations and guidance and to changes in their lives as a consequence of the pandemic. They depict: what people did; where they did it; in what capacity they did it; how they thought about it, interpreted it, gave it meaning; and how they felt about it. In the diaries, we see the strategies and tactics people used to make it through the pandemic and to help others make it through. We see both *how the nation responded* and *the nation who responded*.

Record, archive, museum, exhibition: How to narrate a pandemic?

The rest of this book is made up of extracts from diaries, arranged in chapters or 'entries'. The entries were derived from my initial reading of the diaries. They seek to capture the main topics diarists wrote about on 12 May 2020. The entries are arranged alphabetically, like an encyclopedia, to avoid imposing my own hierarchy and classification on these topics, and to allow for a multiplicity of connections or 'cross-references' between them. The extracts making up these entries were selected to illustrate the range of ways diarists treated each topic. Many extracts are therefore necessarily short in order to accommodate the full range within the word limit, but some are longer, either because such length was needed for them to stand alone and make sense to the reader, or because they include description and interpretation that seemed particularly important to the humanizing purpose of my account. Within entries, the extracts are arranged numerically by the code given to diaries by MO (based on the order in which diaries are received and processed) – again, to avoid imposing my own hierarchy and classification, and also because doing so worked to set up associations and juxtapositions I may have otherwise missed. I have included a small number of images where they were used by diarists to illustrate text included here as extracts. For readers interested in a fuller treatment of the many images collected by MO during the pandemic, I recommend the work of Annebella Pollen, professor of visual and material culture at the University of Brighton.[18] Finally, regarding the diarists and extracts, I've labelled them using the highest level of metadata collected by MO: age group, gender, region and occupation. MO does collect more detail about individual diarists (e.g. locality or age to the nearest year), especially when they are panellists for the MOP (for which MO collects marital status and living arrangements too) – and this detail no doubt would help readers to make their own interpretations of the extracts – but publishing diary extracts from just a few years ago, and from a traumatic period for many people, demands a cautious approach to research ethics. I have erred on the side of redacting any details likely to identify individual diarists, in order to preserve their anonymity as much as possible.

More justification for these editorial decisions is provided in the rest of this introductory chapter and in the concluding essay ('Presenting everyday life'), but now let us turn to the following question: If the rest of this book is made up of diary extracts arranged in such a way, then what kind of book does this make? What is it trying to achieve and by what means? At its simplest, this book is a record of what people wrote about when they wrote about everyday life during the pandemic. It is a record of what they found notable at the time. In this regard, some themes of note are perhaps unsurprising, for example funerals or grief. Other themes, however, were perhaps less predictable, for example birdsong or luck.

This book might also be approached as an 'archive of feelings'. The term comes from Ann Cvetkovich, director of the Pauline Jewett Institute of Women's and Gender Studies at Carleton University in Ottawa. She documented the experiences of, ways of thinking about and responses to sexual trauma found at sites of lesbian public culture in late twentieth-century America.[19] She did this partly to stop these responses from being lost or misrepresented, to keep them alive, to make them visible. The book she produced from that project, *An Archive of Feelings*, is both an archive itself – an assembly of texts and associated practices that act as repositories of the feelings and emotions making up queer cultures – and an analysis of that archive. Similarly, the present book, *Everyday Life in the Covid-19 Pandemic*, aims to archive experiences of, ways of thinking about and responses to the pandemic (found in diaries kept for MO) – not least to stop these responses from being lost or misrepresented – and to provide a first, light-touch analysis of this archive. As historian and MOA trustee Clare Langhamer has argued, using MO to generate an archive of feelings, or treating MO itself as an archive of feelings, is appropriate.[20] Throughout its history, in both its original and contemporary forms, MO has asked contributors to write about their feelings at least as much as their actions or thoughts. Researchers have then used MO materials to access the emotional worlds of ordinary people, including individual experience, its narration and the emotional norms and styles of particular historical moments or periods. This book aims for something similar: a portrait of the emotional worlds of the pandemic, including its emotional norms and styles. In Raymond Williams's terms, it aims to capture the pandemic's 'structure of feeling': its lived experience, practical consciousness and emerging style (language, keywords, manners).[21]

This book might also be approached as a museum or exhibition of pandemic 'civilization'. The model here is historian Karl Schlögel's recent book, *The Soviet Century*.[22] He was interested in the Soviet Union less as a political system and more as a civilization: a lifeworld; a set of values, practices, routines, manners, styles, biographies and institutions. His methods were those of the flâneur and the archaeologist. He followed clues, rescued objects, catalogued fragments. *The Soviet Century* is a mosaic, a picture of the Soviet world, created from these fragments. It contains sixty individual studies covering such topics as bazaars, medals, tattoos, graffiti, wrapping paper, perfume, cookbooks, doorbells, toilets, kitchens, parks, books, borders, parades, queues, athletes and telephones, arranged in eighteen sections covering such categories as signs, interiors, landscapes, rituals and bodies. Schlögel's aim was to present a museum or exhibition of Soviet civilization. He sees the book as 'an invitation; people can follow their curiosity, inclinations, their own interests. Visitors roam around autonomously, more as if through a labyrinth than in a linear fashion.'[23] My own aims are similar. I'm interested in the lifeworld of the pandemic; its values, practices, manners, and so on. The present book is a catalogue of fragments from the pandemic; a mosaic; a museum or exhibition of pandemic civilization – in which readers might 'roam around autonomously'.

Record, archive, museum, exhibition. Most importantly, this book aims to provide an account of the Covid-19 pandemic as it impacted the lives of ordinary people in the UK. The book, we might say, is an attempt to narrate the pandemic; to tell its story. Narrating a pandemic, though, is not a straightforward exercise. The book, therefore, is an experiment in doing this, inspired by a tradition of experimental writing about pandemics.

In *Pale Rider*, her book about the Spanish Flu of 2018, science journalist Laura Spinney wrote:[24]

> The First World War dragged on for four long years, but despite its name, the bulk of the action was concentrated in European and Middle Eastern theatres [. . .] The war had a geographical focus, in other words, and a narrative that unfolded in time. The Spanish flu, in contrast, engulfed the entire globe in the blink of an eye. Most of the death occurred in the thirteen weeks between mid-September and mid-December 1918. It was broad in space and shallow in time, compared to a narrow, deep war.

Her point is that pandemics are not easy to narrate. The dead are not easy to count – unlike war, where they tend to be uniformed, wounded and confined to the battlefield. The experience for most people is mundane: a mild illness. Pandemics lack narrative structure – again, unlike wars with their declarations, acts of bravery, truces, and so on. Whereas wars tend to be geographically focused and unfold over time, so tend to be narrow and deep – a particular shape that lends itself to narration – pandemics tend to be global in scope and relatively fast in pace, so tend to be broad and shallow (a shape less compatible with narrative story-telling). Political scientist Ivan Krastev has developed this point:[25]

The relationship between the epidemic and war resembles the relationship between some modernist literature and the classical novel. The strangeness of the pandemic experience is that everything changes but nothing happens. We are asked to save humanity by staying home and washing our hands.

The challenge posed by Spinney and Krastev is this: How to account for – to construct an account of – a pandemic that lacks conventional narrative structure and where so much experience is mundane?

Experimental, non-linear accounts of past pandemics

To account for such a pandemic, inspiration can be taken from experimental, non-linear accounts of past pandemics. An immediate example is provided by Spinney herself. Her account of the Spanish flu covers how it emerged, swept the planet and receded, but pauses frequently to consider how it affected particular communities. Her 'biography' of the pandemic is built from a series of 'portraits' depicting communities and their experiences. Other examples are provided by some of the most influential accounts we have of pandemics – whether actual historical events or fictional plagues used as allegories. In her introduction to the Penguin Classics edition, Cynthia Wall discusses the non-linear structure of Defoe's *Journal of the Plague Year*:[26]

This work has been often criticised for its apparent wanderings, its 'non-linear' plot. We are constantly distracted by the Narrator's digressions: he begins one story only to tell another, and then goes back to the first. But two patterns emerge that make sense of this wandering. First, we see H. F. [the narrator] in search of meaning, looking for reliable *signs* – signs of plague, signs of wellness, signs of truth, signs of streets. How do we know what we know; how do we know where we are? How do we learn to *read*? By going back over the signs and the stories – and over and over again. Second, the way H. F. tells his story echoes not only his own movements – shutting himself up, wandering out again insatiably, shutting himself up again nervously and darting out again – but *also* the behaviour of people forcibly 'shut up' by officials into quarantine and endlessly, ingeniously escaping, *and* the movements of the plague itself, swelling and ebbing, encroaching and retreating.

Defoe provides 'the most reliable and comprehensive account of the Great Plague that we possess',[27] but he does so by unconventional means. He captures the *feeling* of the plague by wandering over it, back and forth, just as it wandered over London. As Anthony Burgess noted in his introduction (to an earlier edition – the Penguin English Library edition), Defoe also captures the feeling of the plague in writing that 'interposes the thinnest fabric between the reader and the event'.[28] Loose sentences accumulate, not knowing when to finish, piling up 'a succession of events', giving the effect of 'the real world taking control'. These lines from Burgess remind us of David Pocock's comment on Jennings and Madge's *May the Twelfth*: the style, with its purposeful lack of analytical commentary, 'has the effect of putting the reader there'.

Another example is provided by Camus's *The Plague*. The narrator chronicles events drawing on his own testimony, that of others, some written texts and especially the notebooks of one character, Jean Tarrou:[29]

> His notebooks also constitute a sort of chronicle of that difficult period – though this is a very peculiar type of chronicle in that it seems to adopt a deliberate policy of insignificance. At first sight you might think that Tarrou had gone out of his way to view people and things through the large end of the telescope. In short, in the midst of this general confusion, he determined to become the historian of that which has no history. Of course one may deplore this bias and suspect that it derives from some dryness of heart. But the fact remains that, as a chronicle of the time, these notebooks can give us a mass of details which are none the less important. Indeed, their very oddity will prevent us from being too hasty in passing judgement on this interesting character.

Tarrou viewed events 'through the large end of the telescope'. He was 'the historian of that which has no history' (the mundane experience – the staying home and washing hands – that characterizes pandemics for most people). He compiled 'a mass of details', including via 'a minute description of one day in the plague-ridden town, so giving an accurate idea of how our fellow-citizens lived and spent their time during that summer'.[30] Here, we cannot help but think of MO's day-surveys, including the day-diaries kept on 12 May 2020. In doing all this, for Camus's narrator, 'Tarrou was the person who gave the most accurate picture of our life as it was then.'[31]

In his afterword to the Penguin Classics edition, Tony Judt agrees that Tarrou's notebooks, and by extension *The Plague*, provide an accurate picture of pandemic life, even when in service to Camus's allegory (indeed, the allegory works so well precisely because pandemic life is depicted so convincingly).[32] Judt reminds us that Camus wrote *The Plague* just after the Second World War to puncture the myths already solidifying in French society regarding the German occupation. An official version of events was in the process of airbrushing uncomfortable memories. A myth of glorious national resistance was being cultivated by politicians and the compromises of the occupation were being forgotten. In this context, Camus wished to push beyond the myth of heroism developing in post-war France. He 'abhorred the tone of moral superiority' of the Resisters. One purpose of writing *The Plague* was to show up the moral ambiguities of the situation. Camus's chosen structure and style helped in this regard. Myths, official versions of events and rushed (moral) judgements were difficult to sustain in the face of Tarrou's 'mass of details' and 'minute description'.

A final example of non-linear writing about pandemics (or epidemics), from which I've taken inspiration, is American writer Jan Zita Grover's 'AIDS: Keywords'.[33] Grover, of course, was inspired in turn by Raymond Williams and sought to identify the neologisms, adaptations, alterations, extensions and transfers that appeared at the straining points between old and new relationships during the 1980s in relation to AIDS. These 'keywords' would tell of such straining points and relationships, acting as indicators of social and historical shifts.[34] Recently, inspired by Grover themselves, John Nguyet Erni and Ted Striphas have suggested some 'COVID keywords' (as editors of a special issue of *Cultural Studies* on 'The cultural politics of COVID-19'):[35]

> *antibodies; Asians; asymptomatic; balcony; Black; border; boredom; care; China; conspiracy; climate change; contact tracing; community; coronavirus; cross-species transmission; droplets; essential; flattening the curve; freedom; gym etiquette; hate speech; herd; home; immunity; isolation; isopropyl alcohol; lockdown; long COVID; mask; N95/KN95; pandemic; personal protective equipment; police; quarantine; rapid testing; race/racism; remote; resilience; r-naught (R0); SARS-COV-2; shame; social distancing; solidarity; superspreader; supply chain fragility; toilet rolls; touch; vaccine (nationalism); variant; ventilator; virus; wet market; work from home; Zoom; zoonosis.*

Note the overlap between this list and the contents page of the present book (work from home, Zoom) but also the variation between the two. Such a comparison emphasizes how portraits of the pandemic express particular perspectives (in the case of this book, a perspective from the UK, perhaps from MO and perhaps from myself as author/editor), while at the same time, to some extent, capturing something more universally relevant.

In writing this book, I've sought to apply lessons from all these examples. I've sought: to capture the pandemic's broad and shallow shape (by focusing on experiences from across the UK of just one day: 12 May 2020); to interpose the thinnest fabric between reader and event (by including extracts from diaries with little surrounding framing and interpretation); to include a variety of testimonies, a mass of minor details and the compromises and moral ambiguities of the pandemic (in the spirit of Camus); and to identify my own set of Covid keywords (from 'anxiety' to 'Zoom').

To be clear, I view these examples as exemplars: models of experimental writing about pandemics, guides to the narration of pandemics, containing elements worth imitating. I am claiming this tradition as inspiration. I am not claiming a place in this tradition for the present book, or at least more than a very minor place. The same applies to the tradition of experimental writing discussed in the concluding chapter, from which I've also sought to apply lessons: non-linear accounts of everyday life. This latter tradition takes influences from psychoanalysis and Surrealism and includes modernist literature of the 1920s; avant-garde social and cultural studies of the 1930s and 1940s; experimental literature of the 1970s and 1980s; experimental history, geography and related studies from around the turn of the twenty-first century; and recent attempts to advance and reflect on such works. The concluding chapter is an academic essay using everyday life studies to clarify the present book's contributions and limitations. Here, in the next two paragraphs, let me briefly state the lessons I've taken from non-linear accounts of everyday life:

When selecting diaries and extracts, focus on a single day to emphasize simultaneity. Focus on daily life, the everyday, the ordinary, the banal. Focus on the street level and the unofficial view. Include the usually ignored, overlooked, forgotten. Include events, actions, thoughts, feelings. Include sights, sounds, smells, tastes, textures. Include multiple voices and testimonies. Include contradictions and paradoxes. Include the serious and the playful. See 'flatly' – inclusively, democratically, without hierarchy.[36]

When composing selected extracts, don't aim for a single image, narrative whole or coherent argument. Don't privilege a particular voice. Write flatly, with a weak authorial voice – with minimal analytical commentary, in-depth interpretation, mediation between reader and extract – to put the reader there, to achieve graphicness and vividness, to communicate feeling and experience. Choose presentation over representation, surface over depth. Choose showing over telling. Let the extracts be the main work. Present a chorus or cacophony of voices; a democracy of voices. Allow fragments, moments and images to capture the crystal, signature or essence of the total event (as 'illuminations').[37] Allow the material to build, but also to disrupt arguments. To set up vibrations, use the devices of Surrealism: montage, collage, juxtaposition, close-ups and long shots. Use the devices of encyclopedias: multiple entries, arranged non-hierarchically, connected by cross-references. Aim for the collective, cubist poem read by Highmore in M-O's original *May the Twelfth*.[38]

User's manual

If M-O's original *May the Twelfth* is one model for this project, then another is Hans Ulrich Gumbrecht's *In 1926*.[39] Gumbrecht begins his attempt to conjure the worlds of 1926 – a random year, chosen for experimental purposes – with a 'User's Manual' addressing such topics as 'Where to start'. In doing so, he doesn't cite Georges Perec, but the connection suggests itself. Perec's *Life: A User's Manual* begins on the stairs of 11 Rue Simon-Crubellier, Paris, before taking us into the different apartments and rooms of that single building (via ninety-nine chapters in six parts), before offering us other ways through the book in a series of appendices: an 'Index', a 'Chronology', an 'Alphabetic Checklist'.[40] It therefore seems appropriate to finish this introductory chapter with my own user's manual for the present book.

How should readers use this book? I recommend starting where you want, with whatever entries interest you the most, following the cross-references between entries and finding your own way through the book. I recommend choosing your own balance between coherence, provided by summary paragraphs at the top of each entry, and incoherence, or the voices of the diarists, which can stand without my summary paragraphs.

I recommend reading across the entries and extracts for the general feel of the pandemic as it affected the UK, but also pausing on some of the close-ups, in which particular experiences illuminate this general feel. I have in mind here the diarist who reports a row between her partner and son, which develops into a row between her partner and herself, which ends with her 'sitting in the bushes in our local park, weeping' (1979). Or the diarist, aged thirteen, who spends lockdown following the nesting of a swan at the local canal and reports the arrival of cygnets in ecstatic terms (3552). Or the diarist 'trawling the internet for jokes' to send her friend's little boy who cannot be told his birthday is coming up because he wouldn't understand why he couldn't have a party (4688). Or the diarist who describes attending her Great Aunt's funeral on Zoom and then being suddenly back in her living room, 'which is also my office, kitchen, dining room, laundry room, and yoga studio, by turns. I found the emotional whiplash of this very intense. So I cried for a little longer and talked aloud to my Great Aunt' (1940). Or the diarist who writes at length about her grandfather's funeral, the social distancing required, what was allowed and not allowed, the effects on her family and letting the dog out of the car 'so that my nurse sister could hug her, since she didn't have another person to comfort her' (4269). Or the diarist grieving his wife who died of Covid-19 only four weeks ago (759). Or the publican who recounts how one of her regulars came to the pub during lockdown because his sister had just died, he needed company and comfort and didn't know where else to go (1352).

I also have in mind the diarist grieving her daughter-in-law who died of Covid-19 – praying, feeling guilty, 'walking to' the corner of the university garden where there's a bench tucked away so no one walks by to disturb my thoughts', crying (1602). And the diarist, aged twelve, whose mother has Covid-19, who is waiting to hear the results of her mother's CT scan, who wants to cuddle her mother and tell her everything will be alright but is not allowed near (3009). And the diarist who describes her day as a community health worker, driving from client to client, repeatedly washing her hands, eating her lunch on the road, getting paid by the minute (3569). And the diarist suffering from long Covid, who describes her suffering in detail (3150). And the diarist who can't visit her husband in the nursing home, who can only waive to him through the window, before walking on the local beach and crying (4054). And the diarist arguing with her husband, who is meant to be shielding, about whether relaxation of lockdown means he can play golf or not; worried about him and feeling guilty both for worrying too much and not worrying enough (529). And the diarist who writes about the sexual health clinic she runs and the people who come for treatment having broken lockdown rules, used online apps to meet sexual partners and put themselves at risk of unplanned pregnancies, sexually transmitted diseases and Covid-19 (1426). And the diarist whose grandad has dementia and keeps visiting, forgetting there is a lockdown and who has to resist the urge to rush downstairs, from where he keeps a safe distance, to give his grandad a hug (1451). And the diarist who argues with her neighbours over the garden fence because they are breaking lockdown rules, hosting guests and putting herself and others at risk (3890).

I recommend reading across the entries and extracts for similarities and differences; the familiar and the strange; and for juxtapositions that vibrate, illuminate and arrest any fall into humanistic cliché. There are juxtapositions between alphabetically arranged entries, for example between 'Key workers' (often busier than ever) and 'Lockdown projects' (undertaken by diarists with more time on their hands due to furlough, or new working from home arrangements, or the 'stay home' instruction). Then there are juxtapositions within entries between numerically arranged extracts:

Under 'Lockdown projects', the clinician working longer hours (2721) is followed by the museum educator working shorter hours and using the extra time to read all 'the great political novels' she's put off reading for the last half century (2722), and someone participating in their family's 'lockdown art challenge' (4610) is followed by someone for whom work is busier than ever and who confesses to being sick of hearing about other people's lockdown projects (4756). Under '(new) Normal', we find someone for whom lockdown is a welcome break from their usually hectic, stressful, appointment-filled life (4001) next to someone for whom lockdown feels like a continuation of life before the pandemic – a life shaped by disabilities that largely confined them at home anyway (4125). Under 'Stay alert', we find someone worried about the relaxation of lockdown rules and the risk of a second wave (1927) next to someone excited by the prospect of finally meeting a new friend face-to-face (1942); and we find someone who has no intention of leaving home once lockdown rules are relaxed (2030) next to someone who cannot wait for the change of rules – to the extent they 'jump the gun', travelling to the seaside the evening before the rule change comes into force (2143). Under 'Stay home', someone who walks with their friend on the beach because their friend lives alone and is lonely (1451) is followed by someone who claims their family, locked down together, have 'followed the rules properly' and 'not put a foot wrong' (1491).

Ultimately, I hope this book will be used to remember the Covid-19 pandemic and its impacts. Life moves fast. Events move on. Before the pandemic was fully over, it was followed by Russia's invasion of Ukraine, a 'cost-of-living crisis', Monkeypox (another 'Global Health Emergency', according to the WHO). The diaries from 12 May 2020 help us to recall the novelty and strangeness of everyday life in pandemic times. They were written at a time when many aspects of pandemic life were not yet taken for granted. They were written by people who noticed such aspects: being stuck at home, listening to birdsong, starting new projects, walking the neighbourhood, learning to use videoconferencing software, practising the new etiquette of social distancing. The diaries also help us to recall how difficult pandemic life was for many people. Its moods included gratitude and hope, but anxiety, fear, grief and guilt were central to many experiences.

I also hope this book will be used to unsettle myths of the pandemic. Such myths have been settling quietly since early 2020. One is the myth of national unity: that Covid-19 was 'the great leveller', placing everyone 'all in this together', eliciting a (Blitz-) spirited community response. Another is the myth of national disunity: that Covid-19 provoked 'panic buying' and 'lockdown fatigue' among self-interested and psychologically frail citizens.[41] Another is the myth of Covid the disruptor: an event that 'changed everything', leaving world history divided into BC (Before Corona) and AC (After Corona), in the terms of historian Peter Hennessy.[42] Another is the myth of Covid the multiplier: an event that, if it changed anything at all, did so by multiplying existing patterns and trends.[43] The mass of details in the diary extracts – and the contradictions, paradoxes and ambiguities they capture – disallows such grand claims. Indeed, before we get to these details, the list of entries – the contents page – does its own disruptive work. Anxiety, deliveries, WhatsApp, working from home and Zoom may all have been multiplied by the pandemic, but other entries demand a different frame: clap for carers, furlough, home schooling, key workers, lockdown projects, shielding.

I hope this book will be used to generate new frames or will prompt new frames by generating associations between entries and extracts. For example, there is plenty to be thought and written about gratitude and luck during the pandemic, and the cultural work they do in contemporary British culture, both as a conservative force allowing people to justify the status quo and as a progressive force or potential, ripe for mobilization by political work. However, in the spirit of the previous discussion, let me stop before I start my own mythologizing. Let me stop, allowing readers to find their own way.

ANXIETY

Twenty-first-century British society was already characterized by anxiety, but – like so many existing characteristics – the pandemic multiplied this anxiety. In lockdown, while introverts felt less pressure to go out and mix, and some furloughed workers felt less job-related stress, many people found they had more time to think, fewer people to think with, fewer distractions and much to think and worry about. They worried about their own health – the slightest cough, which could indicate the disease, which could be mild or deadly. They worried about the impact of their own illness or death on dependents. They worried about the health and well-being of family, friends and colleagues – especially those considered 'vulnerable' and 'high-risk', including 'key workers' on the 'frontline', but also children at risk of 'falling behind', missing exams, losing places at university. They worried about risky situations – going to the shops, returning to work or school, using public transport. They worried about doing the right thing, following the rules correctly, applying the guidance appropriately. They worried about the future and the consequences of the pandemic for jobs, work, taxes and public services. Anxiety was noticed especially at the start and end of the day, after or before nights of disrupted sleep and dreams about death, graveyards, confined spaces, proximate strangers. It was noticed especially when consuming news and social media. To cope with increased anxiety, people avoided news and social media, especially before bed. They sought comfort and control in familiar foods, books and television shows. They sought escape in fiction, fantasy and sometimes alcohol. They did puzzles and tried to keep busy. And still, sometimes – more than before – they argued and wept. See also Furlough; Home schooling; Key workers; Lockdown projects; Stay apart; Stay home.

Diarist 469 (female, 40s, South East England, farmer)

I feel a bit anxious this morning and it's because I am trying to keep everyone safe, well, healthy, educated, happy, balanced, family, friends and staff. I don't care that my hair is going grey. People are terrified and yet so many different sentiments. I am troubled today that I didn't wash my clothes after going to the shops. I will try and do that more.

Diarist 479 (female, 40s, South West England, clinical pharmacist)

I woke late. This happens a lot at present. Since lockdown started, I have slept better. I think it is quieter at night as people are not out and there is far less traffic than before. I like this situation. I don't want it to change. I have spent time reflecting on this and

I think I feel this way because I quite like staying home and spending time with my family. Sometimes the pressure to go out and 'make memories' is quite strong. There is lots to do each weekend, but I don't always enjoy being in crowds and trying to satisfy my needs and those of the rest of my family at the same time. I think I don't like crowds much anymore. I feel stressed, anxious and struggle to think clearly. When at home I am comfortable and relaxed and as a family we are good at spending time together whilst still doing our own thing. We come together for meals and movies and we play together. If we go out, I find more peace and fulfilment in a long walk or bike ride in the countryside. I like to be outdoors but in peace. I used to be a real extrovert and enjoy going out, meeting new people and getting out of my comfort zone as much as possible. I have lost that sense of restlessness and now feel more at peace with myself. So, for me, this lockdown period is quite enjoyable [. . .] At home in private I have worried. A worst-case scenario would be myself and my husband infected and admitted to hospital and what would happen to the children? We have no family nearby [. . .] protecting the boys not just from the risk of infection but from the consequences of any of us falling ill has been a concern. I like to think that if I was infected, I would experience mild symptoms. However, the truth is that we cannot predict how serious the infection would be and that is terrifying.

Diarist 591 (female, 40s, Scotland, molecular biologist)

All of my staff are anxious about what the future brings. The funding for our group depends on us bringing in revenue from work we do for other groups in the UK, which we have had to pause for the time being. We don't know how this will affect our continued existence in the future. I am concerned about the safety of the people in my team, as well as their mental health and job-security. I have lost sleep over this in the past weeks [. . .] My son is just finishing his first year at University. He is completing all his final assignments and is worried about whether he will be able to return to University after the summer [. . .] We don't know whether to arrange accommodation for him for next year or not. He is thinking about suspending his studies for a year. My daughter is in third year of secondary school. She is coping well with online classes, but it is no substitute for being at school with all her friends. She is a very sociable person and misses that part of life very much. I am concerned for her mental health as lock-down continues. We have started doing a short walk together every evening, when we talk about the day and anything that's bothering her. I think this is helping a bit.

Diarist 746 (female, 40s, London, consultant)

I'm trying to limit my news and social media consumption during this period as I find if you spend too much time immersed in it the situation can become overwhelming. This is unusual for me as I'm normally a politics nerd.

Diarist 901 (female, 30s, London, unemployed)

I wake up first at 00:30, then 3am, then 5am, then 08:30 and finally get up at 9am. Recently due to stress, depression, anxiety and epic levels of boredom, I haven't been sleeping very well so this is quite an achievement.

I make coffee, grab a juice and get back in to bed to read the news for an hour or so.

I notice that my glands in my throat hurt and successfully resist the urge to self-diagnose all current major plagues and diseases – I'm currently on my 9th (?) hysterical self-diagnosis of Covid-19. Thankfully none of these has progressed beyond the stage of screaming at my housemates to 'stay away!!' and them sending me for a nap to calm down [. . .] I'm currently studying [in my room] At some point I get cold. I close my window, retrieve a blanket and retreat under duvet to continue studying. I successfully resist the urge to link this to the glandular pain from this morning as progressing symptoms of plague [. . .] I really hope I can sleep again tonight.

Diarist 989 (female, 60s, retired)

Last night I dreamt of two of the people I worked with closely for years. It was a sad dream as they both died during the dream from the virus.

Diarist 1122 (female, 50s, London, service manager)

My husband comes home complaining of a sore throat and sniffles. This happened a couple of weeks ago and didn't bear fruit but who knows this time it could be IT. I ask him to go upstairs and stay there and take him his dinner on a tray. I mop at the taps and door handle in the bathroom in case he has germy hands. I will be sleeping in the spare room tonight. To help cope with the emerging anxiety, I end the day with another solitary walk around the empty streets, plugged into loud music.

Diarist 1137 (female, 40s, Yorkshire and Humber, psychologist)

I woke up at about 3.30am this morning. I keep waking up in the middle of the night. I looked at my phone. I know that's not a good idea but I can't help myself. I looked at the BBC news website and the front pages of the newspapers: not good news [. . .] Mum and Dad live 200 miles away – Mum has breathing difficulties and Dad is diabetic so they are both high risk and trying to avoid as much contact with others as possible. I haven't seen them face-to-face since Christmas. My younger sister lives near them and is a nurse – not on the front line but none the less it's worrying – she has MS so is higher risk herself. Her partner has been furloughed from his job. He's worried after the announcement yesterday [see Stay Alert] that he's going to be called back to work. He doesn't drive so he'd have to use public transport. He doesn't want to take the risk.

Diarist 1149 (female, 60s, Scotland, lecturer)

I'm in good health although I'm much more aware of my own mortality since the pandemic began. In fact, I've been feeling anxious that neither [my partner nor I] have written a will yet, and we plan to do so soon. We are unmarried and I worry that if I die suddenly, my partner would become homeless [. . .] The beginning of the lockdown was horribly stressful, as I was having to master a lot of new technology for work all at once. Also, more worryingly, one of my siblings and her family caught the coronavirus, and we were terribly worried about my sister as she has a compromised immune system. Meanwhile, another relative's mental health was very fragile as she struggled to ensure adequate care for her paraplegic brother during lockdown. I felt so stressed for the first couple of weeks of lockdown about family and work that I often woke up feeling bleak and tearful [. . .] Tonight we'll watch more of Narcos. Watching Mexican drug wars seems a good way to escape the lunacy happening in the real world [. . .] Overall, I feel pretty happy. I feel lucky that I can work from home and I enjoy my own company, although I feel sorry for those isolating alone (even worse for all those who'd prefer to isolate but can't). I worry about the future though. My parents are in their late 70s/early 80s and I worry I might never see them again. I also worry about my own health if I have to commute again. This crisis has reminded me that nothing is more important than your health, and the love of your family and friends.

Diarist 1205 (female, 50s, Northern Ireland, publisher and volunteer)

The mood in the house has varied greatly today. There were definite moments of humour and laughter but my daughter finds the situation very distressing and her worries become mine. To coin a phrase – you are only as happy as your saddest child.

Diarist 1213 (female, 30s, London, IT consultant)

[Son] has generally been pretty laid back about the whole lockdown thing – he's not really an anxious child, but he has been showing signs of some anxiety, one of them being waking in the night and insisting on coming into our bed. Usually I would strongly discourage this and make him go back to his own bed, but at the moment we've agreed we just have to do what gets us through this nightmare – if [son] needs an extra mummy hug, I'm not going to deny it.

Diarist 1289 (female, 50s, South East England, creative producer and artistic director)

I woke up at 6.37am (why?), wide awake thinking about this terrible situation [. . .] Ruminating on the whole awful mess has become a regular early morning thing, so I've previously tried to get up asap, but not today, I mean, 6.30am!!! So now I'm a mess, feeling awful for a couple of hours & now crying over the keyboard & thinking that I must pull myself together.

Diarist 1341 (male, 60s, East of England, retired doctor)

Like many people we are desperately concerned that there is not a second peak in this epidemic with more fatalities especially to some of my ex colleagues who are part of the front line. My eldest daughter works [. . .] at a teaching hospital and I really feel for her as she is working hard but lives alone and is finding it very tough. Once we come through this illness there will inevitably be a period of austerity and many people will lose their jobs and livelihoods. It is a very worrying time.

Diarist 1375 (male, 50s, Scotland, consultant engineer)

9:00. We all sit watching a rubbish programme on the telly about buying houses [. . .] None of us is interested in bungalows in Derby in 2013. The purpose of this activity is to stop us thinking.

Diarist 1380 (female, 40s, Northern Ireland, librarian)

I woke late as I slept through my alarm. Ordinarily this would cause great panic as we would be getting up for work or school, but as we have nowhere to be I have been trying not to worry too much about a routine and just go with the flow [. . .] I enjoy reading at the kitchen table and then check the BBC news website for the latest news [. . .] I still feel tight-chested and anxious at times, but this has not happened as often as it did in late March/ early April when we first understood the enormity of the changes wrought by the virus.

My daughters sleep even later than I did. Today would have been my youngest daughter's final AS level exam with a long Summer holiday to look forward to. Instead she hasn't seen her friends or boyfriend for nearly 60 days and has only left the house to cycle or make very brief journeys as a passenger in the car. It's hard for her to stay positive and motivated. She feels lonely [. . .] We are all worried about what it will be like in September when they should be beginning their final year of A levels and looking at Universities. Will that even be a realistic option now?

To shake off anxiety and earn my lunch, I walk for 50 minutes or so around the local country lanes, enjoying the sun.

Diarist 1428 (non-binary, 20s, North West England, fundraiser and consultant)

I have a variety of mental illnesses (depression, OCD, anxiety, PTSD) which have to various extents been exacerbated by the general state of the world and by my being out of work. I have a history of self-harm and have relapsed into those behaviours in the past month. I've been finding it really difficult to be motivated to do anything. I played games on my phone for a while and scrolled through social media some more. It's hard not to get caught up in a cycle of checking the news, being scared and angry because of it, clicking on a different app to distract myself, and repeating the whole thing again [. . .] I received some post – my grandparents have been photocopying the newspaper crossword for me so that I can fill in my answers, they can fill in theirs, and we can call each other to try to finish the whole thing [. . .] I hope I'll be able to see them again, but I'm terrified of something happening to one or both of them. I've heard a lot about people not being able to visit dying relatives, and how few people are allowed at funerals, and I can't imagine dealing with something that devastating without the support of your family and friends being there in person, with you. I filled in some of the crossword answers but found it hard to concentrate.

After that, I went for a walk in the local wood [. . .] While I was walking, I listened to a podcast [. . .] I can't listen to anything too serious these days. I find it too overwhelming. It's the same with all media – I've been re-reading Wuthering Heights for the sixth time because it's familiar, and we've been watching a lot of trashy TV and period dramas, because it's soothing to watch things where the biggest concern is about relationships or miscommunications rather than thousands of deaths and the looming threat of your own [. . .] I cooked roasted sweet potato tacos [. . .] While we ate, we watched the final two episodes of the 1995 Pride and Prejudice miniseries. I drank 2 gin and tonics – I've been drinking more during lockdown, which is partially because of living with friends and having a social drink more often, and partly because anything that makes existing in my own head less awful is a good thing right now. As a household, we've been buying a lot of wine and gin and cider. I'm not worried about any of us having a problem, we'll all be able to stop drinking so much when this is over, but it's probably not great for our bodies right now. At the beginning of lockdown, we all had such high expectations of ourselves to exercise more and eat healthily and do lots of projects, and now it's all we can do to drag ourselves through the day without losing our minds. There has been a lot of crying.

Diarist 1456 (male, 50s, Wales, retired psychotherapist)

This afternoon, instead of focusing on the pandemic, I have been trying to read fiction rather than fact, to meditate and rest my mind.

Diarist 1547 (female, 30s, East of England, innovation consultant)

I've limited my news reading to a single check in the morning and in the evening. There is little point in worrying about things I can't control. I've also ruthlessly pruned my Twitter and Instagram feeds [. . .] I decided to watch some escapist TV – an episode of

The Magicians, and Stargate Atlantis. The further from the real world the better at the moment!

Diarist 1574 (female, 40s, Wales, public health practitioner)

I start to help my children to plan their school work for the day [. . .] Probably like most parents I am very worried about their future, for the socialisation and education that they are missing out on and what the future holds. I am concerned that the virus may mutate and that will make a vaccine hard to develop. Whilst so far children have been less affected by the virus, I am concerned that this could change. I am also worried about schools returning too soon and that it will be stressful for children to have to maintain social distancing whilst at school.

Diarist 1691 (female, 20s, South East England, online shopper)

We [. . .] watched the 6pm BBC news which I had been making a conscious effort not to watch during COVID-19, to avoid the many anxious dreams that I was having when I was avidly watching the news three times a day at the start of lockdown. Today however, I watched the news and ended up in tears [. . .] I feel like I have no clue what is really going to happen in the near foreseeable future which panics me [. . .] I know that with a healthy family, employment and a roof over my head I am in a very fortunate position, yet the waves of panic and sadness of my normal life that I am not living still creep in.

Diarist 1692 (female, 60s, North of England, retired teacher)

Tonight I have a slight cold which immediately makes me worry as to whether I have got Covid. I don't have any underlying health conditions but I do worry about dying. I have started to write family stories for my granddaughter and daughters but I can't really bear to think about not being here for them.

Diarist 1710 (female, 60s, London, garden designer)

Woke early again, 5 am-ish. The situation we are in is constantly going round in my head.

Diarist 1711 (male, 50s, West Midlands, geologist)

During the crisis I seem to be listening to The Beatles almost daily. Maybe it is the comfort of returning to something from my childhood? [. . .] We don't usually drink in the week but my wife is so stressed at the moment that she starts drinking G&T as soon as she's finished work. I am worried about the drinking.

Diarist 1815 (female, 20s, Scotland, unemployed)

I woke up at around 8am and sent [partner] to make the coffee [. . .] I felt well-rested and content, which isn't always the case at the moment. We talked about our dreams as the coffee brewed; this is one of those lockdown rituals we've developed over time. Sometimes there isn't much new input on a day-to-day basis, so our dreams give us something new to talk about. My dreams last night were very inflected by coronavirus – for example, seeing a friend and feeling tense because I didn't want to hug her – but, unlike yesterday, they weren't nightmares.

Diarist 1927 (female, 50s, South East England, artist and musician)

I'm trying not to look at the news sites every morning and have whittled down what and who I can see on social media – policing myself as I know I can spend too much time brooding and start losing sleep, which won't help anyone.

Diarist 1940 (female, 30s, Scotland, assistant professor)

Last night I dreamed of exploring a small attic and finding stuff that suggested my Dad was living a secret life. There have been a lot of confined spaces in my recent dreams, not very surprisingly. The night before I dreamed of being in prison [. . .] None of my grandparents are still alive, so my worries are largely focused on my parents [. . .] Their general health is good, but I've still been reminding them repeatedly to avoid taking any risks. One of my worst nightmares is them dying in hospital and not even being able to hold their hands. Even thinking about that makes me cry [. . .] Since lockdown began I've been weepier than I used to be [. . .] There were several weeks when I couldn't read the news at all without crying. Might still be the case, now that I'm avoiding the news [. . .] Although I've stopped reading news articles, I still get exposed to people's coronavirus hot takes on Twitter (and to a lesser extent Tumblr). I would like to spend less time on social media, however this is harder to arrange when I can't just ban myself from the internet or my laptop without it being very isolating. There must be a way to arrange it.

My favourite social media site is Goodreads. I can peacefully post book reviews and read other people's recommendations, without encountering much in the way of current events. That reminds me, I should turn off my laptop and read a book for a while. Reading usually calms my mind somewhat.

Diarist 1971 (female, 60s, Wales, writer)

I managed to avoid the ten o'clock news by going to bed and reading for an hour to calm my brain down enough to consider going to sleep.

Diarist 1972 (female, 40s, East Midlands, communications manager)

We watched the BBC 6 o'clock news to try and help us make sense of what is going on in the world at the moment. There seems to be no other news than that about Coronavirus [. . .] To distract us, we stream a film [. . .] Does the trick for a couple of hours, until we decide to go to bed at around 9:30pm. We both spend a while browsing Facebook and YouTube, chatting and generally reassuring each other that things will be ok, despite neither of us being totally sure that they will be.

Diarist 1979 (female, 60s, South East England, editor and retired nurse)

The nation is extremely anxious, and the day started with my partner refusing to make up an anxiety-fuelled tiff with my son from last night, which has escalated into a furious and irrelevant argument between him and me. I imagine such arguments are probably widespread and it feels as if we have fallen prey to a much wider and deeper fear that we have all tried to stay on top of [. . .] Feeling the fall out of other family members' anxiety is difficult; trying not to absorb it myself, but to understand that they cannot help their reactions and are deeply fearful. I have tried to keep a structured routine to the days to help with this, but sometimes a somnambulance takes over, and I lose track of the time. I know both these men are scared in their own ways. One for his age, which puts him in the high-risk group [. . .] and the other [. . .] who is already on meds for anxiety, separated from his girlfriend and uncertain of his future.

9.45 am So, this morning exploded in fireworks for us and I found myself, instead of looking forward to writing this diary, sitting in the bushes in our local park, weeping.

Diarist 2003 (female, 40s, South East England, housewife and artist/designer)

I'm pretty anxious about the possibility of schools reopening in June [. . .] I suppose I've got to wait and see what measures the schools come up with to maintain social distancing . . . I was having a dream before I woke up that involved school kids and buses and me freaking out that they were too close to each other and me [. . .] I'll check The Guardian on my phone to see what is going on with the coronavirus around the world. I'm a lot less obsessive with the news than I was 8 weeks ago. I've cut it down to morning and night rather than obsessing over it. I feel like I'm coming across as neurotic. I think it's probably hard to find anyone who is chill at the moment though!

Diarist 2041 (female, 30s, Yorkshire and Humber, teacher)

I woke up still feeling rather under the weather from coronavirus symptoms, but yesterday managed to get a test booked so we'll be going to [the local airport] later to have the test done [. . .] So I've been for a test. We drove to the airport which is about 20 miles away. It was well signposted when we got there. We kept the windows up and showed the code I'd been given from the confirmation email and then we went into the marquee area where we were talked through what to do over the mobile phone by a guy wearing full PPE. I had to use the test kit myself, it wasn't administered by someone else. It was put through the window and then we pulled over into a parking space where I could take the test.

It was a little bit tough on [son], the whole situation. He's getting quite anxious around the idea of the virus. So I had to reassure him that everything was ok and that I'm not in any imminent danger. Taking the test was pretty unpleasant if I'm honest. I had to do a swab from the back of my throat around a tonsil area which made me feel really unwell and gag and then have to put the swab straight up my nose as high as possible would go, which was really quite uncomfortable, then pop it in the test tube and package it all up and send it off. The staff at the testing Centre were so helpful and really clear and totally understood that obviously people are feeling quite nervous and uneasy about the whole situation [. . .] I'm back in bed [. . .] I'm just feeling quite emotional and quite drained. I'm quite worried because this is, you know. Hopefully I don't seem to come down with it particularly heavily, if I do have it. It seems to be quite a mild case. Either way, I feel wiped out, but it's still worrying because this is a disease that kills people, has killed over 32,000 people so far in this country that we know about, so it's a worrying time.

Diarist 2070 (male, 70s, South West England, administrator)

So how have I felt? Relaxed because social contact, which I find quite demanding, has been at a level I can easily cope with, but anxious when I think about how some members of the wider family are managing, how our business will survive (and what that might mean in terms of being able to continue to support family members) and what the world will be like in geopolitical terms as (if?) we recover.

Diarist 2164 (male, 40s, London, student)

People report vivid and disturbing dreams: I've had some myself. Even my Mum, normally stolidly resistant to the subconscious, has spoken of dreams staying with her through the day. More to think about and fewer people to think about it *with* means lots circulating in the head.

Diarist 2205 (male, 70s, North West England, retired teacher)

Both daughters are 'at risk' from COVID [. . .] so that worries me all the time. [One daughter] has had to return half time to work as her boss is self-isolating (COVID in house) since last week. She is a manager in a medical practice; though she does not have face to face contact with patients, the environment is a 'tight' one. More worries.

Diarist 2341 (female, 30s, Wales, librarian)

I worry daily about whether we'll make it through this. I worry about making the library safe for the kids and for me. I worry about exposing myself to the virus on the bus. I am so keen to get my life back, but I wonder if that life even exists anymore. Will I always have to worry about this? [. . .] Spent an hour ironing as I've been ignoring the growing pile for over a week. I watched a couple of episodes of [something on Netflix], just to have some background noise. It's much too quiet here this afternoon and the silence sends my brain into overdrive. There seems to be so much to worry about at the moment.

Diarist 2386 (female, 60s, Scotland, coach and charity director)

There is such a long list of things to get done today, as there is every day, and I am thankful for that but whenever a small gap opens up there is space to think. I try to avoid that. It won't be helpful.

Diarist 2388 (female, 40s, South East England, clinical psychologist)

Watched some TV and noticed our need for something humorous and ignoring any current news. Watched an old favourite movie – Night at the Museum which fitted the bill beautifully.

Diarist 2466 (female, 20s, South East England, unemployed)

Before I woke up, I had an odd dream about my teeth falling out. I was on the back of a coach, and they just fell into my hand like candy corn. It is not unusual for me to have strange dreams like this, but they have been happening more frequently of late, including one about a Harlequin dressed in black, dancing around a graveyard.

Diarist 2471 (female, 30s, London, unemployed)

I've been unemployed for just over one month. The longest period I've been out of work since graduating [. . .] And I work in travel/tourism so who knows how long it will be before the industry restarts and recovers to the point where they're hiring again. I'm trying to stay positive but it's quite a Corona-coaster (!) some days.

Diarist 2589 (female, 30s, South East England, actress)

5pm I tried reading my book [. . .] but I couldn't concentrate as I was wondering about whether I would have my old job back or not. I didn't really want my old job back it's just the uncertainty and trying to make use of this time now as much as possible. Money in the bank is going to be needed if I am ever to be able again to pursue acting work and pay my bills. So, I couldn't concentrate on my book so I had a gin, packet of crisps and sat in the garden with my laptop and watched a new comedy programme [. . .] Thoroughly enjoyed it and chilled out. When it got nippy I went up to my room [. . .] Watched an episode of Game of Thrones. I never thought I would watch this show but turns out if there is a pandemic I am all for this fantasy based show. Nice bit of escapism.

Diarist 2627 (female, 40s, Northern Ireland, editor)

I practised the piano in secret for a few minutes [. . .] Starting again at the piano makes me confront one of several failed careers, and a lot of bad memories. I don't want my parents to hear me. But I enjoy playing, even if it means starting again at the beginning, and the advantage of being atrocious at it is that stumbling through the most basic minuet demands total concentration. It gives me a little holiday from the news and my own thoughts, and when my mind starts to run again the next wrong note makes me aware of it.

Diarist 2637 (female, 60s, East of England, potter)

I woke up unusually early today, sobbing in my vivid dream. I dreamt that I was in a queue for the chemist with no one social distancing, which made me incredibly cross. Then I forgot what I went in for and I had lost my credit card and couldn't stop crying. I am not normally a worrier, I thought I had been coping rather well with the lockdown so far, but your body tells you otherwise in your dreams.

Diarist 2705 (female, 40s, Yorkshire and Humber, writer)

This morning my alarm went at 8am and my first thought was that I must stop setting my radio alarm to coincide with the hourly news as it makes for an anxious start to the day.

Diarist 3029 (male, 20s, North West England, editor)

Went for a run. I've always been a runner, but I haven't done much running during lockdown (my first run was last week, and this was only my second). I get anxious about (amongst other things) feeling like I'm in the way, so I get a little paranoid about making sure I can keep two metres away from people while I'm outside – paranoid enough, in fact, that I really haven't been going out apart from my weekly shop. I'm trying to be better about that now, though I do still really wish I had a garden where I could just sit outside without having to worry about other people.

Diarist 3134 (female, 60s, South East England, tour guide)

At present – along with many others, I am 'furloughed' and 'enjoying' an unexpected break from work and most responsibilities [. . .] We are more 'relaxed', feeling 'free' like children with few things to be obliged to do [. . .] Having said this, since my mother has been in lockdown in her Nursing Home since the 18th March and she is two hours away, I am worried for her. Particularly since I got a phone call saying she might have the Covid19 as she had a cough and a temperature. The news reports have been full of the elderly dying alone in care homes with their families unable to visit. I am also concerned for my brother who lives alone and has bipolar disorder so my feelings are very mixed and I feel both elated and terribly sad. My moods are changeable. I had an outburst at breakfast today, I suddenly felt very irritable as I am not sure if I will be able to return to work; at my age they may think I should be asked to bow out. . . . Then, but it calms and becomes contented. The flowers in the verges and hedges are delightful!

Diarist 3513 (female, 60s, South East England, retired teacher)

6.00 am I woke for about the third time. A good night's sleep is non-existent for me – I'm told it's quite common because of the unusual conditions we are living through. I long for a good 8 hours' sleep. When I woke in the night, I resorted to doing word games and crosswords on my iPad. Not good practice but I cannot just lie and fret.

Diarist 3761 (female, 30s, South West England, lawyer)

I awoke early, my fiancé sleeping soundly next to me [. . .] I crept downstairs and prepared my usual breakfast of porridge and fruit (I'm feeling more conscious than ever of the need to look after myself both in body and mind as I feel there is little else I have control over in the world at this time).

Diarist 3789 (male, 30s, Scotland, copy editor)

My mum is vulnerable, and I worry about her getting it – she has problems with her lungs [. . .] My only remaining grandparent is alone in her house, occasionally seeing her youngest daughter (my aunt) plus family at a distance. They are both vulnerable. My cousin, who currently lives with my aunt, is a delivery driver. Her boyfriend has medical conditions that wouldn't be helped by the bug [. . .] My wife's grandfather had surgery on his leg just before lockdown [. . .] My wife's grandmother had a fall before lockdown. Everyone seems more delicate and feels further away than before.

Diarist 4669 (female, 40s, South East England, librarian)

This morning I got up at 7.30 a.m. and listened to [a podcast] whilst dressing. Before lockdown I would have listened to 'Today' on Radio 4, but I've found that I want to limit the amount of time I spend listening to the news during the current pandemic as I find it can become a little overwhelming.

Diarist 4671 (female, 20s, Yorkshire and Humber, carer)

It's nearly time for me to get the kids to bed now. Then I will lay for hours on end dwelling on what will be and what might happen. Feel like a fish in a barrel waiting for my turn to be served as dinner to coronavirus. Awful feeling. Can't wait to just feel safe again.

Diarist 4688 (female, 60s, Yorkshire and Humber, researcher)

Finally the news at 10 on the BBC, never very heartening, and I escaped to read in bed – starting a new book for the book club this month, thriller, pure escapism.

Diarist 4766 (female, 60s, East of England, family support specialist)

I got my clothes and food ready for work the next day. I have stopped using the tube as I felt a little anxious, which is totally alien for me. The tube carriages were full even early in the morning. When I was travelling on the tube one morning, I had a huge urge to cough, so I got off at the next station, coughed, then got on the following train. I knew that coughing on the tube was a big no no.

I now cycle to and from work.

Diarist 4892 (female, 30s, North West England, writer)

I was awake in the night – I find myself mulling over things a lot, particularly the baby's birth as it's all a bit up in the air. I would like a home birth but they're dependent on the ambulance service having capacity, which right now they can't guarantee.

BIRDSONG

12 May 2020 arrived on the back of a particularly warm and sunny spring. Locked down at home, many people found they moved slower, taking more time, through a smaller, more local activity space. They noticed and appreciated their surroundings more – especially the nature found in gardens, parks, graveyards and local woods. Walking, instead of driving or riding public transport, they felt the sunshine. They saw the trees change as the seasons changed. They smelled the flowers. They heard the birdsong. Diarists wrote of 'the positives' of lockdown: less busy roads and skies, peace and quiet, cleaner air, time to chat with neighbours. They wondered if the pandemic had actually changed the outside world – confining humans and so allowing nature to recover – or if it had just changed their orientation to the world, so that now, less busy, they noticed what was always there. Either way, these 'positives' of lockdown were punctured every so often, and frequently in cities, by other sounds of the pandemic – not least the sirens of ambulances. See also Hope; (new) Normal; Stay home; (dog) Walking.

Diarist 421 (female, 60s, South West England, retired)

During my eight years of retirement [. . .] I have painted a great deal but during this last 7 weeks at home I have not really been feeling much like painting. Instead I have been watching. I have been amazed at the intelligence and relationships birds and animals have with us and each other. My gaze has been more intense and my focus longer [. . .] As I have been looking at nature and animals I have moved into a very slow and quieter gear, sometimes thinking I would be happy to live in retreat, how much more peaceful the world feels from here, the sky bluer, the flowers brighter, the birdsong louder.

Diarist 479 (female, 40s, South West England, clinical pharmacist)

I cycle home, a pleasant journey [. . .] I enjoy cycling to work. The weather is pleasant, and lockdown has made my journey much quieter. I hear birdsong in the mornings and raise my face to the sun in the afternoons. My legs feel stronger and I enjoy pushing myself to go faster each time.

Diarist 897 (female, 50s, London, actress)

I miss the travel, the train journeys through the UK and Europe – Edinburgh, Paris, Brussels, Amsterdam, Frankfurt, Madrid, Geneva, Budapest. Those days are gone, I think. I don't miss the flying. It is wonderful to be without the planes. We're on the flightpath into Heathrow here, east to west, and the silence in the sky is a precious unintended gift of coronavirus.

Diarist 1108 (male, 50s, West Midlands, teacher)

The walk around the park next to my house has been a lifeline. Like many people, I've actually relished these days, with their slowness and calm. I've loved seeing the trees turn from bare to bloom to leaf. I've loved the quietness that has allowed birdsong to be heard again. I even downloaded apps to help me learn the birds by their songs and to identify the trees. It hasn't worked, of course. But I'm paying attention and that's the main thing. Most years the blossom can come and go without me even seeing. In the park, everyone is respectful of people's distance. We walk off the path if someone is approaching. We smile. We say hello. Civility has returned. It is as if we see each other again, and respect each other's needs. This is good. I only hope the restart of the rat race doesn't mean we will lose sight of these important lessons.

The hospital is right across the park from my house. At the start of the shutdown, the sound of sirens was regular and it jarred with the peacefulness we were all experiencing and the beautiful warm weather in which it was all bathed. These have been glorious days. The sirens seem to be fewer now.

Diarist 1167 (male, 50s, South West England, insolvency practitioner)

Today the sun is shining, the blackbirds are singing and the bees are visiting my Aquilegia. Sadly, the slugs have visited the young bean plants, so they are so holy they are positively sanctified. I enjoyed a few minutes listening to the birds in the sun. Covid-19 hasn't been all bad. With fewer cars roaring past our house, we've been able to hear the birds this year. I've missed them.

Diarist 1390 (female, 20s, South East England, student)

It's been strange adapting to the sudden change in the speed of life, but I can't say it's all been bad. There were so few cars on the road at first, so few planes in the sky. The world was quieter and the air was so clean. The first few days after I went outside in March and April, I could smell the incredible sweetness and earthiness of flowers and trees in the air, even in more built-up areas. I wondered why I'd never noticed before – if I'd not paid attention, if I'd been too busy going around in cars and on trains, too much in a hurry to get to wherever I was meant to go next. Perhaps. Or maybe it was the lack of air pollution.

Diarist 1410 (female, 60s, London, architect)

We are all thoroughly enjoying hearing the birds instead of the traffic, the weather instead of the inside of an office, walking or cycling instead of the tube. So many positives in the midst of this weird time.

Diarist 1581 (male, 60s, London, office administrator)

After lunch I went out for a walk [...] I stop to have a chat with my neighbours and ask how they are coping. They are not elderly or classed as 'vulnerable', but I find that I am taking more time to chat to them when I see them. This seems to be one of the very few positives to come out of this 'lockdown' – people are taking time to chat and look out for each other. Another is the definite improvement in the air quality. Very few cars, or other road transport and hardly any aircraft flying. I can even hear the birds singing in the morning.

Diarist 1979 (female, 60s, South East England, editor and retired nurse)

The birdsong seems louder than usual, and four foxes visit our suburban terrace every evening. Nature seems to be making itself more comfortable, or maybe I just have time to notice.

Diarist 2164 (male, 40s, London, student)

Everything is so quiet. I can hear the birds singing outside. There was a sense of increased bustle yesterday, but this afternoon it's tranquil, almost hushed. At the back of my mind is the concern that I won't see my family again in person for months, perhaps even next year. It's only 90 minutes but it might as well be the moon. The thought makes me incredibly sad, though there are of course hundreds of thousands of worse stories across the world.
Somewhere in the distance I can hear an ambulance.

Diarist 2463 (female, 50s, North West England, retired police officer)

05.55 I am woken by the early morning chorus of birdsong outside. Since lockdown it has been so quiet I now hear the birds more than ever before. I go to the toilet and then snuggle back into my warm and comfortable bed. I fall back to sleep.

09.02 I am woken by the extremely loud metallic crash sound from outside on the road in front of my house. My first thought is Oh No, I hope my car hasn't been crashed into. I quickly open the shutters to look out of my bedroom window and two houses to the left there is a large rubbish skip on the road. I feel relieved that nothing untoward is happening and wonder what building activity is occurring at my neighbours.

Diarist 2476 (female, 50s, London, personal assistant)

At 7.30pm I went out for a brisk hour's walk [. . .] I did my usual quicky and explored the streets in my neighbourhood that I've never walked down before; you can live somewhere for years and still not know it fully. There are so many lovely flowers and bushes around at the moment, some giving off such beautiful scents, I love it! This strange new world has definitely given time to appreciate the small things.

Diarist 2621 (male, 70s, North East England, retired lecturer)

As it is spring the flora is blossoming: our park is full of the white star flowers of wild garlic and there is a bluebell wood nearby too. The churchyard which I go through regularly is covered in wild flowers at different times and must be a haven for wildlife – I have seen rabbits, but not today. Tree blossom is starting to drop already to give pink snowflakes from the numerous cherry trees by the roadsides. Bird song seems louder given the quiet of the distant traffic and I heard a woodpecker tapping which is a rare event. Perhaps the wildlife is benefiting from us humans keeping out of the way.

Diarist 2637 (female, 60s, East of England, potter)

I go for a walk in the woods and reflect on how things have changed. People are now talking to each other when they are walking past, I feel safe in the woods as so many people are at home and out walking because we are allowed to. We are lucky with the weather, not too hot not too cold. And we have time to revel in nature, hear the birds, see the flowers, and butterflies. I feel like I am a child again, when we used to go blackberry picking, chasing butterflies and dibbling in ponds. Nature is fighting back; sheep, goats, deer are roaming in the towns, birds are nesting on the empty beaches.

Diarist 3552 (female, 13, Scotland)

My mum, my dad and I went for a walk along a lovely canal that we lived really near to. I have been following the journey of a female swan that has been nesting further up the canal since the start of the lockdown [Figure 1] My mum and I have been going daily to

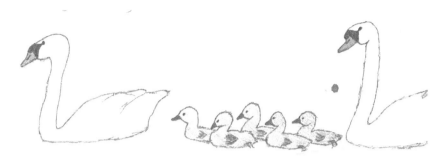

Figure 1 'I have been following the journey of a female swan.' Image submitted by Diarist 3552.

see when the eggs would hatch. As we neared the nest my eyes practically burst out of my head! Inside the nest, lying next to their mother, were four, incredibly fluffy and cute cygnets! I was ecstatic! [. . .] I walked home very happy [. . .] In bed, I thought about how I would normally never have had enough time to see the swans every day, and I would never even have known the cygnets existed! At least that is one good thing that has come out of lockdown!

Diarist 3567 (male, 60s, North West England, retired engineer)

I go for a walk [. . .] The path is bordered with the white flowers of Wild Garlic and in the shade of the trees there is Herb-robert growing. Before Coronavirus I would have hardly noticed these wild flowers, and certainly not been able to name the Herb-robert. Lockdown gives you a different perspective on things. My walk is far more leisurely and I see so much more now.

Diarist 3569 (female, 50s, South West England, community health worker)

Up early to a bright sunny morning, but a definite nip in the air. With the lockdown the lack of traffic is liberating, the air is so clean and sweet. We slept with the window open so woke with the dawn chorus trilling outside. Since this bizarre situation began I've noticed the birds have been louder and louder, a wall of sound greets me at the start of every working day.

CANCELLATIONS

Lockdown and related protections led to many cancellations. Informal gatherings – meet-ups for coffee or lunch – were cancelled. Regular gatherings – at churches or clubs – were cancelled. More occasional events – trips to see music or theatre performances – were cancelled. Holidays were cancelled, sometimes with significance beyond the loss of leisure time or money, because they were also visits to see distant family or long-planned trips to celebrate anniversaries. Exams were cancelled, when students had been preparing for months and years. While young adults missed rites of passage like the celebrations associated with finishing exams, the school prom, graduation and significant birthday celebrations (at sixteen, eighteen and twenty-one), older adults missed or postponed other life events, from long-planned weddings, buying a house and starting a family, to seeing grandchildren for the first time or putting long-awaited retirement plans into practice. Certain cancellations led to knock-on cancellations. A cancelled driving test meant the cancellation of planned trips, including for work. A cancelled job opportunity meant the cancellation of planned expenditure. Cancelled healthcare – surgery, physiotherapy appointments, day centre visits – meant pain, relapse and cancellation of all activities requiring good health. At the very least, these cancellations disappointed the diarists, who wrote of what they 'should have' been doing on 12 May, compared to what they were doing (mostly staying at home). While some diarists received unwelcome reminders of these disappointments from their diaries, calendars and associated – now unwanted – notifications, others bemoaned their newly empty diaries and calendars and found difficulty adjusting to a life without appointments. See also Hope; Stay home.

Diarist 34 (female, 60s, North East England, retired teacher)

Today will be much like others during the lock down. Actually, it is difficult to know what day it is – nothing on the calendar, no friends for lunch, coffee out, theatre visits cancelled long since and church closed.

Diarist 37 (male, 18, London)

Like many of my friends who I keep in contact with on social media platforms like Snapchat and Instagram, I feel like the rug has been pulled from beneath my feet. Had this pandemic not taken place, I would have taken my first history A-Level on Stuart Britain a week from today. In any other year, I would have spent this 12th May in the library at school, attending revision sessions and staying at school late to revise […] We were ramping up for the most intense period of revision of our lives, yet instead these grades are now being decided by our teachers through previous coursework and classwork.

Diarist 139 (female, 15, West Midlands)

Things are being cancelled left, right and centre. I was going on an 8 day service project and international with Girlguiding this summer to Iceland. Cancelled. A week's work experience. Cancelled. Plans to get experience over the summer volunteering at a kennels, rescue centre or stables. Cancelled. Scout camp in the summer. You guessed it, cancelled.

Diarist 602 (female, 50s, Wales, university tutor)

This year is our 25th wedding anniversary – romantic plans made when we married of seeing flamingos in Africa have been aborted – we are healthy that is all that matters.

Diarist 698 (female, 16, North East England)

I am currently in Year 11 (my last year of secondary school), so this pandemic has changed my education quite drastically [. . .] The big changes are that I am no longer doing my GCSE exams. In fact, today I would have had my French and Biology exams. By this point, I would have completed my Art, German Speaking, French Speaking, Computer Science, Religious Studies, French Listening, French Reading, and Biology exams. I cannot say that there isn't a bright side because I am fairly sure that anyone would be relieved to avoid over thirty exams in total; however, I can say that I have worked incredibly hard throughout my education and I would really have liked to prove myself through my GCSE exams [. . .] The thing that the pandemic brought which upset me the most was the inability to properly finish my secondary school career. This includes: a leavers' assembly, leavers' hoodies, Prom, and end of exam celebrations [. . .] The subject I am most sad about is Prom. This is what everyone looks forward to throughout the five years that we spend at secondary school [. . .] I have already bought my prom dress, which was a lot of money (nearly £600!), but my mum assured me that it was worth it because I loved it and had worked hard. Now it all seems like a waste of time and money, plus I will not even get to wear it!

Diarist 1042 (female, 20s, London, medical student)

End of term would normally be doing exams then going out to eat after the last one. But my exam has been cancelled and everywhere is closed.

Diarist 1108 (male, 50s, West Midlands, teacher)

With no GCSE or A Level exams taking place, it is up to us teachers to suggest grades in place of exams. My own son is among this year's cohort. It's hard for them, having prepared so hard for the summer, only for it all to suddenly stop. It's a rite of passage denied. My son is quite happy about not having to sit exams, of course.

Diarist 1289 (female, 50s, South East England, creative producer and artistic director)

I'm feeling down because I spoke to Mum & Dad, via Skype, last night. My Mum has vascular dementia & was doing pretty well, visiting a day centre twice a week & lots of lunches, coffees etc. with friends. That's obviously all stopped since the lock down [. . .] Mum was really struggling to express herself & get her thoughts & words out; couldn't put a story together or focus on a train of thought. It's a devastating drop in 8 weeks!

I obviously knew it was coming, but here it is & I'm completely powerless to help [. . .] Today I'm imagining that maybe I've already hugged her for the last time. It's devastating.

Diarist 1466 (female, 80s, East of England, retired teacher)

I started doing my jigsaw which I've been trying to do for the last three weeks! I spent quite a long time doing that and in between, I sat down and thought about all the things that had and were going to be missed due to this virus.

- My grandson's 18th birthday
- A friend's wedding – cancelled until next year
- An invite to the Victory Club in London for a meal in celebration of 75th VE [Victory in Europe] day
- Watching the celebrations of VE Day at Cineworld
- My Granddaughter's wedding in August
- Our Wedding anniversary party in September, cancelled until next year
- All the football and sport in general that I was missing. I am a season ticket holder for a Premier League football club and I watch practically all sport on TV or live as I go to athletic matches as well
- My other granddaughter's graduation from University.

What a disaster 2020 has been!

Diarist 1473 (female, 50s, North East England, teacher)

I slept fitfully during the early hours of the morning of Tuesday 12th May 2020 because I was in a lot of pain from an old injury to my sacroiliac joint. I have not had my weekly, private physiotherapy treatment since before 'Lockdown' which was 8 weeks ago and I am now suffering really badly.

Diarist 1494 (female, 20s, South East England, student)

I wake up at about 1pm – dammit, I've overslept again. I'm a natural night owl, which I usually try and keep in check, but in lockdown there's quite simply nothing important to get up for! I grab my phone to do an obligatory morning (well, my 'morning') social media scroll. I silence some reminders about now-cancelled events.

Diarist 1521 (female, 60s, South East England, customer service agent)

Today, I am feeling a bit down as we were supposed to go on holiday next week for two weeks travelling in Europe. After a lifetime of looking after the children, we have only just now started to take holidays abroad. I was really looking forward to flying into Prague and taking the train to different places in Europe. It would have been so exciting.

Diarist 1579 (male, 7, Yorkshire and Humber)

I like being off school. I miss my friends a bit though. I would like to go back to school as it's my birthday soon but my mum says I won't be allowed a party so my birthday may not be as much fun.

Diarist 1679 (female, 30s, London, software engineer)

My hobbies are mostly on ice: no swimming club, no band practice [. . .], no karaoke, no pub, no going to random places [. . .] on public transport and tweeting about it.

Diarist 1979 (female, 60s, South East England, editor and retired nurse)

3 pm: Had to cancel our family holiday [. . .] Disappointing as it would have been our first time of more than a couple of hours with my son and his wife [. . .] and his new baby. I hope Airbnb will cough up the refund as I've paid for the cottage in full.

Diarist 2003 (female, 40s, South East England, housewife and artist/designer)

I feel like this lockdown has forced us to live in the present, in the NOW. There's no point looking forward as all the things we would usually look forward to have been postponed or cancelled. Our caravan holiday has been moved to next May, festivals have been cancelled or postponed. All the summer barbecues, camping, rounders on the field.

Diarist 2070 (male, 70s, South West England, administrator)

Today would have been the final day of a 2-week holiday in France [. . .] There would have been a sunny week in a rented property in Provence [. . .] and a three-night stop-off in Burgundy on the way back north. I was hugely looking forward to it.

Diarist 2383 (female, 50s, London, unemployed)

This evening, I should have been going to the National Theatre to see *The Visit*, with the wonderful Lesley Manville. That has been the biggest impact of the lockdown for me – the cancellation of all theatre and music performances. Including tonight's, to date I have missed 18 performances, with as many again cancelled over the next few months.

Diarist 2390 (male, 60s, South East England, customs officer)

So many events have been cancelled and I have almost daily e-mails informing me so. I won't be going to see several bands that I have tickets for [. . .] The All England Tennis tournament at Queens in London is also cancelled [. . .] My local pub has been closed since 20th March (what a night that was) and the annual beer festival at the late May bank holiday sadly won't be going ahead.

Diarist 2517 (female, 50s, London, unemployed)

I have a torn tendon in my ankle. I was due to have a repair surgery on March 19th, but it was cancelled because of the hospitals having to focus on Covid patients. But only cancelled at 5pm the night before . . .

So my exercise options are quite limited.

Diarist 2621 (male, 70s, North East England, retired lecturer)

We had to cancel a visit [. . .] for our granddaughter's [birthday] and cancel an Easter break [overseas]. Who knows if and when the travel insurance will compensate us for the latter? Our claim must be one of millions.

Diarist 2723 (female, 50s, East Midlands, unemployed journalist)

My husband and I are both out of work. He was made redundant at the beginning of the year – the worst timing possible. And my job ended in January. We believed 2020 was going to be a new and exciting year for us. But now I feel quite concerned. We are living off his redundancy money which will run out soon. Both of us are completely shut out of the world of work and unable to get out and network or be involved in projects, as so many things have been shelved or put on hold. Several courses and training opportunities I had hoped to do have all been cancelled. He has applied for 15 jobs which have either been suspended or he hasn't heard back from. I have applied for basic jobs to help the NHS – as a driver, to work in hospital kitchens and as one of the (supposed) army of contact tracers they say they want to recruit. And to work in a farm shop. But I haven't heard back from any of them.

Diarist 2788 (female, 60s, Scotland, retired teacher)

My daughter married [last year]. I danced at her wedding and then 2 months later arthritis caused me so much pain that I was placed on an urgent list for a hip replacement. I was to have my surgery the day after lockdown started and have no idea when this will happen [. . .] [Partner] had a bit of a cough last week and felt a bit dozy. In between dispensing sympathy and cups of tea (I'm not completely disabled) I frantically search – unsuccessfully – for an online delivery slot. No way can I go out and shop, even if my car battery hadn't died months ago. He seems to be improving. Phew. I realise, perhaps for the first time, how vulnerable I am. 7 weeks into lockdown, 7 weeks today since I should have had my new hip. By now, I could be driving, walking unaided, back, almost, to normal. But therein madness lies: I refuse to indulge in *might-have-beens* and *What Ifs*.

Diarist 2806 (female, 30s, Scotland, tour guide)

Six months ago, I kind of had a plan. I've been self-employed for four years now, and for the first time in my life I was making non-minimum wage money. Not a fortune, about £20-23,000 a year before tax, but what felt like grown-up money. We were going to buy a flat at the end of the year and think about having kids. I was going to carry on working this year and make good money from what was expected to be a strong tourist season as always. Now nothing looks certain at all.

Diarist 3029 (male, 20s, North West England, editor)

Around 9:30 I went downstairs to pick up a parcel from the front door. It's my [birthday soon], so my parents sent me some cake pops (apparently it was the closest to actual cake they could get delivered to me while also being sure it didn't have any nuts – I'm very allergic and this isn't exactly a good time (if there ever is one) to make an emergency trip to hospital). I'm not really sure how I feel about my birthday – I'd been really looking forward to doing something fun for it since it's the first time in years that I won't have exams on or around the day, so it'll be a little strange to spend it completely on my own.

Diarist 3367 (female, 50s, South East England, priest and bookseller)

This will be the year that never was. So many sporting events have been cancelled, including the Olympics, the World Cup and Wimbledon. Most theatres have cancelled their full year's worth of productions, and so we are waiting to hear from our local theatre about either a refund or a credit for next year. All weddings have been cancelled.

Diarist 3426 (male, 70s, West Midlands, historian)

If it hadn't been for the pandemic, we would this very day be on a cruise ship [. . .] my wife wouldn't be machining scrubs; I wouldn't be offering to deliver groceries; and the Post Office counter could be open for business.

Diarist 3567 (male, 60s, North West England, retired engineer)

At the start of the year my wife and I were looking forward to a holiday in Japan [. . .] touring the country with a Japan Rail pass, viewing the Cherry Blossom, visiting Kanazawa, Kyoto, Osaka, Kobe – places we had not been to since our honeymoon [. . .] As the months passed and the Coronavirus took hold around the world our trip became less and less likely, then just seven days before we were due to depart the Foreign Office advised against all foreign travel and just like that our trip was off.

Diarist 3569 (female, 50s, South West England, community health worker)

Oldest [son] comes out with me to walk the dog. He has had his life turned upside down. No A levels, driving test cancelled [. . .] He was just about to launch himself into the world.

Diarist 3573 (female, 60s, East of England, humanist celebrant)

I made myself porridge for breakfast, with water and stewed plums [. . .] I managed to lose a stone between January and March, in preparation to feel good in the lovely dress I bought for my daughter's wedding, which should have been in April [. . .] We don't yet know if it will be possible to go ahead with the wedding in the autumn. In the meantime, there are other significant dates to get through [. . .] We had so much exciting stuff planned.

Diarist 3739 (female, 60s, South West England, social worker)

I had a ticket to Tokyo to spend two weeks with [daughter] but the flight was cancelled and getting there/getting back seemed risky. I had all sorts of plans about how to minimise the risk of getting infected on the plane. Those plans all seem ridiculous now. I really did not understand how infectious coronavirus is. I developed symptoms of COVID 19 the day before I would have flown if the flight had not been cancelled. An alternative reality to my plans, instead of enjoying my daughter and being part of her new life, I was in the spare bedroom feeling nauseous and breathless.

Diarist 3944 (female, 30s, London, event producer)

At the beginning of the year I had lots planned – I had a big event to deliver in March (which ended up being postponed), I was due to travel a lot with work & had a few holidays planned with my husband. Now we've been thrown a massive curveball and it's difficult to think long term as there's no clear end to the current situation. As someone who plans both professionally and in my private life, it's been difficult to adapt to.

Diarist 4014 (male, 80s, West Midlands, retired teacher)

Another lockdown day ahead [. . .] My usually busy diary is at the moment empty! A strange feeling after over 80 years of active and organised life! I'm having to take each day as it comes with much more of my time taken up by my garden, domestic chores and painting in my conservatory at home.

Diarist 4688 (female, 60s, Yorkshire and Humber, researcher)

I wrote a letter to my friend's little boy, who [. . .] is very much in lockdown as he has special needs and is waiting for another heart operation, delayed at the moment. He has just turned [one year older] but his Mum kept it quiet as he is not aware of the date, and would not have understood why he couldn't have a party with his friends. He likes having letters, and jokes, so I am trawling the internet for jokes on a different theme each week. Today it's vegetables.

CLAP FOR CARERS

The pandemic generated a wave of gratitude for NHS and other 'key' workers – cleaners, postal service workers, public transport workers, supermarket employees and so on – who continued working during lockdown, providing care, often in risky situations. A social media campaign sought to capture and express this gratitude. People were asked to come to their doors or windows at 8.00 pm every Thursday and clap. The campaign won support from the mainstream news media, the prime minister and members of the Royal Family. 'Clap for Carers' became semi-official. The first 'clap' was on 26 March. They were still happening every Thursday by 12 May. Although 12 May was a Tuesday, many diarists commented on Clap for Carers, alongside similar expressions of gratitude: lighting a candle in the window to mark International Nurses Day (12 May); sewing laundry bags for doctors and nurses to use when changing their potentially infected scrubs; sending food to staff working in hospitals and other NHS facilities – cakes, Easter eggs, pizza; putting notes of thanks on household bins; consciously saying 'thank you' to postal service workers, delivery drivers and shop assistants. Clap for Carers in particular became an orientation point during the first months of the pandemic. Some people embraced it enthusiastically – clapping, cheering, banging saucepans, playing musical instruments, letting off fireworks. Some people engaged with it more ambivalently and critically, wishing to express gratitude and support, but disliking the social pressure to conform and join in, and wishing also to keep the focus on NHS and other key workers (when, over time, the clap became more of a social event for neighbours in some communities), to ensure the focus extended so far as hospital porters and cleaners, and also non-NHS carers, social workers, supermarket workers, delivery drivers, and so on, and to ensure the focus – the appreciation of key workers – lasted beyond the immediate moment of crisis. In this connection, some people refused to join in. They suspected the clapping might distract from what key workers really needed: a better long-term pay settlement and adequate supplies of PPE right now. They charged at least some of those clapping with hypocrisy: clapping having voted for the Conservative Party (the current party of government, associated by many with underfunding the NHS) or clapping having broken lockdown or social distancing rules (so having not 'stayed home' to 'protect the NHS'). See also Deliveries; Gratitude; Guilt; Hope; Key workers; Shops; Stay home.

Diarist 99 (female, 50s, East of England, secretarial assistant)

The NHS have been incredible, working tirelessly in incredibly difficult and trying circumstances and I make sure I take part in the weekly "Clap for Carers" event at 8pm on a Thursday when people stand on their doorsteps or at their windows and clap, cheer and make as much noise as possible to show our appreciation and support for every one of them. Buildings have had messages of thanks and support on them lit up in blue lights. People have finally started to appreciate how lucky we are to have the NHS in this country and I pray that this is remembered when we return to our normal lives.

Diarist 223 (female, 80s, East of England, retired medical secretary)

Today being the 12th May is a very special date. It is International Nurses Day and also the birthday of Florence Nightingale. The whole country is now realising how much we rely on the NHS, from the porters, cleaners and everyone up to the nurses and Consultants. What brave people they are keeping the hospitals open at this time of crisis.

Diarist 470 (female, 50s, East Midlands, child psychiatrist)

I get to work as usual for 8:30. Traffic is still good with no traffic jams [. . .] I work in a mental health unit for young people and we have been open throughout, in effect shielding the young people to prevent them catching the virus SARS-COV2. In reception I walk past the piles of PPE (personal protection equipment) we have to use to work with the children [. . .] Lunch is a home made salad. My colleagues have a "Deliveroo" Taco Bell for lunch. Yesterday there was free pizza delivered by Pizza Hut – too much for the staff to eat. We have had lots of freebies as an NHS unit – we've not long finished the 1000 Easter Eggs Mars donated to the unit.

Diarist 479 (female, 40s, South West England, clinical pharmacist)

My day ends with a brief visit from my Practice Manager. The terms for pay for this financial year have finally been confirmed and I will have a small pay rise backdated to 1st April. This is a bittersweet moment as I am aware that many of my NHS colleagues are facing a pay cut this year [. . .] At a time when a number of key workers are losing their lives due to being on the frontline in the fight against Covid-19, some of them living apart from their families to protect them, the "clap for our carers" every Thursday night rings hollow. The mixed messages the government are issuing to the public to minimise the impact of Covid-19 and the failure to provide NHS staff and keyworkers with the appropriate personal protective equipment to do their jobs safely leaves me feeling really angry.

Diarist 589 (female, 50s, South West England, unemployed)

The things I would like to keep from this period are fewer cars, the friendliness and support of neighbours and strangers, the re-established relationship I have with my son, and the community spirit and support for the NHS and all the low paid key workers.

I think the key workers now need to be recognised financially as well as by, let's face it, fairly useless clapping. Without them the country really does fall apart, they need to be rewarded accordingly.

Diarist 1024 (female, 60s, Yorkshire and Humber, massage therapist and charity worker)

Cook tea and watch Channel 4 evening news [. . .] It is National Nurses Day, apparently and, I think, International Year of Nurses and Midwives. There is a suggestion that we place a light in our windows to mark Nightingale's anniversary and as a mark of respect for all nurses and carers across the country who are under such stress just now.

I light a candle and put it in the most visible of our windows.

Diarist 1107 (female, 50s, Yorkshire and Humber, nurse)

I see many many posts on Facebook celebrating International Nurses Day. Large numbers are from friends and colleagues and I join in by posting my own images and comment. I am always a bit embarrassed by the comments and praise that gets heaped on me when I do something like this. I want to celebrate my profession and my colleagues but struggle with the status we seem to have been elevated to at the present time. I do it because a). it's my job and b). I love my job.

Diarist 1108 (male, 50s, West Midlands, teacher)

It's on Thursday that we all stand on the doorstep and clap for carers. That's been great. It's a little civil ritual. Everyone waves. You can hear the echo of applause from other streets. Fireworks are set off down in the valley. Neighbours come together, all apart. Community has come to this street somehow.

Diarist 1189 (non-binary, 20s, London, support worker)

Nobody ever mentions domestic abuse support workers when they thank key workers. I want to thank all my colleagues who are doing such amazing work helping keep people safe from abuse during lockdown, which is even more difficult than usual. As well as obviously thank all the other key workers – the NHS staff, the cleaners, the supermarket assistants, and all those other jobs people are still doing that we might not think of, thank you.

Diarist 1867 (female, 20s, West Midlands, cabin crew)

After dinner we watch the news and it's all about the new lockdown measures that are coming into place, and also about celebrating nurses as it is International Nurses Day. Me and my family joke about the people on our street that clap on Thursdays for nurses and how if it was International Nurses Day on Thursday instead of today that they'd all be trying to one-up each other with their clapping – we have some right characters on our street that seem to compete to make the loudest noise. My favourite is [neighbour] over the road who comes out with tambourines.

Diarist 1984 (female, 60s, North West England, unemployed)

On to one of the other lockdown projects. I've been sewing laundry bags for the NHS so I tackle the latest batch I've cut out, which will probably be the last (no more fabric). When I finish these, I will have sewn 160. Not perfectly; wonky seams, shonky stitching, but hey, their purpose is to be flung into the washing machine, so they'll do.

Diarist 2357 (female, 50s, Yorkshire and Humber, unemployed)

The bin men have just passed the window, giving me a cheery wave. We have notices on our bins thanking them for the work they have continued to do throughout the pandemic and wishing them safety and wellness.

Diarist 2394 (male, 50s, South East England, unemployed actor)

The Thursday Night Clap. Sigh.

Well, yes – it's something I want to do, or did at first anyway. The first time was wonderful, moving, surprising. Fireworks were let off. People banged saucepans. It felt needed, a chance for us all to express our gratitude and our hope and to experience community. My sister-in-law works in the NHS [. . .] so of course I want to applaud her and everyone like her – not to mention the other less (shall we say) photogenic workers [. . .] the train cleaners, the delivery drivers, the Bulgarian woman who walks along our road daily at 7am to wake and feed the 90-something year old widow at the end of our street, all the people restocking the shelves on a night shift at Morrisons, all the low-paid, formerly despised, usually non-'English' people who do the crappy jobs that we don't like to think about. . . . But after the first few weeks, it's now become a Thing, like the poppy day Thing, a sense of truculent righteousness about it, it reminds me of the applause for Comrade Stalin at the annual party congress when nobody dared to stop too early, it's a sort of signalling of – what? I don't know. But I do know that I feel uneasy – my friend has taken to chanting "PPE, PPE" during The Thursday Night Clap, and I wish I were brave enough to do the same.

Diarist 2408 (female, 40s, London, theatre worker)

I've been watching quite a lot of theatre online via the internet. The National Theatre puts out a new play every Thursday evening at 7 which has to be interrupted at 8pm by the 'clap for carers' which I do out of my bedroom window every week without fail. It always brings a tear to my eye and a lump in my throat.

Diarist 2806 (female, 30s, Scotland, tour guide)

I spoke to my friend [. . .] on WhatsApp [. . .] She talked about how angry she feels during the eight o'clock clap for carers on a Thursday, knowing how many people in her area voted for another Conservative government that would continue to destroy the NHS as they've always wanted. There's a lot of anger on the left at the hypocrisy of those who vote Tory and laud the "heroes" of the NHS; the NHS they voted again and again to underfund and undermine.

Diarist 3192 (female, 60s, East Midlands, retired teacher)

'International nurses' day' indeed. If it wasn't for the pandemic, they would be making no more of it than international – I don't know – make-your-own-compost day. I know, cynicism is corrosive and destructive, but I won't go out and clap on Thursdays either (although I am profoundly thankful for the work of all the health and other key workers). I can't help reflecting how many of those people out banging saucepans not only voted Conservative last time, but probably will again.

Diarist 3569 (female, 50s, South West England, community health worker)

I work for an agency and visit clients in their own homes. I pay my own fuel (through some contorted loop hole in contract) and am paid by the minute for each call (no money for travel time and if you run over it's a fight [. . .] to get anything like recompense) [. . .] We've been elevated from Low Skilled to Key Worker; the nation claps but we still get paid a pittance with no job security.

DELIVERIES

During lockdown, people could go shopping for 'essential' items, but ideally people would stay home and have supplies delivered. In this context, deliveries took on a new significance for people. They consumed time and attention, not least because delivery slots were hard to secure, at least in the first few weeks of lockdown, when some people would get up in the middle of the night to book new slots released by the supermarkets. They were how people helped each other – by sharing delivery slots or making deliveries for vulnerable family or neighbours. They were the highlight of the day, eagerly anticipated when stocks were running low or treats had been ordered. And they were how the virus might enter the home, so deliveries were often received wearing masks and gloves, at a distance from delivery drivers – standing 2 metres away – then washed and sanitized, then quarantined for a period of time. Still, this was better than going to the shops – safer and more convenient – though not in every way. Some people missed going out, seeing others, choosing their own fresh produce. See also Key workers; Shielding; Shops; Stay apart; Stay home.

Diarist P80 (male, 90s, South East England, retired)

10am my neighbour delivered a bag of shopping he'd kindly done for me. I washed it all down with soapy water (as instructed by govt) and left it to dry.

Diarist 102 (female, 60s, South West England, retired journalist)

After breakfast I watch the news headlines and read the *Times* which we now have delivered to our door step. This took a bit of arranging. Local shop stopped taking our subscription vouchers. Another place delivered for a week or so. Then we found a third prepared to do so when hubby over 70 appealed in person. We joined a waiting list.

Diarist 189 (female, 70s, North West England, nurse)

Time for the weekly excitement and decision-making needed to compile our weekly shopping list. Fortunately old friends have been doing this for us, as well as our younger daughter who is entitled to home deliveries as she and her husband are care workers. We have tried to get deliveries ourselves, but have so far failed to get a slot, as although 'old' (over 70) with health problems, we are not decrepit enough to make the government's shielding list. It's hard as a person who usually does the caring to have to ask and be on the receiving end of other people's kindness. I also miss the opportunity to choose for myself.

Diarist 377 (male, 60s, North East England, retired IT engineer)

Typical, I've been waiting for a delivery of gravel and woodchip to complete my landscape gardening project for over a week, the weather has been exceptional for this time of year, and it's arriving today, on a grey, drizzly morning.

Breakfast was the usual home made muesli, with milk delivered by [local farm] and home made yoghurt. (The yoghurt enterprise came around on the back of the coronavirus lock down, a way of not wasting resources.) My daily ritual is to read the FT [Financial Times] on my iPad whilst eating breakfast and drinking tea with lemon.

Ordered more coffee beans and whole leaf tea from Exchange Coffee. Local suppliers have been brilliant during this crisis, and where would we be without the delivery men and women!

The gravel and wood-chip was a little more than I was expecting.

Diarist 484 (female, 60s, Yorkshire and Humber, charity administrator)

Lunch was a bag of crisps as I'd run out of bread. Tesco delivered my online shopping just after 2.00 pm so I was able to have a proper lunch! It's amazing how excited I get over a shopping delivery these days! I'm doing all my food shopping online as it's just too scary to go to the supermarket where people, including staff, tend to ignore the 2-metre distancing rule.

Diarist 530 (female, 20s, London, social media manager)

As I write this today, overall I feel ok. I had a delivery of a t-shirt I ordered, which was a highlight. Just a small treat to give myself a boost and contribute in a small way to the economy (or that's what I tell myself).

Diarist 697 (female, 11, North East England)

My dad came up to tell us to come down to choose what we wanted in our sandwiches [. . .] I chose ham and cheese. My brother, dad and sister had twiglets. We didn't order them in the shopping but they came anyway. I don't like them, none of us do, but as we are in a crisis we still ate them.

Diarist 989 (female, 60s, retired)

A book arrives in the post. We treat it with caution. Should we put it aside for three days until any virus on the packaging is dead?

Diarist 1213 (female, 30s, London, IT consultant)

The school have been publishing daily tasks for us to do with the kids [. . .] The tasks are always one reading/writing, one maths and one 'Topic' which is usually something creative or active [. . .] We didn't do the topic – we were supposed to make sculptured animals out of tin foil, but I didn't want to waste tin foil because it's the kind of thing that might easily be sold out when I do the online shop [. . .] Once I had my little break I started on the tea just after 5. Nothing exciting today: sausages and mash (mine veggie). We are trying to be very resourceful in what we cook, taking even more effort than usual not to waste food. I'm currently managing to get an online delivery every 2 weeks, because I'm alternating with one for us and one for my mum. So I have to make the delivery last 2 weeks to minimise trips to the shops.

Diarist 1310 (female, 30s, South East England, business developer)

Lunchtime: I have a slice of ham and heat-up a tin of chicken and vegetable soup. I'm looking forward to my Tesco's delivery arriving tonight as I haven't got much in the fridge [. . .] At 10pm my Tesco's delivery arrives, yippee, and I spend 20 mins unloading my shopping. I am delighted that I got 12 eggs for the price of 6 but am disappointed that 2 eggs have cracked and the gin I ordered has leaked slightly. Still, on balance, less stressful than going to the supermarket.

Diarist 1346 (female, 60s, Scotland, retired doctor)

Today – and the days in lockdown are ill defined – is the day the fruit and vegetable boxes arrive from a local farm shop. So a frantic appraisal of what is still left from last week – and I make roasted beetroot and orange soup and roasted cauliflower and chickpea stew.

Diarist 1423 (male, 30s, London, auditor)

London has definitely brought out the convenience of big city living in the times of a pandemic [. . .] We've self-isolated 2 times for 14 day periods, and it has little impact because you can get takeaways, shopping deliveries from actual supermarkets who deliver to your door, and now there's even on-the-day deliveries like a takeaway where they go to local shops and bring you stuff. I don't even care that it's got delivery fees, tips, processing fees and then no deals on your shopping, it's just a safe mechanism to ensure we always have the ability to get food in if we are so inclined. As a result, the last time I went to a shop was 53 days ago, and I have not missed it one bit [. . .] Convenience rules.

Diarist 1480 (female, 20s, London, bar worker and sales assistant)

I've currently been furloughed from both jobs, meaning that I'm earning 80% of my usual wages. I should really be saving money here because I can't go to the pub or go out for food or get public transport, but I keep finding ways to spend money, I have a delivery most days! Retail therapy seems to be my new crutch to get me through, now that I no longer have the pub as a coping mechanism.

Diarist 1602 (female, 60s, South West England, school librarian and counsellor)

I walked [. . .] Nearing my house, there seemed to be a whole cluster of delivery vans, Sainsbury's, Abel and Cole and other white vans were parked. It's a sign of the times [. . .] Already today before 7 o'clock, [husband] and I had our regular order from *Milk and More* (today it was milk, butter and soya yoghurt – other days they bring oat milk, cheese, yoghurt and eggs). Later, we'd had an order from the Co-op which comes via Deliveroo with a man on a motorbike (the online Co-op website has a motley array of things you can order so today I had batteries for the garden lights, loo-cleaner and parmesan cheese amongst other things but I was missing dark chocolate – oh the things I see as essential!). On my return, the veg box and fruit box arrived from Riverford and when I went into the garden to empty the rubbish, I found the bag of coffee beans I'd ordered had been delivered, thrown over the garden gate.

Diarist 1651 (male, 70s, West Midlands, marketing consultant)

Whilst supper is cooking, my wife and I go online to buy some presents for our grandson's second birthday coming up at the end of the month. First stop, John Lewis – nothing doing. Then, Boden – definitely nothing doing! Then the Disney story – lots doing! Then over to Argos and Smyths to see if we can buy a garden swing and slide set. We could, but everybody is out of stock. We think that's definitely a sign of the times – housebound parents with young kids buying up all the toys, etc. they can find. Oh well, we'll keep trying . . .

Diarist 1700 (female, 50s, London, piano teacher)

The doorbell went and my shoes arrived (I had been waiting for them for a number of months), followed swiftly by the post and my daughter's next paint instalment. I had to wear rubber gloves to handle every delivery, spray each package and then the contents with disinfectant before handling them and then wash my hands for the required 20 seconds.

Diarist 1710 (female, 60s, London, garden designer)

We had a coffee in the garden and discussed the latest online food orders. We get everything delivered and have managed to avoid going to the supermarket at all. Reports from my sister and daughter are that there is no way you can social distance in the supermarkets in London.

Diarist 1848 (male, 50s, Scotland, broadcast and telecommunications engineer)

Another big shower of snow blew over at 10:20, to coincide with the postman's van arriving. While we're in Lockdown/Shielding the postman knows to simply drop the mail on the seat of [wife's] car – our cars are never locked – so that there's no need to come into the garden or to the front door. Once the postvan had driven off I went out to collect the mail – just a dull letter from my accountant. Nothing interesting.

Diarist 1866 (non-binary, 20s, South East England, student and proof-reader)

Got a glass of water and a pain au chocolat for breakfast [. . .] It was the last croissant in the pack and a bit stale, but we have a click and collect slot booked for this afternoon, so more groceries are incoming (this is a big relief, as we've had genuine concerns, especially at the beginning of the pandemic when everyone was panic buying, about being able to get food for us, my nan, and my grandparents; we've had to rely on digging out the back of cupboards and the freezer for a few meals, and gone without fresh fruit and veg a few times but, overall, we've managed to get a delivery or click and collect slot every week or so and are managing with what we've been able to get without physically going to a supermarket and putting ourselves and, by extension, our vulnerable dependents at risk).

Diarist 1867 (female, 20s, West Midlands, cabin crew)

I eat some ice cream that I had delivered from a local farm because it's a pandemic and when else can you have 4 tubs of ice cream delivered to your home and it be acceptable?

Diarist 1979 (female, 60s, South East England, editor and retired nurse)

I finally managed to book a shopping slot with Asda last week for 18th May, two weeks ahead [. . .] I wasn't able to find a delivery slot for weeks, but our neighbour has a new baby so is up all hours and texted me very early one morning that some new slots had been made available.

Diarist 2205 (male, 70s, North West England, retired teacher)

Breakfast (granola) without banana was a tragedy – albeit minor. The ASDA deliver order was cocked up and I've been without bananas now for about 4 days.

Diarist 2238 (female, 60s, South East England, landscape archaeologist)

Running short of some groceries so checked for online deliveries slots. There are none but looks like I may be able to get a click and collect next week [. . .] It will be pasta tonight for supper. Made onion soup for lunch as I have a surfeit of football sized onions. That is the trouble with online shopping, I ordered eight, thinking they would be medium sized, they are gigantic.

Diarist 2640 (female, 60s, Scotland, counsellor and therapist)

I shop differently now. Asda comes every 12 days or so and brings the shopping to my door [. . .] The man knows me now and has some cheery 2 metres chat in the hallway [. . .] I spray every item with a diluted bleach then after 5 minutes I wash every item. It doesn't feel weird anymore.

Diarist 2723 (female, 50s, East Midlands, unemployed journalist)

After lunch I went to pick up prescriptions for a few people in the village as I have volunteered to help people here. I drive to the local surgery in the nearby town, put on latex gloves, stand outside and hand the masked nurse a list of the patients I'm collecting for. She gets them from inside the building, hands me the medicines and I drive back and drop them at people's houses. I ring the bell, stand well back and either drop the parcels on the doorstep or hand them to the individuals.

Diarist 2764 (female, 14, Northern Ireland)

It seems the highlight of most days is waiting for the post to arrive. I have always loved the thought of getting things delivered without having to leave the comfort of your own home but now that we are in quarantine I have ordered so much more. I have an unusual obsession with film magazines and movie posters. I have to entertain myself somehow right?

Diarist 3284 (male, 20s, South East England, retailer)

Rounded off the day with some videogames with the flatmate while we waited for a food delivery from Iceland. It's very hard to book a delivery slot with any supermarket right now – ours turned up at 11pm, which was the only time available for the whole week.

Diarist 3390 (male, 60s, South East England, retired NHS manager)

One final sympathy card arrived in the post today – my father died of Covid last month and was cremated ten days ago.

Diarist 3426 (male, 70s, West Midlands, historian)

Emailed local community contact to offer to deliver groceries for the housebound tomorrow. I have done this for the last five weeks. It is encouraging to feel that I can be of some use, rather than just a potential liability who might overload the NHS.

Diarist 3573 (female, 60s, East of England, humanist celebrant)

Got up at 7.45am and unpacked my Amazon order, which had been quarantining in the hall for a couple of days. We take this precaution because the virus has been found to live on paper and card for up to 24 hours and plastic for up to three days. There is no evidence that you can catch it from them but, to be on the safe side, we treat everything coming into the house as contaminated and dispose of or thoroughly wash any packaging/containers, even after they've been quarantined. The order included about a year's supply of kitchen bin bags, a small soap to tide us over until the five litre refill bottle arrives and a large E45 moisturiser. My handwashing frequency is excessive, especially considering it's unlikely the virus has even entered our home. I wish it glowed red or green, like a germ simulation in an advert, so we could know whether it's present or not!

Diarist 3808 (female, 70s, North East England, retired school inspector)

7.45 am Breakfast in the kitchen – cereal and fruit and a cup of strong coffee [. . .] Neither of us have been in a shop for the past eight weeks or so and rely on getting our food by supermarket delivery [. . .] Eating up fresh food in date has become our obsession.

Diarist 3987 (female, 70s, South West England, milliner)

It seems that even ordinary simple activities have suddenly become very difficult. Shopping is almost impossible if you are staying home. On-line shopping slots are fully booked. There has been a supermarket shopping frenzy for basic necessities. Food, cleaning materials and even toilet paper have rapidly become unavailable. I did manage to book one delivery in April for my Mother and one due on Friday for myself. I have also ordered a few luxury goods and some wine from specialist online suppliers. Fortunately, I contacted [local] Mutual Aid, and now a young Veterinarian collects my prescriptions from the pharmacy and manages my weekly shop [. . .] The postman arrived as usual before lunchtime. It will be my birthday tomorrow, so there are cards and a parcel to be quarantined and sterilised in the garage before they can be opened. We are told the virus remains on paper for up to 72 hours, so to open items for my birthday I shall have to wear gloves and a face mask.

Diarist 4008 (female, 70s, South East England, retired caterer)

I go to bed between 9 and 10 [. . .] I have to get up at midnight to book a slot for Tesco delivery, 4 weeks in advance. It is the only way to get a slot. I do this once a week. I do miss shopping myself. It is exercise, you see people. I live opposite a Tesco Express, and know all staff by name. I take them home made cake occasionally [. . .] I will continue to do this after we are released!

FEAR

If one mood of the pandemic was anxiety, another was fear: dread, horror, terror. People didn't just have anxiety dreams. They had nightmares. Many people were scared of an invisible threat perceived to be stalking them. They were scared of catching the virus, getting ill, getting a novel illness about which little was known, dying – especially if they were 'vulnerable' or 'high risk', and especially if they lived alone with no one to look after them. Fearful of catching the virus, they were scared of going out, crowds, confined spaces, proximate strangers. They were terrified that vulnerable loved ones might get the virus and die before they could see them again. So they washed their hands and cried. Such responses were rational and justified. Government briefings and news media reported alarming statistics for infections, hospitalizations and deaths. Some diarists wrote while suffering symptoms, fearing they would get worse. Some diarists wrote while family members were being treated for serious breathing difficulties. See also Anxiety; Shops; Stay apart.

Diarist 14 (female, 30s, London, film producer)

I suffer from Obsessive Compulsive Disorder (OCD) which was largely under control until the pandemic hit. I've regressed considerably, with a flare-up of contamination OCD – a fear of the invisible threat of coronavirus which I try and mitigate through extensive rituals around hand-washing, food preparation, clothes washing etc. It's exhausting, and the frustrating thing about OCD is that it actually exacerbates anxiety in the long-run (even as it tries to soothe it), so I'm struggling a bit with some physical and psychological symptoms of anxiety most days. A tight chest, mostly, which feels fittingly Freudian given the symptoms of covid-19!

I fear for my loved ones, which adds not only to the anxiety but also the OCD behaviours – I have rituals which I feel I have to do in order to keep my family safe. It's called 'magical thinking' OCD, and it makes some day to day activities much harder to do. For me, the rituals get worse around bedtime, so it can sometimes take me an extra hour to get into bed and turn the lights off.

Diarist 200 (female, 30s, London, visual designer)

Mum is classed as vulnerable [. . .] And my little sister seems likely to be back at work in June [. . .] I'm so scared and sad and concerned for my family's future, more than my own right now. I found myself in a moment yesterday where I didn't even know how to feel anymore. I sat in the bath and cried so hard I couldn't breathe.

Diarist 486 (female, 80s, Midlands, retired)

As I write, the future seems very uncertain and for the moment quite scary: will we ever be rid of this virus? Can I, as one of the 'vulnerable', ever feel free to go out and about as I used to, without a mask and a level of anxiety that I might get infected? Will all the little shops and businesses in our town reopen, will the pubs and restaurants survive? Will I ever again be able to catch the train [. . .] with friends and go to a live concert [. . .]? I try not to think of such things – 'one day at a time' is still my rule. We are where we are and we must do the best we can.

Diarist 542 (female, 60s, East Midlands, retired accountant)

I started listening to the daily briefings from Downing Street and reading the news on my phone constantly. The result was that I became depressed and frightened of going out. Facebook posts by others seemed to make it worse and it was difficult to determine what was true and what wasn't. By the end of the first 3 weeks I was trying to concentrate on doing my jigsaw puzzle and I found that I became upset. This was not living, just existing.

Diarist 884 (female, 50s, London, psychotherapist)

Throughout lockdown my moods have changed swiftly. I would say I am generally coping with it ok, but then I read something, or think about my parents and I tear up . . . I find not knowing when I may see them again painful. My mum was very upset on the phone when we last spoke, unsure she'd ever get to see people again. Both parents are [older] so I have dreaded them getting Covid-19 and being unable to see them again [. . .] I am fed up of being alone, weeks and weeks of being alone . . . I find things like Zoom and messaging too much, make me feel more lonely not less . . . at the beginning of lockdown I was afraid of being ill and having no one to look after me . . . I do have good friends but none live nearby . . . my neighbour and I made a pact, if either of us got sick we would shop etc. for the other . . . luckily it didn't happen . . . not to date [. . .] I have frozen food I bought in case I got sick.

Diarist 1150 (female, 80s, London, retired teacher)

I decided to take a walk before preparing breakfast and although I have been shopping online and avoiding going to the shops, I had no eggs so combining exercise with buying eggs seemed like a good idea. It was quite quiet on the streets around my house and it was pleasant noticing the different ways in which my neighbours are acknowledging the NHS and VE Day last week – rainbows in windows and chalked on the pavement; hand painted signs and flag banners draped over trees.

When I hit the 'mainish' road at the top it seemed that business was back to normal – lots of cars on the go, although not too many people on foot. I am not enjoying the fearfulness that I am beginning to experience and when I went into a small supermarket at the top of the road one of the staff sneezed and I didn't like my reaction to that which was to get out of the shop as quickly as possible.

Diarist 1390 (female, 20s, South East England, student)

I cooked two veggie burgers in the oven, from Tesco. I had leftover salad from earlier and my mum had sweet potato fries. She's just come out of hospital after having coronavirus symptoms and pneumonia, and they discovered a potential heart problem too, but they let her out for now and she has to go back for tests. But it seems like we might have to wait for ages as things are so overwhelmed right now in the NHS. It was very scary – for about 24 hours we all really had to face the possibility that she might not make it. She was struggling to breath and to move.

Diarist 1451 (female, 60s, Northern Ireland, retired teacher)

My beloved and I would have spent a few days at the Cork International Poetry Festival in early March had it not been for this virus. We went last year, had an Airbnb and I managed three or four poetry events a day while he went birdwatching in the daytime and joined me for the bigger evening readings. Seems unthinkable now. Crowds! Sociability! Horror film music. . . . Imagining the scene makes me nervous, I am now so conditioned to see proximity as dangerous.

Diarist 1456 (male, 50s, Wales, retired psychotherapist)

This morning I awoke at seven thirty, feeling slightly disturbed in the aftermath of another lucid Lockdown dream. The dream had an atmosphere of 'Film Noir', set in a dark and satanic landscape leaving me haunted by a feeling of menace, a quality pervading a lot of my dreams at present.

Diarist 1940 (female, 30s, Scotland, assistant professor)

I am terrified of coronavirus, both catching it myself and any of my loved ones catching it. Initially it didn't seem quite as frightening for me specifically, as I am not in any higher risk group [. . .] However in the last month I've read a couple of news items about the potential longer term effects that coronavirus can have on people who only had a mild case [. . .] That scared me so much that I stopped reading the news [. . .] At the moment, my flat feels like the only safe place in the world and every other human being feels like a potential threat.

Diarist 2341 (female, 30s, Wales, librarian)

I had a flare up of my autoimmune condition last year and spent the best part of [late 2019] in the hospital. Recovery is going well but when the lockdown started, I was told my infusions of Tocilizumab would have to be suspended. I was having them every four weeks and have missed two but it's unlikely they'll be restarted anytime soon since it's an immunosuppressant and would increase my risk of catching the virus even further. It's a little bit scary, because I know how quickly a flare up can manifest. If it happens, I'll need a lot of help with the day to day things like getting dressed and preparing meals, but I won't be able to lean on my family in the way I have in the past.

Diarist 2627 (female, 40s, Northern Ireland, editor)

The virus has a hold on everyone and everything now. Numbers of deaths in Northern Ireland are relatively small but they hurt in a big way. When I feel fear and anger and sadness and despair, I can't help thinking of Covid-19 as having the personal qualities of a stalker, an assailant, a terrorist.

Diarist 2640 (female, 60s, Scotland, counsellor and therapist)

I caught a bus 4 weeks ago, it was empty but filled up enroute and I was not safely distanced. It was suddenly very frightening until off the bus.

Diarist 2957 (female, 50s, North West England, careers consultant)

I've been signed off work with depression for a few weeks, something I do suffer from occasionally [. . .] I'd been managing the anxiety, stress and uncertainty of the last couple of months reasonably well, with a few ups and downs obviously, until about 3 weeks ago when I had a bit of a 'crash', crying a lot, feeling incredibly anxious and slowing down considerably. So I spoke to the GP who signed me off for 3 weeks, I'd already had one week at that point. We'll have to see how I go, it's a wait and see situation and there are no quick fixes for this illness, just rest and medication in my experience, plus counselling, which I've not needed this time. I feel quite detached from this description as I'm writing, as it doesn't fully convey the fear, dread and horror I've been experiencing the last two months.

Diarist 3562 (female, 50s, South West England, garden designer)

I started to feel unwell the first weekend of the lockdown with virus symptoms. I was lucky. Though I've felt very poorly, I didn't need to go to hospital. My main symptom throughout has been a tight chest. I can feel the congestion in my lungs and that symptom has continued long after everything has got better. I am resigned to taking time to recover, but in the back of my mind is a fear that this has done some longer-term damage. No-one knows what this disease is or what it does. I didn't really want to be a guinea pig.

Diarist 3789 (male, 30s, Scotland, copy editor)

Woke with a bit of a sore throat. That it is not a scratchy feeling, and that it is accompanied by dry eyes, suggests allergies or dry air as the cause, but in these troubling times there is the niggle that it is coronavirus, 'the bug' (we almost dare not speak its name).

Diarist 3906 (female, 40s, London, hospital worker)

Today is no ordinary day. I am very scared and stressed. I am self isolating for 10 days. I cannot go to a job I love because I may have a virus, covid-19. I work with premature babies at the local hospital [. . .] and I have a rash, high temperatures. My husband and I are both at home. We got tested 2 days ago and are awaiting results. I keep checking email but no answer.

Diarist 3987 (female, 70s, South West England, milliner)

09:30 My partner managed to persuade me to go out for a walk, exploring some local footpaths I had not visited before. I do not usually go out for a walk these days, as I am increasingly frightened by the proximity of others. The experience leaves me feeling uncomfortable, as there appears to be too much risk until this time of contagion has passed.

Diarist 4564 (male, 16, East of England)

My day began with some household chores like washing and then I sat down to complete some work for College [. . .] In between doing work and making lunch, I was able to

FaceTime my Mum who was in hospital and had been in there for four weeks (3 in intensive care) with COVID-19. She was able to give us the great news that on the next day she would be able to come home. I was elated! I missed her so much and was so scared at points that she may have died.

FUNERALS

According to the Office for National Statistics, there were 43,796 excess deaths registered in England and Wales in April 2020. This was in addition to the 44,242 deaths predicted by the five-year average (2015–19). Some of these people died alone in care homes closed to visitors. Some of them were buried or cremated alone in direct funerals. The rules and guidance regarding funerals varied over time and between jurisdictions and providers, but commonly placed limits on the number of mourners and required people to keep at least 2 metres apart. Many people couldn't attend the funerals of loved ones because of limits on the number of mourners, or difficulty travelling, or their own vulnerability. In this context, new rituals arose. Hearses were clapped through the streets by those unable to attend. When those who could attend arrived, they did so to seemingly empty chapels or graveyards – where open-air burials were common. Mourners were unable to comfort each other with hugs or handshakes. They were unable to touch the coffin – to 'carry in' the deceased or 'lay flowers'. Short services, dictated by the high demand, were led by funeral directors in facemasks, doing their best while also worrying about exposure to infection. Services with no singing were followed by no wake – no opportunity for mingling, reminiscing, communing. For those mourners who couldn't attend, service endings could be tougher still. After watching live online, in the click of a mouse they found themselves alone at home. Mourning alone mirrored dying alone. See also Grief; Stay apart; Zoom.

Diarist 101 (female, 30s, London, funeral celebrant)

Most people think funerals are always miserable – but they aren't; they can be uplifting and joyous as people come together in solidarity to celebrate a person they loved. But in these strange times there is an additional shadow of sadness cast over everything . . . no hugs or shaking of hands, everyone sat apart, no touching the coffin or carrying in. Funerals have a hollowness like I have never experienced before [. . .] Everyone is trying their best but it is heartbreaking to say 'no' to simple requests like laying a flower or pall bearing when a family is devastated.

Diarist P293 (female, 30s, London, hairdresser and account manager)

Nanna's funeral is next Tuesday. In her 90s, we expected it at some point but it seems so cruel that no-one could be with her at the end. I feel deeply sad that I couldn't say goodbye in person. She was frail, especially in the past few months, but no-one would have guessed that it would be Covid-19 that would bring an end to her life.

Diarist 746 (female, 40s, London, consultant)

My Mum updated me on the family news. My Aunt, who had cancer, died from coronavirus in the early weeks of the crisis. My cousin, who was at home to help his parents, has had 5 weeks in hospital with it. He was in intensive care on a ventilator and has been very lucky to survive. He found out about his mother's death via a text message in hospital. He's just home now and is on the long road to recovery. It was his mother's funeral yesterday. They were allowed 10 people, all sitting 2 metres apart. No hugging.

Diarist 779 (female, 60s, East of England, publisher)

Today I awoke with a nervousness – a sense of the inevitable – for today was the funeral of my mother-in-law. She passed away at the age of 85 having been a little unwell, but ultimately a victim of the dreaded Covid19.

My husband, one daughter [. . .] and I set off to the crematorium for a 10am service. With printed 'order of service' tucked under our arms and the sun shining on our backs, we gathered our strength. On arrival we were met by the warm smiles (but no hugs allowed) of our other daughter and her partner and we noted the bizarrely attired crematorium staff and their black top hats, tails and face masks. What strange times we live in.

Restricted numbers meant we were a congregation of just five in a chapel built to accommodate 150 mourners. We anxiously awaited the hearse and noted the back-to-back bookings for this day in both chapels. Strange times, busy times.

Diarist 916 (female, 60s, South East England, retired teacher)

I walked from my house into town [. . .] I had a big surprise when I got home. A knock on the door and an enormous box of flowers, sent by my daughter. That's so kind of her – she sent them because my favourite aunt died a few days ago from a stroke. None of the family had been able to see her for two months, because she lived in a care home. This dreadful Covid-19 means the home was closed to visitors. A death is always sad, but seems more so when you know the person was not able to be with their family at the end. I plan to buy a rose to plant in my garden as a memorial. She loved gardening, and roses.

Diarist 1310 (female, 30s, South East England, business developer)

My mother-in-law rings me in tears to tell me she is having her dog [. . .] put to sleep tomorrow [. . .] I offer to go with [her] to the vets [but she] explains that because of social distancing the vet will do it in the boot of the car and then [she] can say her goodbyes. Then the dog will be taken away and cremated. Even if I was there, I can't give [her] a hug afterwards.

Diarist 1364 (female, 60s, East of England, solicitor)

My beloved brother died of the virus some six weeks ago, only 64 but he had asthma. He was the loveliest of men, a brilliant scientist, a wonderful husband and father, the kindest brother, the best company, I miss him dreadfully. My sister in law and nephews are still in shock, we all are. I wake every day still in disbelief. The funeral was brutal, just 6 of us and no wake, no hugs, no reminiscing. So, in some ways this enforced seclusion has suited me, meeting other people is too difficult at present.

Diarist 1451 (female, 60s, Northern Ireland, retired teacher)

One of my first thoughts when all this started is how glad I was not to have my mother in a nursing home at this dreadful moment. I am pleased she didn't have to die alone in such fear and that she could have a proper funeral. My husband and I (this makes anyone who says it sound like the queen's Christmas message) have been discussing what we would like if we became very ill with Covid 19. We would not want intensive care unless we were very likely to survive it. We would prefer to die as gently as possible, with palliative care in our own house, and be with each other. We have been writing death plans.

Diarist 1700 (female, 50s, London, piano teacher)

My husband's brother died in the middle of March. He died in the bathroom in his home after being ill with Coronavirus symptoms for 7 days [. . .] There was no testing to see if he definitely had it and they wouldn't test when he was dead [. . .] His death certificate says: 'Virus related death'! [. . .] He couldn't be cremated until over 6 weeks after his death. His funeral was on Zoom and my husband and his remaining brother could not even go to comfort their elderly mum who has been isolating all alone with no company at all. Simply awful.

Diarist 1940 (female, 30s, Scotland, assistant professor)

I am tired and slow this morning. I think in part because yesterday was rather emotionally exhausting. I attended the funeral of my Great Aunt, who I loved very much, via Zoom. That was a new experience and a very strange one. I had so little notice of when exactly it would take place that I couldn't take the day off, so had an ordinary working morning, had lunch, then at 2pm was grieving with my family at a distance [. . .] There were more than 50 people in the Zoom call, watching the vicar say prayers and a handful (four or five?) family members do readings next to my Great Aunt's coffin. The service took place at her home. I hope that I can visit her grave once it's safe to do so.

The oddest thing about the funeral was that while it was happening it really felt like an actual funeral. I could see my family's faces on video and hear the emotion in the voices of those reading. I cried through most of it. Then it ended suddenly after 45 minutes and I was back in my living room, which is also my office, kitchen, dining room, laundry room, and yoga studio, by turns. I found the emotional whiplash of this very intense. So I cried for a little longer and talked aloud to my Great Aunt, saying the things I hope she knew about how much I loved and appreciated her. Then I did some domestic chores that didn't require much concentration. What I missed about a normal funeral was the mingling afterwards, sharing the loss with family and comforting one another. I felt very alone.

Diarist 1953 (female, 50s, North West England, bereavement services manager)

Earlier burial today so I leave at 10. Check the grave and lead the funeral directors to the right place. The funeral was intimate with 12 immediate family attending and around 30 people stood at safe distance away. The streets had been lined with other people clapping to show respect as they took a route around the town before arriving at the cemetery. There's a big sense of community in this particular town.

Everyone keeps their distance around the grave which is hard to watch as people are upset and naturally want to comfort each other but under the guidelines it is not permitted/recommended for fear of spreading the virus. I find my role more difficult and emotional. It is near impossible to stay 6ft away from the [Funeral Director] or minister as some conversations that we need to have need to be quiet and not heard by the family. The family place a multi coloured rose into the grave before leaving. I just hope that I don't catch it or that symptoms will be mild for me if I do. I sanitise my hands before getting back in my car. I listen to the radio to take my mind off the burial.

Diarist 1984 (female, 60s, North West England, unemployed)

My father-in-law died a fortnight ago – he would have died soon anyway, Covid19 just brought it forward – but as daughter and I couldn't go to even the cremation, she has come up with a patchwork quilt idea. A community quilt, asking around 'the local community' for contributions [. . .] [She] fancies donating the finished result to the care home where [he] died, but I suppose it would have to be washed at 90 degrees to be safe first.

Diarist 2640 (female, 60s, Scotland, counsellor and therapist)

I had a long telephone video call with a close friend who is at her father in law's funeral tomorrow. My Mum died last year and we gave her the most beautiful funeral send off [. . .] I feel more gratitude – to think of having her die now, with the very limited possibilities for gathering, having a Zoom funeral service for relatives, no hugging, no hand holding, the very essence of love at such times forbidden, just so very sad. I have 3 friends who have had a Covid family funeral, 10 mourners maximum, all spaced out by 2 metres unless they live together. 30 minutes at the crematorium. No wake.

Diarist 2723 (female, 50s, East Midlands, unemployed journalist)

There has been lots in the news recently about the number of deaths in care homes attributable to Covid and also evidence of a dramatic increase in deaths apparently from non-Covid related issues. I feel quite upset about this as my mother died [in April] in a care home. It had already been in lockdown for nearly three weeks (earlier than the government imposed lockdown) so I hadn't seen her. I don't really know what happened. I was allowed to visit her the day before she died and she was unresponsive with very laboured breathing. I don't know if she knew I was there.

We faced lengthy delays after her death as the doctor referred it to the coroner, basically because no medical professional had seen her for a few weeks before she died. We couldn't register her death and my brother and his family could not come up to see us. We were in limbo for weeks. Finally we were able to hold her funeral, under all sorts of restrictions, last [week]. My family came up and, as the weather was beautiful and warm, they had a meal and we all sat in the garden. Technically we were breaking lockdown as two of my sons who are living [elsewhere] also came up. So lots of households mixing. But I think you are allowed to do this for funerals so long as you maintain distancing (which we did try to do). I had warned the neighbours as I didn't want to cause concern and there have been incidents of people reporting their neighbours to the police if they think they are breaking lockdowns to socialise.

Diarist 2869 (female, 60s, East of England, retired teacher)

I text my sister [. . .] to see if she wanted a chat in the garden. She lost her partner to cancer on Thursday and it still hasn't sunken in. Her son and daughter are staying with her to arrange the funeral and to sort out all the paperwork. We sat outside for a cup of tea and a chat. She is seeing a solicitor this afternoon with her son. We discussed the funeral arrangements, which are difficult because of the corona virus. The only car allowed is the hearse, and only 10 to 20 guests. It will be hard to congregate beforehand, or afterwards because we are all meant to be social distancing. There are 3 people in the house, including my sister, who are social isolating because they have serious health problems. They are not meant to go out at all and no one should go near them. They will wear masks at the funeral and gloves, but it will be very hard to keep 2 metres apart from everyone.

Diarist 3086 (female, 30s, London, archivist)

Earlier this afternoon I started writing a will – nothing formal, just a note of what songs I'd like played at my funeral and what bits and bobs I'd like to leave to my friends. I've always been mindful of death, but now it feels closer to everyone.

Diarist 3367 (female, 50s, South East England, priest and bookseller)

Funerals after 23rd March have been limited to no more than 10 people, and they have to be immediate family, and if the family want a churchyard burial the whole service has to be at the graveside, with no singing. Interestingly the funeral I took the week after Easter, with just the children and grandchildren of the deceased, was actually really intimate and meaningful for the family and they sent a lovely card saying how much it meant to them.

Diarist 3404 (female, 60s, South West England, retired curator)

My cousin [. . .] died in a care home two weeks ago. Today is her funeral. She died of old age and dementia, not the virus, and her physical and mental decline mean it is hard to feel grief for her death – just regret that she could not have family around her, and that she can't be cremated with family around her. She is in [South East England], her nieces and nephews and cousins are spread across England. So it is a direct funeral, no family present, and we will meet later to celebrate her. One of her nephews suggested that we should all stop at noon to remember her, so we sat in the garden with tea, and thought about her and her husband, who died a few years ago and to whom she was devoted. Others in the family did the same in their own space all over the country.

Diarist 4054 (female, 70s, North West England, retired teacher)

Yesterday I went to stand on the pavement outside a pub and clap the hearse of a friend on its way to the crematorium because only 10 people were allowed at the funeral.

Diarist 4269 (female, 20s, South East England, editor)

Tuesday 12th May was the date of my grampy's burial. He [. . .] died from Covid [. . .] in a care home [. . .] – he had dementia and had been in a nursing home for just over a year. When it became clear that he had just a few hours left to live, the care home said that a family member could briefly visit (with PPE on, and sitting at a distance). My granny couldn't go because of her age and the associated risk of contracting Covid, and nor could my mum [. . .] Mum made the difficult decision to support Granny instead (as clearly she couldn't visit Grampy then be with Granny, because of the risk of passing on the virus). However, my brother, a trainee GP, is exposed to the virus anyway through work so went on behalf of the family and was able to sit with Grampy for 20 minutes or so. Grampy was more or less unconscious but my brother played him his favourite piece of music [. . .] on his phone, and did a WhatsApp video call with Mum and Granny, which they found very comforting. Lockdown prevented us having the kind of service Grampy had requested in his will, but we were given permission to have a very small, brief, open air burial on 12th May so long as we complied with social distancing [. . .] [Sister and I] pulled up in the car park next to the church at 2.00 and my aunties and their families were already there in their cars. My other sister was also there [. . .] and my brother and his fiancé soon arrived, having come straight from a hospital shift [. . .] Under normal circumstances we'd all have got out of our cars and hugged, but we didn't – most people stayed in their cars until 2.15, even though it was a beautiful day.

At 2.15 we got out and said hello to each other, kind of awkwardly and warily, keeping much more than 2 metres apart [. . .] Mum appeared, pushing granny in her wheelchair, and we all stood at the side of the car park as the hearse drove down it, following the funeral director (I presume?) who was smartly dressed with gloves and a top hat. My nurse sister and my brother and his fiancé stood (separately) much further than 2m away from everyone, given their close contact with Covid patients at work.

The funeral director said socially distanced hellos to Granny and her daughters while we waited for the coffin to be taken out of the hearse and put on a wheeled frame – the pall bearers weren't allowed to put it on their shoulders because of the Covid risk, and had to use straps to lift it on and off the frame. It was then wheeled to Grampy's plot at the bottom of the graveyard, followed by Mum and Granny [. . .] and then the rest of us, each household keeping a significant distance from the others. I turned around as my sister and I walked in and saw our other sister, the nurse, walking at the back of the group by herself and sobbing. She never usually cries [. . .] The service was incredibly sad but also quite beautiful, perhaps even more so because of the small number of people, the social distancing (which somehow underlined how much you'd naturally have wanted to be close to people and touch them), and the very simple outdoor service. The sun was shining and there were buttercups on the common [. . .] After the service, we all stood around at the edge of the common and talked for a bit, still distanced. People walked by staring at us, which was unsurprising as it's so rare to see a group of more than 4 people at the moment, but they clearly realised it was for a funeral. We let the dog out of the car so that my nurse sister could hug her, since she didn't have another person to comfort her.

FURLOUGH

Lockdown meant entire sectors of the economy were temporarily closed. To bridge the gap until they could be opened again, the UK Government provided various kinds of support, including the Coronavirus Job Retention Scheme, which initially supported businesses to furlough employees on 80 per cent of their salaries (up to a limit of £2,500 per month) and the Self-Employment Income Support Scheme, which initially provided self-employed people with grants worth 80 per cent of their average monthly trading profit (up to a limit of £7,500 over three months). The diaries from 12 May capture experiences of people furloughed since March or in the process of applying for self-employed income support (applications for the first round of this latter scheme opened on 13 May). They capture a sense of anxiety. While some people qualified for support, or thought they would, others didn't, or thought they wouldn't. While some people could still live comfortably on 80 per cent of their previous income – or had that figure topped up by their employer – others couldn't. While some people were relieved to still have a job, which they hoped to go back to once protections had been lifted, others felt like they had been made redundant and worried that redundancies really would be made by their employer if the pandemic continued beyond the support schemes. The diaries also capture a sense of drift. Without work, people felt lethargic and lacking in motivation. They felt no sense of purpose and struggled to sleep after days lacking accomplishments. They felt unimportant and surplus to requirements. While some welcomed the freedom of furlough and the more relaxed and leisurely lifestyle it allowed, others quickly became bored and felt the need to fill time and establish new, productive routines involving training courses, voluntary work, gardening, DIY. See also Anxiety; Lockdown projects; Stay home.

Diarist 913 (male, 20s, London, regulation officer)

I'm going to be furloughed for the whole of June, but my work have been good and are topping up everyone's salary to 100%. Effectively, a free holiday! I'm hoping to use the time productively and revisit my French language skills.

Diarist 1133 (female, 40s, South West England, receptionist)

I [. . .] have been furloughed and as I work in the hospitality trade will be one of the last sectors to return to work.

Today started like all the other days since lockdown began. Not having a reason to get up in the morning means even though I may wake up around 8am, I have not been getting out of bed till at least 9:30. I have given up wearing make up or making an effort with my appearance [. . .] I scrolled through Facebook and the news, procrastinating as always. I then went to the shop for bread with express instructions from my daughter to get some snacks, no wonder I have put on weight since lockdown began.

Diarist 1157 (female, 40s, London, archivist)

I was furloughed on April 15th [. . .] This was a blow to me as the message I have taken from my employers [. . .] is that they don't see the importance of archives or archivists. I am disappointed and angry by this decision. My daily routine has quickly adapted to finding new ways to occupy my day. I am doing an online digital archives course, a small amount of voluntary work for another archive, reading (badly) and tending to some plants [. . .] I drove to [the local park] for a longer than usual walk, lovely sunny day, more people out than usual and I was lifted by the birdsong, rhododendrons and goslings. Especially after hearing the 1pm news and the government announcement that the furlough scheme will be extended until the end of October. This made me depressed at the thought of not getting back to the office in some shape or form and further months of endlessly filling my days.

Diarist 1250 (female, 60s, Wales, sales assistant)

Got up around 6am. Still get up early even though I'm not currently working. Took [dog] for a walk in the forest. Five minutes' walk from my house takes me onto beautiful forest tracks. Enjoy the early morning peace and tranquillity with just me, my dog and the birds [. . .] Came home [. . .] fed the dog his breakfast. Made a cup of tea [. . .] When I'm working I usually rush off to get ready after this. With being on furlough a new routine has happened. Now we relax a while and catch up on the news.

Washed, cleaned teeth etc. then we went downstairs and ate breakfast with a nice cup of fresh coffee. Working means we only have time for instant coffee. We spent a while doing a jigsaw. We have one out all the time while we have this extra time off work. Then we went outside. My partner worked on building a cover for the new raised vegetable planters he built in the back garden. He built these since we've been off work but a pesky squirrel has been stealing the seedlings [. . .] I did some other gardening, weeding, trimming and earthing up my potatoes. I did a bit of training with my young dog, just fun stuff.

We sat outside and ate our lunch on our decking underneath a pergola that my partner built last week. Another extra project we've had time for recently.

The afternoon was spent in a similar way. My partner built a low table to go in the pergola from a log and a piece of wood that he cut into a hexagon [. . .] My partner had a doze in the sun. I planted out some veg.

Diarist 1369 (female, 40s, West Midlands, housewife)

This crisis is costing us financially. [Husband] stopped working, literally, overnight, and our income dropped by about 70%. [Son and fiancé] are staying with us, which is fortunate because otherwise they would be living on her furlough salary of about £500 a month while they wait for [son] to hear how much he will be getting from the government as a self employed person. He will hear tomorrow. He is anxious. If they were paying rent on their house they simply would not be able to afford to live. It is a very worrying time for them [. . .] There will be a lot of cloth cutting for all of us after this.

Diarist 1428 (non-binary, 20s, North West England, fundraiser and consultant)

My sleeping pattern has been all over the place recently, so I didn't wake up until 10:30am today, at which point I texted some friends, scrolled through social media for a bit, and fell back to sleep by accident until 1pm. I ate some leftovers when I got up – egg, bacon, sausage and ketchup in a bread roll – and put my bedsheets in the wash.

It has been hard filling my days since I've been furloughed.

Diarist 1458 (male, 20s, North West England, television director)

I haven't been able to do my normal full-time job as a freelance assistant director on TV commercials since 17th March, just a few days before the UK entered 'lockdown'.

A significant proportion of my day was spent making a small shelf between a new storage unit and the wall. It is the perfect size to house vinyl sleeves while the vinyls are being played on my turntables.

Diarist 1480 (female, 20s, London, bar worker and sales assistant)

I normally work part-time in a pub and part-time in a shop, but have been furloughed due to the Covid-19 pandemic.

Today started the same way that my days in isolation always do. I woke up at around midday, after ignoring my alarm that I set for 10:30 the night before. I've been staying up late most nights, until around 4am and not sleeping until the birds are singing – I think I can blame my lack of routine there. I scrolled through Twitter and Instagram for a while, responding to messages from my friends about the prospects of McDonald's opening their drive-thrus again, finally choosing to get out of bed at around 1pm [. . .] I crawled back into bed at about 1:20pm, I've felt sad all day and just wanted to be lazy and have a little cry at this point. After some time, I dragged myself out of bed, had a quick bath, and did a 20-minute yoga video. I've been trying to do a 20-minute session every day, but sometimes I just can't be bothered. I tidied my room a little bit and made a smoothie [. . .] I read outside for a little bit. I'm trying to make my way through all the books on my shelf that I hadn't been able to commit to before.

Diarist 1867 (female, 20s, West Midlands, cabin crew)

Normally for work I am cabin crew [. . .] but due to coronavirus there's no flights and I've been furloughed for about 2 months now [. . .] I love my job and today I found out that my area of the company are starting consultations to make redundancies. As I'm fairly new to the company I will likely be one of the first to be cut. I will be devastated. The job market has disappeared due to the virus so I don't know what I will be able to do or how I will be able to make a living.

Diarist 2341 (female, 30s, Wales, librarian)

I really should get out of bed and start my day. That's the thing about being furloughed though, you drift from moment to moment with no real sense of purpose [. . .] There's nothing to get up for but I know if I stay here, sleep will elude me tonight, and the cycle will keep perpetuating. I'm trying hard to keep myself in some kind of routine so that when I can return to work, it's not completely overwhelming [. . .] There is no sense of accomplishment today and that's something I have been struggling with. When you come home after a day at work, you feel like you've achieved something. You might not have managed to get through everything on your list, but you know you've made some sort of difference. Your participation in the events of the day mattered to someone at some point. What difference have I made today? None. Does it matter that I got out of bed? No. Would anybody have noticed if I didn't? Probably not. But even though it feels completely futile, it seems important to keep going through the motions.

Diarist 2394 (male, 50s, South East England, unemployed actor)

The governmental financial assistance scheme, once it was announced (after a few very anxious weeks wondering whether any attention would be paid to the 5 or 6 million self-employed workers rendered redundant by the virus shutdown) has meant that I became aware that a huge psychic burden had been lifted for the first time in 35 years – the endless nagging worry about where I'd find the money for the next bill payment. It has been really extraordinary for me, this – to realise how much this has shaped my life, the constant underscore of fear and anxiety, like the sound of distant traffic or aircraft noise, not consciously noted perhaps but when it stops suddenly because of this virus… what a silence!

Diarist 2408 (female, 40s, London, theatre worker)

I was furloughed 2 weeks into lockdown, along with the majority of my colleagues. So for the first time since being on maternity leave 13 years ago I am being paid NOT to work. It is so strange. At first it felt like I was being fired and was surplus to requirements and felt awful, but I've got used to it now. All I care about is that we have an industry and jobs to go back to at the end of this, and if being furloughed means that can happen I will keep calm and carry on!

Diarist 2707 (female, 40s, South East England, painter and decorator)

I am a self-employed Painter and Decorator, and during this Covid lockdown I am unable to work due to the social distancing restrictions. This means I am spending my days much more leisurely than I have ever done since being of a working age! Even with the restrictions of not travelling or socialising in person, this time feels like the freedom of the long summer school holidays of my childhood!

Diarist 3284 (male, 20s, South East England, retailer)

I work for a fairly large company that acquires second-hand items and lists them for resale online. Due to the coronavirus, stock dried up and I was sent home on furlough, which means the government pays the cost of my wages to my employer. It's a relief to still have a job, and I can get by comfortably enough on 80% pay. At the time of writing, I am on my eighth week of furlough.

I got up at around 9:30, which is my 'new normal' [. . .] Life on furlough began as a welcome opportunity to relax, read, and do some proper cleaning, but lethargy set in after about three weeks. I often feel becalmed and useless, and I sleep poorly without work to tire me out!

Diarist 3562 (female, 50s, South West England, garden designer)

Like many freelance and creative people I know, I've fallen through most of the cracks in terms of support. I haven't been self-employed long enough to prove my income and benefit from the new self-employed income support scheme so I've had to sign up for Universal Credit. It's been sobering to realise how poor our benefits network has become, how punitive the state is to those who need help.

Diarist 3944 (female, 30s, London, event producer)

I work as a freelance Event Producer working on live music and Arts events. Due to COVID-19 all of my summer contracts have been cancelled, so I have no work during

Lockdown and my next pencilled job isn't until October 2020. My husband is currently furloughed from his role [. . .] I sleep fitfully until finally waking up around 10am. Sleep patterns and routine have gone out of the window since lockdown began. We typically go to bed anywhere between midnight and 2am, and get up any time from 9am-11am, much to the annoyance of our friends with children. We have no responsibilities, no work, no routine, so why not?

Diarist 4610 (female, 30s, South East England, maternity nurse)

I woke up before the alarm [. . .] I went to make the all-important first cup of tea and let the dogs out [. . .] We drank our tea in bed, [wife] read the news and I mostly stared into space. I'll be glad tomorrow when I can file my claim for the government self-employed grant. Being at home is more than lovely, but earning no money at all at the moment definitely weighs on my mind.

GRATITUDE

Reflecting on their situation, many diarists listed things they missed or worried about during the pandemic, but then quickly moved to another list. For some, this other list was actually something they'd learned to produce in their everyday lives, as a means of keeping perspective in the face of anxiety. They'd learned to 'count their blessings' by listing things for which to give thanks, either mentally before sleep or by writing in journals or notebooks. For others, this way of structuring reflections must just have seemed right when writing their diary for Mass Observation. At a time when life seemed especially precious, it served the purpose of identifying the important things in life – health, family, company, safety, security – and also the 'small mercies' that make life joyful, whether today's sunshine or last night's favourite television programme. It also allowed diarists to acknowledge their position and recognize the different positions of others. They wrote of gratitude for their own position and the 'worse problems' of others: people without nice houses with gardens in which to be locked down; people without company during lockdown and suffering from loneliness; key workers unable to stay safe at home, at risk on 'the frontline'. In this way, many diarists not only wrote about their own day but also made broader observations and interpretations in the tradition of Mass Observation. See also Anxiety; Clap for carers; Luck.

Diarist 14 (female, 30s, London, film producer)

The pandemic has definitely proved a good moment to evaluate where we all are in our lives. It has certainly made me appreciate some of the things I have, and mourn or question the things I don't have. I feel incredibly lucky to live so close to my parents and sister and niece (the light of my life!), and to be able to see them in the flesh, even if we can't hug. I am hugely fortunate to still have a job, and to have been able to pay off my mortgage last year, so I don't feel an immediate financial pressure. But as much as I enjoy my own company, and love my flat, I feel sad not to share my flat with someone I love. I miss the family I don't have, if that makes sense [. . .] So as I look forward to life after coronavirus, I mostly imagine selling my flat and buying a house, with a garden. I think about that house being full of people – my sister and niece, or my partner, or maybe a couple of kids I've adopted. Maybe all of the above. In the meantime, though, I am thankful for what and who I have, and try to take things a day at a time [. . .], cherishing the people and things I hold dear, hoping for good outcomes for all, helping where I'm able to help (which, right now, is by staying at home as much as possible), and trying to put my best foot forward every day.

Diarist 486 (female, 80s, Midlands, retired).

My daughter taught me to write, before I turn off the light, three things I am thankful for from the day. It is seldom difficult to find them, even if it is something fleeting or inconsequential like the pleasure of a tv programme I enjoy, a rose coming into flower, the sun warming us up, a happy video call with a friend or family member. So I count my blessings.

Diarist 1089 (male, 40s, South East England, chaplain)

This has been a fairly good day in lockdown. It's frustrating that I can't really see [partner] except on Skype, and the social distancing and other restrictions are quite difficult, but I also have in mind that I am relatively lucky compared to some. I have enough money and food to survive, and for that I am grateful.

Diarist 1547 (female, 30s, East of England, innovation consultant)

I have a daily diary where I keep a work to-do list and have recently started using it to keep a gratitude list [. . .] I write down 10 things every day that I am grateful for. Today's list was:

1. [Boyfriend]
2. The cats
3. The house
4. The garden
5. My job
6. My health
7. My family
8. My friends
9. Bread
10. My noise cancelling headphones.

Diarist 1661 (female, 13, Wales)

I got ready for bed; got changed into my pyjamas, crossed off the day on my calendar, wrote down something I'm grateful for in my bullet journal (the postal service), brushed my teeth [. . .] I went to sleep quite easily, on my side as usual.

Diarist 1815 (female, 20s, Scotland, unemployed)

I was putting on my running clothes when [partner] got out of the shower. We rough-housed a bit: he bit my shoulder, I punched him in the chest, and we ended up on the bed laughing and kissing as we caught our breath. I felt full of love and gratitude to have someone with me 'in this ongoing situation' (one of the many euphemisms I've seen on shop signs) [. . .] As lockdown days go, this was a pretty good one. I've had many days where I was more stressed, or received bad news, or felt lonely or caged up. I recognize that I have a lot to be grateful for. This night I went to sleep thinking: I am safe, I am loved.

Diarist 1971 (female, 60s, Wales, writer)

Our world has changed. Our boundaries reduced to the few square metres of house and garden, without which I would be in a much darker place, mentally. Our lives revolve around meals (and snacks), permitted exercise and television. For me, books, writing, photography and gardening take up my day. I am immensely grateful that I have unlimited access to all of the above.

Diarist 2160 (female, 40s, South West England, mental health nurse)

I am relieved and grateful at the things I have in my life at the moment: touch wood good health of myself and close family and friends – and a meaningful job I love (even though it is hard, stressful and tiring) – great colleagues, and a place to live where I am very happy.

Diarist 2640 (female, 60s, Scotland, counsellor and therapist)

I feel profound gratitude many times a day that my children are not working on the front line risking Covid.

Diarist 3513 (female, 60s, South East England, retired teacher)

Today has a much better feel about it than yesterday. My hair is clean, my house is clean and tidy. The sun is shining and the fierce gusty wind of yesterday has gone. Thank goodness for small mercies.

Diarist 3761 (female, 30s, South West England, lawyer)

I return to study at my desk. I enjoy the view of our garden from my makeshift desk/ kitchen table and I feel grateful that I have my health and the support of my fiancé to get me through this bizarre time. I keep reminding myself that I have so much and that I shouldn't feel downtrodden by the weight of the whole global crisis and the feeling of collective anxiety around if and when and what the world will look like when we emerge again.

I also remind myself that although we have had to cancel our wedding in July because of the pandemic that there are far worse problems in the world to have and we will have so much more to celebrate when things begin to improve. But I also allow myself to have a little cry or feel a fraction of self-pity at times just because I think maybe it's ok to grieve over the carefully laid plans that have been unravelled.

Diarist 3808 (female, 70s, North East England, retired school inspector)

10.45pm Lights out. As usual, as I settle down, I wonder how many days will have to pass before I see my daughter and her children, when I will be able to go to a football match with my son or spend time with his wife and when we will feel safe meeting friends. I also feel thankful that I am not one of the very vulnerable 1.5 million who because of medical conditions have been told to stay indoors or at very most confine themselves to their gardens and that I am not living alone.

Diarist 4256 (female, 60s, South West England, retired doctor)

Despite everything there's a lot to give thanks to God for – my Mum's long life and the fact that her illness was short and with such good care; the fact that I'm not in lockdown alone even if [husband] and I have words from time to time; we have a small garden so can be outside; we have great neighbours and a WhatsApp group that started long before the lockdown; we can experience the fantastic weather and wonderful spring season.

Diarist 4766 (female, 60s, East of England, family support specialist)

I feel such gratitude to all the people who are working to ensure we have food in our bellies, water in the taps and the rubbish off the streets. I placed a notice on my dustbins today thanking the refuse collectors.

GRIEF

There was a lot to grieve during the pandemic. People grieved all those things lost, missed or cancelled due to lockdown. They grieved for family and friends who died before the pandemic, because news of deaths and funerals brought it all back, and grief does not disappear quickly anyway. And they grieved for family and friends who died during the pandemic, whether from Covid-19 or not. So people woke up after disrupted sleep and were hit each day anew by their grief. Lockdown made one or two aspects of grieving easier, in that it gave an excuse for withdrawal from society, if that was desired, but it made most aspects of grieving harder. People could not hug those from other households. They could not attend face-to-face grief counselling. Many of the events and activities people usually lose themselves in, to take their minds off things, were cancelled. People faced practical difficulties sorting out paperwork with organizations now working in different ways due to the pandemic. They found the many online condolence messages and calls exhausting and overwhelming. Unable to protect loved ones from the virus, or to be with them when they died, or to attend their funerals, or to fulfil their funeral plans, people felt guilty. While some people struggled to cope, those able to cope felt guilty for being able to cope. So people hugged those in their household, and they cried alone – in bed, in the shower, at the park and while writing their diaries for Mass Observation. See also Cancellations; Funerals; Guilt; Stay home.

Diarist 759 (male, 30s, East Midlands, student)

I have recently become a widower as my wife passed away from Covid 19 [. . .] Like the last four weeks since my wife died I wake up either thinking that she is still alive or knowing that she is dead. I wake up and already everything is different, not like it was in March, no one to ask me how I slept and I them, no one to ask if they would like a cup of tea [. . .] Today I changed my routine of the last few weeks and showered and got dressed. Something very weird about having a shower, it instantly makes you cry. I've never cried so much in my life since she's died. Sometimes it is silent tears, sometimes howling and sometimes I just want to shout at the top of my lungs [. . .] After I've had my shower I walk through into our living room, past the urn containing my wife's ashes. The memory of having a funeral of 10 people, not allowing limos, not being able to hug my Mum and Dad and not fulfilling one of my wife's only wishes of being carried by pallbearers. Because death in coronavirus is something else, all of the 'widower jobs' requiring you to call up these companies who are working from home so they have a series of call centre numbers and hold music [. . .], the last 7 weeks seem to be grim challenge after grim challenge [. . .] I think the thing about my Tuesday is that I never expected I'd be a widower sitting here in the middle of a lock down, not really knowing where my future will lead but I guess no one else does either. I wanted to talk about my older brother, younger sister, parents, other family, friends and interests but my life has taken a devastating turn and so I need to share about the truths of living after someone dying of Covid 19.

Diarist 989 (female, 60s, retired)

I take the dog for his second walk [. . .] I get back in time to watch a bit of the government coronavirus briefing. More virus, more death. My father died nearly two years ago now but all this tragic loss of life – so much death – so many sad stories, many gone before their time, has revived my desperate feelings of loss. I go to the church yard with my dog but my father cannot comfort me. I hug my husband and sometimes the dog. He is not so keen – the dog.

Diarist 1033 (female, 40s, South West England, author)

I slept right through the night for a change, and woke up at a much more appropriate time than 2am or 3am.

5am is really good for me. My first thought before I'd even opened my eyes properly was the same as it has been for the last six months and three days: *my Mum died.* Grief is such an enormous and invasive thing, it even permeates what you hope will be peaceful sleep when you get it – grief never lets you rest properly. I did what I always do on waking: went to the bathroom, had a wee, and then used a damp cloth to wipe away the salt from around my eyes. I guess I cry in my sleep. I guess that's why we aren't sleeping in the same room at the moment. One parent at least should wake up fresh every day [. . .] I got some tea and checked the news online, caught up with the latest 'advice' and 'rules'. Felt sick all over again. It's fuzzy, but I suppose probably easier for me than many other people, because being a writer I work from home anyway, and being a person who has been in this awful stage of grief for some time, I was 'self isolating' for ages before all this happened. I hadn't been out much at all apart from school runs, I was avoiding seeing people. So for me more than others, I think not seeing anyone at all is a new normal that I'm kind of used to. It's okay, apart from how much I miss my sister now every day at the moment, because she has been my solace, and me hers. She was the person I saw outside of this house, the person I hugged tightly.

Diarist 1137 (female, 40s, Yorkshire and Humber, psychologist)

I headed out for a walk into the local woods. They are beautiful and we are so lucky to live close by [. . .] It was good to spend some time alone although it set my mind thinking about the situation. I've not given myself much time to think about it since this all started really. Partly because when I think about it all too much I get upset. I miss so much –

people, friends, family – doing normal things – going to the cinema, pub, being able to head to the seaside for the day.

Diarist 1157 (female, 40s, London, archivist)

Last week I unexpectedly lost a very dear friend following a heart attack, possibly Covid related. We await the coroner's report [. . .] I woke around 8:30 and was instantly confronted by the loss of my friend. This was an enormous shock and has dominated the past few days. Today, I felt overwhelmingly sad and struggled to get up and deal with the situation [. . .] I bathed, lots of time for baths these days. Drank tea but couldn't face food. I then dealt with the endless condolence messages and various WhatsApp messages, ignoring all calls. I just couldn't face them this morning. To lift my spirits, I watched a short BBC archive film about London in 1955. Charming and distracting [. . .] I am exhausted, sad and overwhelmed by my friend's death but also the need for everyone to contact me and express their own loss and anxiety. I don't feel strong enough to deal with this right now. Not my best day under lockdown.

Diarist 1352 (female, 50s, East of England, publican)

The dog barks. I see one of our customers, an old boy, heading to the patio. He lives alone. My husband and I drop off essential supplies (beer) to his house a few times a week. He is going out of his mind with boredom. What brings him here? Should I wear my face mask? He is three metres from my back door when he sits down on the bench. I greet him barefaced. (I am aware that the dishwasher has reached temperature. I really want to be left in peace for once. Is he going to ask me for a beer?) Then I sense a need and respond instinctively, I ask him what I can do for him. He tells me his sister died this morning. Cancer. He appears lost, bewildered. He has some time to wait before catching a bus. I bring him a half of beer and discuss his sister.

Diarist 1494 (female, 20s, South East England, student)

It's now early evening [. . .] I end up watching an old documentary filmed at Cambridge in the '80s [. . .] I watch students at dinners and tutorials and in bars and mourn the term – my last here – that I'm missing out on.

Diarist 1602 (female, 60s, South West England, librarian and counsellor)

Today I woke up slowly, aware of the radio. I could hear that it was *Farming Today* on Radio 4 and they are talking about picking potatoes at a safe distance from one another. I drifted in and out of sleep for the next hour, hearing the latest news about the government's plans for us to *Stay alert*, whatever that means. I can hardly bear to listen to the news anymore. This time of pandemic has not been kind to our family. Our daughter-in-law died of Covid-19 on Easter Saturday and each morning I wake up, the enormity of our tragedy slaps into me, and I become aware again of our new reality.

I move downstairs to make our breakfast [. . .] We move from the kitchen to the front room where the sun is shining in and call [son]. Since [son's] wife died more than 4 weeks ago, this is something we do daily [. . .] We usually have long conversations with [son] which meander between so many things; his wife [. . .], how she didn't deserve to die so young [. . .], how he doesn't think he'll ever be happy again [. . .], what he's going to say to friends and colleagues when he does finally meet them again for the first time after this endless lockdown, how he predicts that he will bring the mood down of any gather of friends he's part of, how he feels guilty that he is managing to eat and function when he reads about other people who have been widowed not being able to get out of bed for months at a time [. . .] In the week before [daughter-in-law] died, as she lay in the ICU we sometimes gathered as a family on Zoom for a Quaker Meeting for Worship. As Quakers, we say that we are holding someone in the light and I was most definitely holding [her] in a pure golden light. After she died, I fretted that I might not have been praying hard enough or in the right way or not asking God hard enough to keep her alive and let her recover from this terrible virus, *Please don't take her yet, we're not ready for her to go.* But it didn't work and during the first days following her death I started to feel anxious that things might have turned out differently if only I'd prayed harder [. . .] Today was the first time I'd tried to pray alone on a day that wasn't Sunday. There are Quakers who do spend time during the week in quiet contemplation but I have never before made time to do this. Today I focused on a few lines from the bible. *To every thing there is a reason and a time to every purpose under heaven. A time to be born and a time to die* (Eccl. 3:1). This made me cry and I could feel the tears flowing down my face. I asked *Why was it time for [daughter-in-law] to die? Why has [son] been left to face the world alone? Why was their time together so short?* Gradually I started to feel calmer. I said the Lord's Prayer to myself [. . .] I decided to go shopping [. . .] Walking back up the hill, my shopping bag on wheels feels very heavy and I notice that I'm breathing more heavily than usual. Before lockdown I walked everywhere and I kept myself reasonably fit but now I don't always exercise every day even though the government said it's OK to do so, sometimes I just want to stay at home. To start with I didn't mind walking round the streets, but I began to grow tired of walking for the sake of it. The university gardens are nearby and I've walked round there more times than I've ever done in all the [time we've lived here]. In the first weeks after [daughter-in-law] died, I sometimes walked to a corner of the university garden where there's a bench tucked away so no one walks by to disturb my thoughts. I would sit crying and thinking about [daughter-in-law].

As I walked through [town] from my trip to the food shop, I could see two people ahead. They seemed to be waiting to go into one of the flats, maybe to clean it as they had a vacuum cleaner, mops and brushes in their hands. The young woman called out brightly to me, saying hello and I said hello back. I wondered if I looked sad with my head bowed, as I pulled the heavy shopping bag along [. . .] Before [daughter-in-law's] death I was counselling clients on the phone or by Zoom. Now, of course, I have had to stop for a while. I'm not in the right place to counsel anyone. My own grief has been raw and supporting [son] from a distance has been unbearably sad. Although we did manage to attend [daughter-in-law's] funeral, unlike some families who have not been able to do so, not being able to even hug [son], only being able to watch him from a distance as he was supported by [his sister] felt so desperate. All this has been completely overwhelming for me.

Diarist 2205 (male, 70s, North West England, retired teacher)

My wife died [last year], and following this I have had a long period of depression, inability to concentrate, withdrawal, the usual grief, etc. I am taking anti-depressants which are helping considerably. I was seeing a counsellor regularly, but this stopped in early March with the COVID lock-down. Fortunately, by that time, I had made some recovery, and the onset of Spring has helped me re-focus. I had also joined the U3A and was doing regular tai-chi, but all such activities have stopped dead. Just before lock-down, I also managed to make my first trip away from the house to visit an old school friend and wife [. . .] This was the first real 'away day' I had had since last Spring, and I really had to **fight myself to make it happen**. I hope that, by the time COVID has run its course, I will still feel myself to be in the same outgoing frame of mind. It wasn't easy to make the first 'jump', and I really do hope to sustain it. At the moment, I'm still hopeful [. . .] Grief is a very difficult process, but the worst bit is handling all the dual (shared) memories, sometimes quite mundane, from which a relationship is constructed, realised, and constantly being re-formed [. . .] Virtually anything will stir a memory, and – depending on my mood that day – I will either dismiss it cheerily, quite often ruefully, or (inevitably) sadly.

I *have* to get by with something of a stoical attitude (what are the choices?), though I am still completely raw underneath. (*Writing this now, I am flooding with tears.*)

Diarist 3150 (female, 50s, West Midlands, unemployed)

I checked the latest news on my phone. A probable total of 50 000 people have now died in the UK (the latest 'excess deaths' figure) [. . .] I don't know anyone personally who has died, but I feel for everyone who is grieving – 50 000 deaths could mean half a million or more currently grieving a loved one or friend.

Diarist 3739 (female, 60s, South West England, social worker)

My father [. . .] died [in April, from coronavirus]. If my account of 12th May sounds downbeat I suppose it is because I am bereaved and working through grief in the strange virtual way we do in lockdown. I was not with him when he died, there was no funeral, I do not know when I will get his ashes back, I have cleared his bungalow in defiance of lockdown because I could not stand the lack of reality surrounding his death anymore.

GUILT

If those grieving loved ones felt guilty – for not protecting loved ones, or giving them the death they deserved, or not grieving well enough – then so did others. Some felt guilty for not grieving the dead who they didn't know personally, but who were fellow human beings. Some felt guilty for taking risks and spreading the virus, which may have led to illness or death for others. Some felt guilty for 'doing nothing' while others were ill, dying or taking risks on 'the frontline' to care for those ill or dying. Some with good pensions, or able to work from home on full pay, with nice houses and gardens, in good health, felt guilty for enjoying lockdown – for relaxing and having fun – which seemed indecent and indulgent, given the circumstances. Some with such privileges felt guilty for not enjoying lockdown – for not even being capable of feeling the contentment supposedly appropriate to such privilege. It seems that some people were able to recognize that staying home, caring for oneself, family and friends, was not 'doing nothing', but rather was making an important contribution to government of the pandemic. Nevertheless, some felt the need to supplement this basic contribution – driven by guilt and presumably other forces – by calling people locked down alone, sending care packages, giving to charity, volunteering. See also Grief; Home schooling; Key workers; Luck; Stay home; Working from home.

Diarist 200 (female, 30s, London, visual designer)

I've reached out to friends. I've sent care packages of food and money to those I know needed it. Tried to find something to help each day pass quickly. And whilst I do this, I feel guilty. **I'm lucky, I realise this** [. . .] I work from home as a visual designer; I live in a flat I rent alone. I'm still on full pay and my health is good (as far as I know). My biggest battle is loneliness and accepting I can't help those I want to.

Diarist 422 (male, 70s, South West England, garage forecourt worker)

Feeling a little guilty as lockdown for us in rural Devon is not so bad. With a garden and an allotment, neither of which have ever had so much attention before, and surrounded by glorious countryside, what's not to enjoy.

Diarist 1027 (non-binary, 30s, Scotland, unemployed)

I'm [. . .] struggling to forgive myself for my own lack of action. The pandemic is terrible, but it is an opportunity to radically shift social power away from the state and toward the people through mutual aid efforts, and I'm simply not doing enough because I'm too depressed. [Partner] made some test baygls for a mutual aid effort we're doing where we bring food to our local community on a pay-what-you-can basis, so people can pay nothing if they need. This will hopefully not only alleviate the burden people are feeling, but my guilt for not doing enough. He's a great cook and they were delicious.

Diarist 1042 (female, 20s, London, medical student)

I am bored and I feel guilty for feeling bored. I am a medical student, I could be helping but I'm not sure how. A few weeks ago I was applying for jobs through the NHS jobs website but I never got a reply. I think my mum is relieved though. She was worried about me getting exposed.

Diarist 1122 (female, 50s, London, service manager)

I am waking and getting up later during lockdown than pre-Corona. This is one of the benefits and for me so far, there have been definite up-sides to this situation [. . .] I daren't admit to liking lockdown in any public arena however as it feels so wrong when people are dying in their thousands. I am also something of a magical thinker so take the view that I will get my comeuppance if I am too bright and breezy. There have been some nightmares and moments of rampant anxiety to balance out the days when I have enjoyed the simplicity of this new constrained existence.

Diarist 1331 (female, 30s, Scotland, restaurant worker)

There is a BBC1 fly-on-the-wall documentary called Hospital showing and it is very sobering. It follows the day to day lives of the doctors and nurses dealing with the COVID-19 response and I am crying from the moment I watch it. It has been quite easy to forget that people are risking their lives and fighting for their lives due to this brutal virus when you are living in a nice big flat, with no money worries and a green garden. Whilst we watched the programme so many people died and seeing the effect this had on the doctors and loved ones really brought things home.

After watching the show, I realise I have been living in a bubble pretending things aren't as bad as they are. I feel like I have maybe been treating this as a big holiday, drinking wine and having fun Zoom calls with my friends on the weekends because I have been lucky enough to not have anybody I love or care about die. I feel very lucky about this but watching that show makes me feel powerless and lazy. People are working frontline and I am doing nothing to help anybody else's life but my own. I feel very down.

I come to bed, where I am now, to write this. My cat joins me and so does my boyfriend and for a while things don't seem quite so bad [. . .] I think I need to try not to beat myself up for not doing enough and just be happy with dealing with my own psychological state as well as my partner's and try and be happy with just that currently. We are all in a fragile place and it is ok to just need to deal with that. I just need to remind myself how lucky I am and lucky to have my partner and cat – I could be alone.

Diarist 1494 (female, 20s, South East England, student)

Grocery shopping [. . .] To my absolute delight, I run into two friends of mine as I'm walking home [. . .] We have a socially-distanced chat for about half an hour (what? We haven't seen anyone in weeks!) and it feels like drinking a hot coffee or the first sip of beer after a long week. I never thought just seeing someone else I know in the flesh could be such a viscerally joyful experience, but this encounter really is enough to put me in a great mood for the whole rest of the day. I'm a natural extrovert and have been doing lots of video calls with my friends, but it's just not the same. The only tinge of sadness is seeing people looking at us talking as they go by. It's not that they're angry we're talking; their faces are wistful. I feel guilty rubbing it in by laughing so freely in broad daylight; it feels sort of indecent when the streets are so quiet.

Diarist 1574 (female, 40s, Wales, public health practitioner)

It is difficult trying to focus on my job and help my children with their school work. Both of my children cried today because they were finding maths hard. I try to help them, but all the time I know that I should be working. I have a supportive manager and have a lot of flexibility but I still feel guilty and strained.

Diarist 1679 (female, 30s, London, software engineer)

I don't pay much attention to what's happening out there [. . .] I mute the words 'Boris', 'COVID', and 'coronavirus' on Twitter and try not to think about how many people have died. If I think too hard, I find myself feeling guilty that I don't care enough about people I don't know. I find the blitz-spirit public service broadcasting (and weekly clapping) unnerving rather than comforting. It's like the BBC was waiting for a national crisis to wheel out this feelgood stuff, but it's not working and everyone is still angry. People are doing their best in a shitty situation on the frontlines, meanwhile I'm staying out of the way. If I let myself get angry I'll fall apart, and I'm no use to anyone then.

Diarist 1927 (female, 50s, South East England, artist and musician)

I'm a woman in my 50s, living [. . .] with my husband and my mother. My husband and I run our own graphic design and print business and my mother is retired [. . .] I'm an artist and musician and am currently furloughed as an employee from our own business (graphic design and print), with 80% of my wages being paid by the government, which is small but more than we would have coming in as all of our work dried up at the start of the lockdown. Our finances are bad so we are all three of us relying on my mother's pension to pay the bills and put food on the table. This feels so wrong and makes me feel incredibly guilty every day.

Diarist 2290 (female, 30s, Scotland, historian)

My husband gets up, grabs some cereal and shuts himself in our bedroom for the day to work [. . .] He started working from home on 13 March and I started on 17 March. We have been at home social distancing since then. My son's nursery closed at the same time, so up until late April I was working part-time in the sitting room with him in the background. It was a challenge, but my boss was very understanding and didn't expect me to be at peak productivity. [In late April], I started maternity leave [. . .] At least I no longer have to try to do work on top of being heavily pregnant and looking after my son. I was feeling very guilty. My son and my work were only getting half of my attention; I felt like I was neither a good parent nor a good employee.

Diarist 2473 (female, 60s, South West England, retired)

Woke up just after 7 am and looked out of the window to see clear, blue sky and sunshine – knowing that the weather is nice would usually make a really good start to my day, but now it does not always help me to feel positive; I know it will basically be very similar to the many days which have passed since lock down; I am truly grateful that my situation is so much easier than that of millions of people, yet feel guilty that this is not enough to make me feel content with life.

Diarist 2627 (female, 40s, Northern Ireland, editor)

In the weeks before the lockdown I went to London, on a ghost of a trip for a book fair that had already been cancelled. Starved of their company from across the Irish Sea, I was so desperate to see precious people that I put them at risk to do it. I think of myself as diffident and stilted in my contact with others, but social awkwardness did nothing to help me maintain social distancing. I was so thrilled by their nearness to me that I missed the moment when I could have stopped myself. I have been so afraid of spreading the virus and felt so guilty about the risks I visited on others that I have not been able to stop distancing since I got home. It has been two months now and theirs are still the hands that last held mine.

Diarist 2750 (female, 40s, South East England, heritage collections manager)

I started a new piece of work [today]. It's been hanging over me during the lockdown and I have been guilty, if that's the right word, of prioritising the family's needs instead of knuckling down.

Diarist 3051 (female, 70s, London, retired stage manager and personal assistant)

After lunch I made chocolate cake, and sorted out some ideas for this week's dinners. We have enough food, which makes me feel rather guilty given the hardships others are suffering. I give money to charities but I can't shake the feeling that we are being protected while others wait on us. I know the reason is so that we don't overwhelm the NHS, given that we are among those more vulnerable to the virus, but it still seems indulgent.

HOME SCHOOLING

Schools were closed during the first lockdown of 2020, but schooling continued with teachers setting tasks for completion at home. The diaries capture perspectives on home schooling from teachers, students and parents. From the perspective of teachers, home schooling could lack the camaraderie of the classroom. From the perspective of students, it could be intense with class after class online, task after task to complete, deadline after deadline to meet. It could be hard to concentrate when surrounded by distractions: siblings, pets, toys, gardens, games consoles, television, friends online. It could be hard not seeing friends previously seen face-to-face most days of the week. Alternatively, it could offer quieter students a quieter space for study, away from the noisy classroom, and also a more relaxed morning routine, better breakfasts and lunches, and the opportunity to wear more comfortable clothes. From the perspective of parents, there was a desire to help teach their children and stop them 'falling behind', but also a recognition that times were hard psychologically for children (and parents) – that snuggling on the sofa or escaping to the garden might constitute appropriate responses to a pandemic. The experiences of parents varied. Those on furlough found themselves with time to help with home schooling. Those working from home found themselves juggling home schooling and work while feeling guilty that neither was being done well. One thing common to all three groups – teachers, students and parents – was the struggle for motivation while home schooling. Also, kids say the funniest (and most devastating) things. See also Anxiety; Furlough; Guilt; Stay home; Working from home; Zoom.

Diarist 8 (female, 14, East of England)

Today I woke up at 8:00 AM to go to online school [. . .] I had chemistry, english and PSHCE [Personal, Social, Health, and Citizenship Education] in the morning and in the afternoon I had french, history and maths. Most lessons we spend revising for the end of year tests ☹.

Diarist 46 (female, 40s, East of England, teacher)

I have spent my day trying to work from my desk at home instead of in my classroom. This has included today teaching a lesson online using video conferencing software, assessing student work completed by them at home and sent to me by email, [and] speaking to parents of children who are increasingly struggling with the school closure and other 'lockdown' conditions, with a commensurate impact on their engagement with school work.

Diarist 53 (female, 13, East of England)

The first lesson was Chemistry: where I learned about something new and burning fossil fuels. After that I had English where we did the word study task to help with our end of term exams. After that it was break where I had to go and deliver something to a friend of my parents. After break we had games where I did some cricket skills, then it was lunch and I had pizza. After lunch it was Spanish where I did a poster on quarantine. At last break I didn't really have much to do so I just talked a bit to my brother and then got ready for my History lesson [. . .] After History, I will have Maths which is where I am learning about simultaneous equations. After Maths, it is the end of school, so I am going to have some peace and quiet.

Diarist 59 (female, 9, Scotland)

I am learning from home and it SUCKS. Normally, I'd be asleep at the back of the class but now I can't do that because the schools are shut thanks to coronavirus!

Diarist 60 (female, 30s, Scotland, school clerical assistant)

Today I woke up, showered, got dressed in comfortable trousers and a zipper hoodie. The girls started their school day by practising maths using worksheets sent by their teachers via an application on their tablets (iPads). I started responding to work emails and taking calls. While working and helping the girls, I inadvertently sent an email out to the whole school, which made me feel so inept + incompetent. My partner reminded me that mistakes happen, especially when juggling different tasks at the same time. I include this in my diary because I think that many people right now are struggling to juggle work + home schooling + staying sane + staying efficient + being happy.

Diarist 61 (male, 30s, Scotland, engineer)

I have enjoyed being cloistered with my two daughters [. . .] very much. So too have I enjoyed teaching them. This is where the coin flips to frustration: I am unable to teach them all I want to and am perhaps unreasonable in my aims.

Diarist 141 (female, 10, East Midlands)

My dog has been licking my arm on and off all morning [. . .] It's a nice interruption from home schooling which can get very tense as we are expected to hand in assignments. I try as best as I can to stick to my timetable as I am constantly worried about falling behind [. . .] I'm looking out the kitchen window. It isn't as sunny today as it has been, which in some ways is helpful as I don't want to go out in the garden as much as I have wanted to when it is really hot. Although right now I would love to curl up on my sofa and watch a movie with my brother. He keeps going upstairs to play with his toys and my mum is trying to get him to do his spellings. It's hilarious (not for my mum though).

Diarist 235 (female, 14, Scotland)

French has been the worst to learn from home – it's all textbook and vocabulary, textbook and vocab, textbook and vocab. Très ennuyeux.

Diarist 236 (female, 19, Wales)

I am studying acting and stage combat. Before corona, this was the perfect course, that I loved and enjoyed dearly. But now because of corona I am being taught acting and combat online [. . .] We are stuck in an electronic state. I have 8 hour lessons almost every day, and most of these involve me and my class mates staring at a screen. This term we should have been learning group fights, doing 2 week improvisation projects and all the other incredible, important aspects of the course.

Every lesson our teachers ask us 'how are you?'. More and more they are being answered by a sigh or a shrug. Our mental health – as a nation – is not doing well. Today, when asked how she was, my teacher was close to tears. We should have been doing once in a lifetime lessons, learning things that you can't learn anywhere else, and, as teenagers, making experiences that will shape our lives. Not staring at a screen or being stuck in a house unable to train and therefore achieve our full potential as drama students [. . .] I feel lost and I now sometimes struggle to feel motivated to do the course that I treasured 8 weeks ago. I'm also struggling because I feel like a wimp – banging on about drama school. But our training is like no other. It is hard to explain our lessons, which I find has distanced me from my friends as they cannot ever understand what I am mourning and missing out on (this is not their fault, of course). In times like this, everyone turns to tv or film – our future industry. Last week an actor was on the radio and tried to discuss the negative impact of corona on theatre and theatre training, but the radio host swiftly interrupted her and changed the subject – this really helped to boost my spirits! I feel so honoured that I got into the school and experienced the training I have had, but this only makes not having it even more painful. Even today, I sat in my garden, hunkered down against the strong winds, and tried to hold back tears as I thought of what could have been if not for corona.

Diarist 479 (female, 40s, South West England, clinical pharmacist)

My husband has been working from home for 10 weeks now. It is the first time since we had children that I have been leaving the house to go to work and he has been left in charge of the children. I enjoy this role reversal. He is adapting slowly. When he complains of the pressure to get his work done and supervise our youngest, I gently remind him that at least he is doing this at a time in our sons' lives when they can speak. I had to push through the crying/screaming phase twice plus the toddler tantrums, nappies; the list is endless. My oldest son is pretty self-sufficient and has work sent online from his school. He has a good work ethic and does not need to be reminded to get his schoolwork done [. . .] My youngest is the complete opposite. He does not want to do schoolwork. We have tried all manner of approaches to get him to study. Bribery, manipulation, threats, treats, crying, shouting. Nothing works. I have finally conceded defeat. I have explained to him that it is for his benefit only. I have already been through the school system. I cannot make him work but he may have quite a lot of catching up to do. The compromise is to do a minimum of some maths, times tables, spellings and reading each day. If he does not want to study, he must do chores. Sometimes he does chores and sometimes schoolwork and most days he tries to spend as much time watching television, playing on his tablet or playing on the Xbox. We sometimes switch these devices off. This is not well received.

Diarist 755 (female, 11, East Midlands)

At the moment my favourite part of the day is lunch because I can take my mind off work and think about the more positive things in life.

Diarist 927 (male, 20s, West Midlands, student)

Today has been stressful. This whole lockdown period has been stressful, but today more so than usual. I submitted my dissertation this afternoon, and whilst I am relieved, with it comes the sudden terrifying realisation that I am, in essence, no longer a student. No more assignments, no more lectures. Now what? Not that it's felt like I'm a student; during the Covid-19 pandemic, my university (like most) has moved its teaching and resources online, meaning that I have been studying in my living room instead of on campus for the last nine weeks. Not quite how I imagined it would end, but that's just the way it goes. Hopefully I'll get a good grade. Hopefully.

Diarist 960 (female, 30s, North West England, quality auditor)

April started with our work putting my partner and I on the furlough scheme. This helped massively with the childcare, home schooling, failing working from home situation. Our daughter [. . .] is missing her friends so much. Our son is [. . .] not missing school one bit.

Diarist 1005 (female, 19, West Midlands, student)

By ten past seven I was writing revision notes and trying not to get too stressed-out by all the work teachers are dumping on us. I can't be too mad; teachers are people and they're probably under just as much pressure from their bosses and the education system to keep us up with our studies. I didn't think keeping us up to date involved a thousand essays, though.

Diarist 1033 (female, 40s, South West England, author)

We didn't do too well on home schooling today. The school has been amazing supplying work and activities for the children to do at home, but I can see sometimes it's just really not 'going in'. The weather was lovely, warm again, so the children played swing ball and helped their dad in the garden, planting out some seedlings. They played with the puppy. They talked to their friends online [. . .] Now it is 9.28pm and almost dark. The puppy is asleep on my bed, the children are up far too late watching a film we couldn't afford to buy but did anyway, because they needed a treat and some fun and some popcorn. I suppose home school won't be so great tomorrow either. As long as they are happy – life is too short, and this lockdown is too short to worry so much about decimals and fractions and frontal adverbials.

Diarist 1305 (female, 40s, Wales, diplomat)

I work until about 6 pm and then start a WeChat conversation with two of my female colleagues. We are all finding the whole 'working full time, home schooling full time' challenge a bit, well challenging.

Diarist 1401 (male, 50s, West Midlands, vicar)

Woke the boys so they could start homeschool at 9am.

Took [dog] out for a walk [. . .] Got in just after 10:30. Youngest son was playing SIMS instead of working. Older son still asleep in bed!

Diarist 1557 (male, 40s, Wales, teacher)

Today has been dominated by online teaching and marking in the midst of the lockdown. This is a largely frustrating and soulless process dictated by the effectiveness, or otherwise, of the technology. Remote learning lacks the professional satisfaction of communicating ideas face-to-face, challenging pupils' assumptions and supporting their progress. The camaraderie of classroom and staffroom are missed too. The weeks wear on and wear down interest in a job I usually love being now reduced to e-mails and conference calls. However, I find organising my very messy files on the school network strangely satisfying – like I'm investing time in a better productivity in future. It tells me that I will get through this.

Diarist 1573 (female, 40s, North West England, analyst and programmer)

Got a coffee and checked on things downstairs – my daughter has made an origami whale and is arguing with my husband about his summary of the plot of The Snail and the Whale. Son is doing Art and is worried about deadlines – told him they were all arbitrary and not to worry. Not sure really how arbitrary the deadlines are but surely all the children must be working at different rates. Trying not to worry about both kids falling behind as they aren't lucky enough to have a non-working parent focused on them most days. They are still probably better off than a lot of kids, hopefully, and aren't in key years so hoping the effect on them in the long run won't be too bad [. . .] Finished meeting at 1115, then my son came in to ask about work – he doesn't like the English work set by the school as it's quite tedious. Normally he loves English and I don't want him to get put off so I asked him to write a poem instead.

1150 and son has come back with 3 sad poems about death and homelessness.

Diarist 1579 (male, 7, Yorkshire and Humber)

I had to do maths. It was fractions. It took a long time.

Diarist 1580 (female, 50s, Yorkshire and Humber, administrative assistant)

Initially, my son was quite enthusiastic about doing work from home. Now the novelty has totally worn off and it is becoming increasingly difficult for us to get him to concentrate. Trying to do work while explaining fractions and not entirely understanding them yourself is a challenge.

Diarist 1583 (female, 10, Wales)

I am enjoying doing work at home. It's nice because it's not as noisy as being in a class room.

Diarist 1612 (female, 17, Yorkshire and Humber)

Today my alarm woke me up at 8 o'clock, much later than I would have woken up on a school day two months ago. Being able to sleep in a bit is definitely one of the few advantages of lockdown. All I have to do before attending online school is make breakfast and get dressed. Today I made myself a fried egg sandwich because I was feeling like a treat and filled up my hot water bottle to keep in my lap during my morning's lessons; I've found that it's important to find small ways to comfort yourself during this time.

Diarist 1751 (female, 30s, South West England, finance manager)

I read the school home learning activities for the week [. . .] Most of it looks manageable but motivation to make it happen is lacking to say the least. Kids will be very reluctant too if last week is anything to go by [. . .] Husband will work until 1.30pm whilst I home school the kids. We'll swap after lunch and I'll then do 5 hours work, plus an hour more for us both in the evening. It's hard work and very intense going straight from childcare to home school to work with no break in between. At times I feel stretched very thin and like I'm not doing a great job of any of it.

Diarist 1908 (female, 16, East Midlands)

Today I woke up at 8:30am as school makes us sign in via Microsoft Forms before 9. I find this annoying as it means I must wake up early, although it is better than normal as I must wake up at 6:30am to go to school normally.

I had a call with my art teacher at 9 so I got ready and signed into Microsoft Teams before breakfast. I wore my oversized red hoodie with my normal PJ bottoms because it is comfy but looks okay on video calls. My art call was on our new project to capture how we are feeling in isolation [. . .] I did two charcoal drawings of famous scenes without any people.

Diarist 2003 (female, 40s, South East England, housewife and artist/designer)

We started 'school' just after 9 [. . .] We have been doing maths this morning [. . .] Arghhhh it's a struggle to keep them focused and interested in what I'm trying to get them to do. I don't know how the teachers manage a whole class of them . . . I've just got the two to contend with [. . .] English was partially successful. It was the eldest's turn to be reluctant to write today. They are like a box of ferrets that keep popping out of the box when you try and get them back in. I long for the day that I can get them both engaged and happily working at the same time (there was a day last week, I think).

Diarist 2354 (female, 30s, South East England, lawyer)

Today was not a great day. I feel we're usually coping pretty well in lockdown, but I felt quite tired and overwhelmed today. I usually work 3 days a week and have been finding that quite hard to do alongside looking after children [. . .] and managing homeschooling. My husband works full time and has been very busy, his job feels quite insecure with redundancies of colleagues and furloughed staff so all the childcare is falling to me at present as I'm part time and work in the public sector. I'm very fortunate to have a very understanding employer but it's still been quite hard. My husband is very stressed with it all. It's just how it has to be, but I am missing the support [. . .] Today is supposed to be one of my working days, but I got very little actual work done today. I find it very hard to concentrate when I'm with the kids even when they're occupied doing something else [. . .] My daughter has work set on an app by the school. It's been quite hard to get her to engage with it and I was not very good at insisting on it today.

Diarist 2408 (female, 40s, London, theatre worker)

After a bit of faffing and procrastinating school work begins. Since being furloughed my mornings are now focused on supporting [son] with his work. He is intelligent but easily distracted and prone to cutting corners, so I stick around when he is working to help him and get things set up and submitted properly [. . .] He's studying Macbeth in English which I am loving! It's taking me back to my school/University days of properly analysing a play and the characters. He's not loving it as much as me!

Diarist 2705 (female, 40s, Yorkshire and Humber, writer)

My son and I have invented a game in which we recite times tables whilst bouncing on the trampoline and throwing a ball. It's the easiest way to get him to learn and to exercise. He does not like the work set by the school and neither do I. It feels so dry and removed from our reality at the moment. The temptation is always there to just give up and snuggle under the blanket on the sofa.

Diarist 2750 (female, 40s, South East England, heritage collections manager)

Our lives are currently a rather ineffective patchwork of home schooling and trying to work. In some ways I feel more aware of exactly what my children do and don't know in terms of Maths and English etc. But I also worry that they will be so behind with their learning when they do eventually go back to school. I know it's not just them, and there is some comfort in that, but it's impossible to know exactly how much or little other kids are achieving at home.

Diarist 2762 (male, 50s, East Midlands, events manager)

Home school while the schools are closed can be trying. We are attempting to manage 3 lessons/activities a day. Today we only had 1 traumatic maths lesson!

Diarist 2764 (female, 14, Northern Ireland)

Logged onto my computer to do some school work. There was an email from my Maths teacher saying I hadn't got enough Maths done. I replied and apologised to them and then began working to get caught back up. To help it not feel so dreary and boring I put on Spotify and listened to my favourite playlist.

Diarist 2772 (female, 14, Scotland)

Nearly all my friends [. . .] have all said how much they miss going to school and seeing their friends but I actually prefer having a bit more control over when I need to wake up, when I can eat and other things like that [. . .] It's also been nice not having too much homework being set, usually at school homework would be around 30 minutes to an hour every day but (some) teachers are reluctant to give extra work now – since our eyes are strained on the computer enough as it is. Some days I do have a bad headache just from staring at the screen for 6 hours straight.

Diarist 3062 (female, 30s, East of England, nurse)

Time to get the laptop out and print off today's school work for the boys. I have to sit with the boys and go through the work with them at the kitchen table, otherwise it wouldn't get done!

Diarist 3245 (female, 30s, South West England, painter and decorator)

My daughter wakes up and we start chatting. She gets up to go to the toilet and shouts from the bathroom that she plans to play SIMS. I immediately get annoyed with her, she isn't doing enough school work as it is, she has fallen way behind with assignments, although in her defence a lot of parents are reporting that their children are also struggling with the current system that the school has adopted, which consists of uploading lesson plans onto an app with the same regularity and intensity of a school day. As an adult that often works from home, it can be hard to find the focus and motivation to go post a letter let alone adopt [a] method of self-teaching at the age of 12, and yes I could become a teacher, I have worked as a teaching assistant, but I never taught my own child, the dynamic is totally different and she is a wilful child, we clash. But there's no way I can just let her spend another day playing SIMS.

Diarist 3742 (female, 14, Northern Ireland)

I woke up, threw on my fluffy robe, ready for day 51 of the COVID19 lockdown in Northern Ireland. I came down the stairs at around 8.30am and ate my breakfast at the kitchen table [. . .] Reluctantly I began checking my emails from my teachers because although schools are shut, online schooling must continue.

Diarist 3797 (female, 40s, South East England, teacher)

The students are trying their best at home, but I know that they must be struggling with motivation to work. I know I do!

Diarist 4671 (female, 20s, Yorkshire and Humber, carer)

School work has taken a back seat to just simply getting by, getting through the day. I'm no teacher, never proclaimed to be, never wanted to be if I'm honest. Slightly jealous of those who seem to have their lives together at this point.

Diarist 4702 (female, 13, East Midlands)

I am on lockdown which is NO fun at all because I miss seeing my friends and hanging out and having a laugh. For me it feels strange not sitting in a classroom with all my classmates that make a lot of noise.

HOPE

In their diaries, correspondents took the opportunity to look forward. They described what they hoped would come next. These hopes ranged from grand hopes that the pandemic would be a moment of societal reset, when people would realize how much we depend on each other and the natural environment, and push for change, greater equality, more environmental protection; to modest hopes for a return to normal – to hugging family and friends, celebrating birthdays and weddings, dancing with others, going to the pub or café, visiting the shops without having to follow so many rules and guidelines, going to church, taking holidays; to desperate hopes that a CT scan on the lungs does not show blood clots and for a time when treatments and vaccines would allow people to live without fear of the virus. Some of these hopes were acknowledged for their naivety, but hope – grand hope, modest hope, desperate hope – is what kept people going during the pandemic. See also Birdsong; Cancellations; Clap for carers; Fear; (new) Normal.

Diarist 81 (female, 15, North West England)

Being in year 10 during this pandemic is nerve racking. Will I be able to take my GCSEs? Will mocks still be on? How will this affect my future career? [. . .] I got upset the other day. I didn't get my Chemistry assignment. Being selected to do triple science is quite the honour, so I worried I would fall behind and get moved down to dual. But no! I'm going to work my socks off (is that the right expression?) and 2020 will be my year (although maybe not for boys)! [. . .] Next year will be great! I'll (try) to ace my exams, see my friends, and celebrate my 16th with a small family get-together. I can't wait.

Diarist 119 (male, 60s, South West England, retired teacher)

The crisis is showing the undeniable truth that people who can't work from home are overwhelmingly our poorest and lowest paid who are more likely to depend on public transport, to live in densely populated areas, to be disproportionately BAME [Black and Minority Ethnic] and therefore at highest risk from Covid-19. It is also undeniable that the lockdown has shown how much we all rely on these workers. I hope that one of the effects of the crisis is that there will be a long overdue rebalancing of society and the worth we place on those who enable us to live our lives.

Diarist 200 (female, 30s, London, visual designer)

Today makes it 58 days since I've seen the face I love in front of me. I never counted the days before; it was just a given I'd see him on the weekend and we'd have a nice weekend in our bubble away from reality.

He doesn't even know I love him; well I think he does. But we've never said it out loud. But we have our ways. I actually now daydream about telling him in person, because I think after all this, we should allow each other that.

Diarist 564 (female, 13, Scotland)

I went to the shop today with my Mum. As we walked, we talked about the way things used to be, and all our plans for after this is over. We want to travel to the Maldives to celebrate my Dad's [. . .] birthday (obviously not possible at the moment due to the travel bans). So, to get us through this hard time, we dream about sandy beaches and clear blue waters.

Diarist 776 (male, 20s, South East England, journalist)

Here are a few things I'm looking forward to once the lockdown ends:

- Driving the car across the Severn Bridge just to visit my old Gran, kiss her on the cheek and chat about nothing in particular with her over a cup of tea.
- Looking out from the top of a mountain caked in my own dried sweat and panting.
- Eating a McDonald's late at night with friends in a lamplit car park.
- Drinking a pint in a pub garden at the end of a warm day.
- Hugging my parents, my brother and sister, my family dog, my friends.
- Lying out in a field watching the bees and the clouds.

Diarist 901 (female, 30s, London, unemployed)

I drop into the grocer's [. . .] I get chatting with a man   he tells me he's fucked off with the lockdown and just wants to go raving. He says the minute this is all over, he's going to grab some whatever, get all his mates, run to a field, throw his hands in the air and dance all night.

Diarist 1005 (female, 19, West Midlands, student)

When we come out of this, I have the feeling the world is going to make some very important decisions – decisions I hope will mean change for the better. I hope by the time someone reads this we'll have made plans to protect our environment, support our healthcare systems (and have a more definitive meaning of what a hero is), be kinder to our fellow humans, and remember all of the good we've done during this pandemic was done through compassion and global teamwork.

Maybe I'm being naïve and romantic for thinking like that, but at this rate believing in our future is all I can hang onto.

Diarist 1013 (female, 70s, Yorkshire and Humber, retired teacher)

I do feel anxious about the future and wonder if we will ever manage to live a different life to the one we have at the moment. I hope I will be able to be with my family again, have holidays with them and return to some of the activities we did with our friends.

Diarist 1086 (male, 30s, London, doctor)

For all the horror of this virus, it has opened up some space, slowed things down and provided time to reflect, learn and grow as individuals and as a society. When space arises, consciousness increases and there is increased compassion and togetherness. The climate is also benefiting. Despite the darkness of COVID19, I hope some of these positives can be its legacy.

Diarist 1150 (female, 80s, London, retired teacher)

I feel that currently the future looks very grim unless we are able to control this virus, not to mention the work needed to get the economy up and running again, however slowly. I do so want to be able to move around without fear and anxiety and meet up with friends again and hug each other freely. Reading about the hardships that so many families are suffering makes my own circumstances pale into insignificance in contrast. I do so hope that whichever Government is in the House will begin to acknowledge, address and rectify the huge differences and inequalities that exist currently and if they don't then I fear for the future of our society.

Diarist 1213 (female, 30s, London, IT consultant)

The lockdown is certainly the oddest on-going experience of my life. I sometimes have moments where I forget about it, but am brought back to reality fairly quickly, because the virus has infected and destroyed every aspect of life as we know it. I suspect that by this time next year we won't actually be back to normal. I don't think we ever really will be. I just hope we can be with our extended families. I don't care about going to restaurants, parties, the cinema etc. (although I don't wish those places to be out of business). More than anything I just want to hug my friends and family and tell them face to face how much I love them.

Diarist 1582 (female, 50s, West Midlands, office manager)

WhatsApp chat to [friend] – he's just doing minutiae for work and is bored to tears. He and his colleagues in the engineering company have had an enforced 10% pay cut. And one to [another friend] too. He was wanting advice on the red pepper and goat's cheese soup recipe. Really good to catch up with friends! All this never really happened much when we weren't in lockdown . . . I hope it lasts but I doubt it. People will go back to their busy lives.

Diarist 1692 (female, 60s, North of England, retired teacher)

I read the newspapers online, the Guardian and Times and the FT articles and graphs. The scientists and statisticians are the most reassuring aspect of this crisis and the work being done by them to find treatments and vaccines. They provide hope.

Diarist 1692 (female, 60s, North of England, retired teacher)

I am looking forward and hoping that in 2021 we will be able to celebrate my father's [. . .] birthday all together and my daughter's postponed wedding [. . .] I want to be able to collect my granddaughter from nursery in September as we planned!

Diarist 1940 (female, 30s, Scotland, assistant professor)

Let me think of some things worth looking forward to: Hugging my parents. Hugging my friends. Hugging my friend's children. Going to the library. Going to the seaside. Seeing the new Wonder Woman movie. Taking a bath (as my flat only has a shower). Sharing a meal with other people. Feeling calmer and happier.

Diarist 2056 (female, 50s, Scotland, communications manager)

Read a bit of a travel book [. . .] It is getting exceedingly harder to deal with this lockdown thing. I want to travel, I want to see my mum and mates, I want to go to the pub and I want to drift around the supermarket without a list and not be told which way to go.

Diarist 2315 (female, 80s, South East England, retired lecturer)

What am I missing? Seeing people face to face, being able to go to the shops and choose things myself, to go out for a cup of coffee, or for a drive, go to church, go to art group [. . .] This is what I shall enjoy when lockdown and self-isolation finally ends – and we might even go on holiday!

Diarist 2394 (male, 50s, South East England, unemployed actor)

A vast and dense fog of unknowing about the future, how we will all resume our lives, what form this will take – whether we will be able to return to the world we knew in 2019 or whether – and I hope this may happen – there will be a new impulse towards greater responsibility for each other, and for the world we live in and on. My kids say they don't think anything will change – I am a naïve optimist so hope for better things to come.

Diarist 2426 (female, 30s, South East England, office manager)

I've been monitoring my temperature daily as I'm sure many people are, and keeping my fingers crossed that we all stay healthy and that soon we can see just a few more people. My wish list right now would pretty much just be my parents, brother, niece and my best friend. Most of my favourite things in the world (trees, long walks, good food, home cooking, keeping my garden nice) are still available to me, but to have some others here to share the food and garden would be lovely.

Diarist 2476 (female, 50s, London, personal assistant)

[Friend] called me and we chatted for an hour or so which was lovely. Am so looking forward to the time when all this is over and we can go out together with all our friends, play records, go to gigs and dance!

Diarist 2597 (female, 30s, North West England, security services worker)

Will we return to life as we know it or will the impact of the last few months leave a lasting impression on humanity and society as we know it? I sincerely hope it is the latter, people are more receptive to others and a true sense of community spirit has emerged. People talk to each other in the enforced socially distanced queue for the supermarket and recognise the importance of key services and workers.

Diarist 2721 (female, 40s, North West England, clinician)

I'm looking forward to seeing my family again and being able to travel. Discussing a potential yoga trip [. . .] with a friend in November . . . surely by then.

Diarist 2806 (female, 30s, Scotland, tour guide)

Maybe there are things we can fix out of this, like working together more, like tackling climate change and trying to make some kind of sustainable future for Earth and for humanity. Nothing I've seen in politics in my entire lifetime has given me any reason to think that will happen. But you probably couldn't carry on if you didn't let yourself have a bit of hope.

Diarist 3009 (female, 12, London)

It was weird waking up and my mum not being here, but I know she's in the best place for her to get better. She's having a CT scan on her lungs this morning to rule out any potential blood clots. I hope and pray all will be clear. The weather looks dull and grey outside, a bit like how I feel inside. For breakfast I had a bowl of coco pops and a fresh orange sliced up. It was just before lunch when my dad got a call from my mum. She hasn't got blood clots but she has been told she has COVID-19 and has to self isolate. She can come home and for the next 10 days the local healthcare team will look after her. My dad went and picked her up from the hospital and as soon as she got in she went straight to bed, she looks really weak. Me and my dad then did a family Group FaceTime call with my grandma who is still in Somalia [. . .] A person from the home healthcare team just came and dropped off a pulse oxygen monitor and a thermometer for my mum with some sheets that she has to keep records of her results on. They said a doctor will call her later [. . .] I'm sad that I can't go near my mum when all I want to do is cuddle her and tell her all will be ok. Some photos my mum had ordered and got printed arrived in the post this afternoon. They were of my grandad who died [. . .] whilst in Somalia from COVID-19. I was so happy to see his face but then that turned to sadness and tears because I realised that this is the only way I will ever see his smiling face again. I really hope things get back to normal soon as I'm missing my family and friends and my usual routine but mostly I want my happy, healthy mum back.

Diarist 3104 (male, 50s, South East England, trainer and author)

To bed [. . .] praying (but not religiously, we're all devout atheists) that the football season can restart for at least two games and Liverpool can secure the four points they need to be crowned Premiership champions.

Diarist 3245 (female, 30s, South West England, painter and decorator)

I get a WhatsApp message from a mechanic I met on Tinder [. . .] I think I'm a bit in love with him. It's been hard to type this and stop myself from texting him a billion times a day [. . .] I said I would send him pictures of my van conversion [. . .] I send him the van pics, looks fucking fantastic he says, wish he thought the same about me. Maybe he will come away with me in the van when lockdown is over? I want to go away all the time after this.

Diarist 3367 (female, 50s, South East England, priest and bookseller)

This afternoon I have to record a Q & A Zoom session for the parish [. . .] The focus is on what the New Normal will look like. There is so much talk at the moment, following the Prime Minister's statement on Sunday [see Stay Alert], about slowly coming out of lockdown and what that will mean for individuals, businesses and of course the church, so I want to get people thinking about what they have gained from this time, and what they have learnt. I hope people will come out with a greater appreciation of each other, an understanding of how the whole world is so connected, and how there is so much that unites us, more than divides us. I also want to focus on Eco matters. The way nature is reclaiming places like the canals of Venice, how mountains are now visible from 100s of miles away in India because there is no air pollution, is something that should inspire us to be far more careful in how we use, and abuse, the world and its resources.

Diarist 3524 (male, 70s, Scotland, retired IT specialist)

My generation was born at the end of WWII and we grew up to see a better UK [. . .] Is COVID going to be a defining moment that will see change? I don't know. I hope so.

Diarist 3562 (female, 50s, South West England, garden designer)

I am an optimist by nature and sincerely hope that we can use this strange time to reset society. Can we come out of this crisis with a more compassionate green agenda that redistributes wealth more fairly? I am old enough to be cynical but I live in hope.

Diarist 3860 (male, 60s, South East England, electrician)

The lockdown has been quite good for me and allowed a slowdown of my life. I am hoping for a much-needed return to a better community spirit and civilised lifestyle with a greater awareness and respect for all that is around us. Still a bit of hope left in the old hippy that is me.

Diarist 4651 (female, 30s, South East England, GP receptionist)

I find the weekends the hardest at the moment as these are the times I want to be out of the house having a nice time with family and friends. I look forward to the time train travel will no longer be only for essential journeys and we can have a long jaunt out to the forest exploring.

Diarist 4756 (female, 40s, Yorkshire and Humber, academic)

When all of this is over, we hope to be able to keep our holiday booking [. . .] at the end of July [. . .] and the image I keep in my mind is of walking along the seafront with the wind in my face, with all four of us happy and healthy, and Covid-19 a distant memory. Keeping everything crossed . . .

KEY WORKERS

During the pandemic, the UK Government published a list of 'key workers' who would be needed to keep society moving while most people were confined at home. This list included workers in health and social care; education; justice; security; other emergency services; other essential government services; food production, distribution and retailing; transportation; utilities; public service broadcasting; religion; and management of deaths. Some of these workers can be heard elsewhere in this book. In this entry, we hear from doctors, nurses, midwives, community health workers, carers, pharmacists, scientists, teachers, chaplains and supermarket workers. We hear from key workers who are proud of this new designation ('key worker'); touched when people say 'thank you' or send gifts; relieved still to have jobs – and the income, camaraderie and normality jobs provide. And we hear from key workers who are busy, stressed, tired; who are working hard to implement new ways of working; who have been redeployed to the Covid 'frontline'; who are dealing with anxious patients or customers; who are struggling to social distance at work or when commuting; whose bodies are marked by constant hand washing and wearing of PPE; who are terrified of catching the virus themselves or bringing it home to family; who have colleagues currently off sick with the virus; who are living separately from family or, if not, following strict routines of quarantining, washing and sanitizing when returning home from work; and who, in many cases, are not paid enough to carry such burdens for the rest of society. See also Clap for carers; Deliveries; Fear; Shops.

Diarist P84 (male, 50s, South East England, doctor)

Yesterday was a hard day at work. Today slightly better. Lots and lots of phonecalls to patients, talking also with staff about their anxieties as we start to have a few patients coming in for essential blood tests/cervical cytology. Camaraderie is generally good amongst staff. We've become quite a close 'family' unit. Some COVID patients are taking a long time to get better. By the end of the day (12 hours) I had a stinking headache. Didn't drink enough fluid? Head in funny position all day and looking at screen and webcam [. . .] Time in the garden looking at the vegetable patch before supper was good. Tired.

Diarist 132 (female, 50s, West Midlands, supermarket worker)

Only a few months ago I regarded my job as tedious and unimportant but I am now regarded as a keyworker [. . .] These are definitely strange times. Our lives have shrunk. We cannot go out except for shopping or exercise and we cannot see our friends and families. But there are a lot of good things happening. People are helping and supporting one another in many ways. We have come to value people previously thought of as unskilled – people like care workers, supermarket staff, postal workers, transport workers, dustmen etc. [. . .] Work is different. We are trying to maintain social distancing but some people disregard it, even mock the notion. Most people have got used to queuing and behave reasonably. We don't have any panic buying anymore and no serious shortages. Many people are shopping for others. And many of our customers thank us and even give us little gifts. Yesterday a small boy said that all supermarket workers should be given medals!

Diarist 328 (female, 10, Yorkshire and Humber)

My dad is a consultant cardiologist [. . .] This means he specialises in hearts. He is seeing patients with covid 19. This is why I'm not able to see my dad.

Diarist 407 (female, 30s, South West England, nurse)

My department in a hospital [. . .] until two months ago was an acute medical department seeing a very broad range of conditions. Now we are the respiratory emergency department, taking any patient who presents with a cough or temperature or any one of the many symptoms we are seeing with Covid-19 [. . .] Despite my fears a couple of months ago we have seen nowhere near the numbers of patients we were expecting to see. Less than three months ago it was common for every one of my 34 beds and 6 trollies to be full, patients bedded in areas never intended for them and up to 5 queues in corridors around the emergency department. It was hellish for the staff and brutal for the patients. We were on our knees and most of us facing burnout [. . .] This period has been real respite for us, however there has been an underlying unease as we are in a perpetual brace position. I now have a deep fear in me that the numbers of patients coming in will again become great, that they will be very unwell, and we will be pushed harder than ever.

Diarist 479 (female, 40s, South West England, clinical pharmacist)

I really love my job and the people I work with. I have been going in to work early in order to catch the daily huddle. As the Covid-19 situation is changing rapidly and there are daily updates [. . .] we are finding that we keep having to reassess the services we provide and the way in which we provide them in order to keep our staff safe and ensure that our patients receive the care that they need in spite of the current Covid crisis. All this intensity has brought us together as a team and I feel that we are really caring for each other in a way that did not exist before the crisis [. . .] I think that we all appreciate being able to leave our homes and come to work. In some way this has created a sense of camaraderie that could not flourish before. I could work from home. I was recently given a laptop that enables me to connect to our patient records system. However, part of my role is to support our reception team, and this is done better face to face than over the phone or via direct messaging. Social distancing at work is not easy. I work in a consultation room alone, but the tearoom is small so making drinks and heating food for lunch means mixing with others. Assisting colleagues with prescription queries on screen is impossible from a distance of over 2m so we all accept that we do our best as much as we can [. . .] I am never sure what challenges the day will bring when I head to work. Last week I sent out a letter to all patients currently receiving Vitamin B12 injections to inform them that for the foreseeable future we will not be administering injections and that they will need to buy vitamin B supplements until we are able to resume this service. The majority of patients will be fine for up to a year without anything. However, it appears that our reception team have been on the receiving end of quite a few agitated patient calls and the way some patients have reacted to this news leads me to think that B12 injections may be the middle-class equivalent of crack cocaine! [. . .] One of my worries at present is the situation in our care homes. I have been trying to speak to a nurse in one of our local care homes for more than a week. There is a patient at risk of malnutrition and the staff keep requesting nutritional supplement drinks. It is not clear why the patient has lost so much weight and I am concerned that an extra 200 calorie drink per day is not going to meet their nutritional needs. I cannot speak to a member of staff to discuss and the receptionist who answers the phone sounds like she's had enough. I have tried to call on the support of the community care homes dietician only to find that he has been re-deployed elsewhere due to the Covid crisis. I am concerned and have made plenty of notes in the patient record but still have not found a resolution. As we face the extra pressure that Covid-19 brings, my worry is about the normal everyday healthcare that still needs to be maintained. I worry that this care home is short on staff or have so many patients unwell at present that they are struggling to cope [. . .] When I get home, I say a quick hello to my family and have a shower. After each day I need to put my clothes in a bag and leave them for three days before washing them and then shower to reduce the chances of Covid infection. I shower using plenty of shower gel and shampoo and then dress in clean clothes and join my children to catch up on their day.

Diarist 485 (female, 8, Yorkshire and Humber)

I woke up at 8:15 and started to do my school work. I am living at my Nanny and grandpa's since my mum is a nurse. For breakfast I had fruit with strawberry yoghurt and granola and after that I had bread, Nutella. Then I got dressed into warm and comfy clothes. I FaceTimed mummy while she was at work.

Diarist 591 (female, 40s, Scotland, molecular biologist)

I walk to/from work to get my daily exercise and it helps to clear my head and give me some peace. I have devised a route that takes me off-road as much as possible. I walk through local woods and a large park and often see red squirrels and deer as I go. I listen to comedy or poetry podcasts, or music. I quite often find myself in tears brought on by something I'm listening to in combination with the situation we find ourselves in [. . .] I am conflicted about continuing to go to work. I am pleased to be occupied and able to contribute something to the global scientific effort, but at the same time I am conscious of the added extra risk to myself and my family. I have been given a letter of authorisation to be travelling to work in case I get stopped by the Police. That hasn't happened yet, though I continually see many police cars/vans pass by [. . .] When I arrive at work I check in with security. Under normal circumstances, several thousand people would be arriving to work in the building. Currently, the whole place is in lockdown except for a small number of us who are authorised to continue to work. I put a surgical glove on one hand to allow me to safely open doors [. . .] There are other people from different teams in the laboratory and we are working together on several coronavirus-related projects [Figure 2] Some are research and diagnostic-test-related, and some are vaccine-related. We try to give each

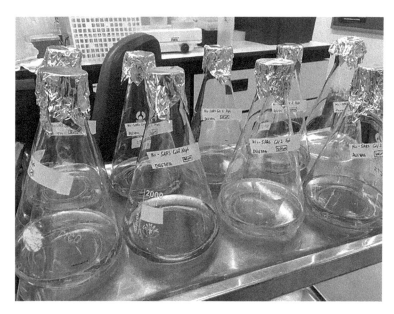

Figure 2 'We are working together on several coronavirus-related projects.' Image submitted by Diarist 591.

other space in the lab, but it is not always practical. The corridor that runs up one side of the lab is less than 2m wide. There has been a good feeling of teamwork and everyone is feeling the urgency of the situation and working hard to complete all the projects quickly.

Diarist 698 (female, 16, North East England)

My mum is a nurse, so she was on a night shift for the past two nights in a row. She is extremely tired and (even though I am not worried about my own safety) she is close to people who have coronavirus and I am worried about hers. She must come in through the back door and immediately shower and wash her clothes, so that she does not pass on the virus to my brother, sister, and me.

Diarist 699 (female, 40s, North East England, nurse)

I'm at work, sat on a unit that I do not usually work on. It's a totally different environment, different client needs, different staff team. It's OK, I will get used to it! You see, because of coronavirus I have been moved from my current job as a nurse to support another team. It can be scary. You don't know if people have the virus. It's invisible, until the symptoms start showing. We have some protection. I put on my face masks, gloves and apron, hoping that this will protect me from catching this evil virus. I can't bring it home to my lovely family. We all have to look after each other, protect each other. At the end of the shift I drive home. The roads are very quiet for this time of day. It's usually bumper to bumper with cars, everyone usually rushing to work. I phone home to let them know I'm on my way. My husband opens the side gate, back door, even the washing machine door ready for me to remove my clothes, putting them straight into the washing machine to stop the spread of infection. Before going to bed I check the news [. . .] the numbers of virus deaths are still very high [. . .] it is so sad. I go to sleep hoping that this will end soon.

Diarist 1107 (female, 50s, Yorkshire and Humber, nurse)

I have a day off work and so I managed to lie in until 0800hrs [. . .] My day, despite being a day off, has been structured around 3 virtual meetings, 2 planned calls and monitoring my emails.

I keep a regular check on my work email as I have volunteered to go and work at one of the Nightingale Hospitals if it is needed [. . .] I have been for my induction training [. . .] Early dinner tonight 5.45pm as I have a call to make at 6.15 followed by another [. . .] conference call from 7-9pm.

Call made and conference call completed early so [. . .] am now typing this watching a programme that started last night following the impact of COVID-19 at the Royal Free

Hospital in London. To a health care professional like me it is alarming. I cannot imagine how lay people are feeling. It is very very frightening.

It is now coming to the end of the evening. I can't say that any day at the moment is a normal day. Life is not normal. But it is a reflection of how many of my so called 'days off' are at the moment.

Diarist 1247 (female, 60s, West Midlands, NHS worker)

Today we are in the midst of the covid 19 crisis. I have been redeployed to a community-based service that aims to keep people out of hospital if they have been discharged and prevent admission for people who are at risk of admission through deteriorating health.

I woke slowly at 6am. I needed to iron uniforms as I had washed them on my day off and left it late to iron them in advance. I washed and showered, ironed and put today's uniform in my travel bag. I wore my travel clothes [. . .] I called goodbye and drove my Dad's car known as the Covid Mobile as I have agreed to use his car for work during the crisis. No one else will go in there while we are shielding ourselves from the virus. At work I met my colleagues and went to change into my uniform putting my travel clothes safely on a peg [. . .] I called the patients. One is a woman in her 70s [. . .] I do not know that I have the knowledge and skills to help her so feel a mixture of dread and dismay that yet again we will not meet. I am a pain specialist physiotherapist and have limited rehab skills in this area. I do not know any system or individual who can help me. I worry about being out of my depth and just hope I can wing it until I find an answer.

Much of the day was spent discussing this conundrum; all the staff I am with have been redeployed from areas they have spent years developing specialist skills in specific areas, only to find ourselves in a new area facing some very poorly people who could be helped out of the worst if we get it right.

Diarist 1338 (female, 40s, South East England, hospital consultant)

I got up this morning and got the children ready for school. Life feels more relaxed as there are no pre-school clubs for the kids and no traffic on the way to school. I cycle into work, seeing only a handful of cars in the deserted streets [. . .] I feel like I'm one of the only people going to work (and I probably am). Many of my friends locally are furloughed from work or have lost their jobs. At work it all feels different, though I'm glad I'm not stuck at home, trying to homeschool the children and potentially juggling work from home as that would definitely be worse.

I phone my patients for clinic, everyone appears to be expecting my call, as I contact most on their landlines. Many are elderly and find the isolation of the new normal incredibly difficult, some have had shielding letters from the government telling them not to leave the house even to go shopping. Many say thank you, far more than usual in clinic and are grateful for the care offered within the hospital. I do some paperwork, attempt to answer emails, there are some that I cannot answer with any degree of certainty, we know so little about COVID 19.

Diarist 1490 (female, 50s, Yorkshire and Humber, nurse)

By profession I am a Registered Nurse. I am working during the pandemic, assessing patients over a video link. Until last year I was an Emergency Department nurse. Because of this I felt guilty about not being on the 'front line' and being in physical danger at the start of the pandemic, but after a while I realised I am doing an important job helping to look after people in Care Homes and the work has been quite stressful because of the way the pandemic has affected the Care Homes and the large numbers of deaths. Also, working has in itself not been without danger because in our open plan office about 20% of the staff have been off sick at various times with Covid-19.

Diarist 1585 (female, 60s, South East England, therapist and chaplain)

My morning starts early as my husband had to leave for work at [the local hospital] where he works as an engineer keeping equipment maintained and adjusting appliances for the children who use them. He is classed as 'vulnerable' at present, as he is diabetic, and had to wear a specially fitted face mask at work and have no contact outside of the workshop. He has travelled up to work on his motorbike in order to avoid meeting people on public transport where social distancing is impossible. I make him a packed lunch as he cannot go out to eat.

Diarist 1691 (female, 20s, South East England, online shopper)

My day started at 3.20am as I got ready for my 4-8am shift at [. . .] Sainsbury's, working as an online shopper. I spent most of the shift rather tired, talking to the other employees about how tired we are.

Diarist 1700 (female, 50s, London, piano teacher)

I worry about my husband going to work [as a Civil Enforcement Officer] on a bus and a train but there is nothing we can do – we need him to work and he is a key worker so he has to work (no furlough for him). He has a routine that when he comes home, he takes his clothes off outside and leaves them under a porch, he sanitises his hands and then comes in and goes straight into the shower – his clothes will be collected and will be washed every few days. He wears gloves on public transport and all day and now he will be wearing a mask. Nothing more we can do.

Diarist 1874 (female, 40s, South East England, GP)

There were 3 GPs in today covering 9000 patients. We all currently pick calls off a triage list, phone patients, or sometimes video consult through a rather clunky mobile phone app which is not ideal with the elderly, and bring some non Covid patients into the surgery if they need to be seen. There must have been about 120 calls today and I saw about 8 patients face to face. We wear masks all the time we are in the surgery and plastic aprons and gloves when we see patients [. . .] In the past 2 weeks the number of phone calls we have had has at least doubled. Patients were happy to keep away from us at the start of this pandemic but are now realising this is going to be a long haul and are rightly now seeking our help. However the day was exhausting. I left the surgery for 30 mins at 2pm to eat my lunch in the car and walk around the block before carrying on with the list [. . .] I got home at 7.30 completely shattered.

Diarist 1913 (female, 50s, East of England, nurse)

6.30 am Woke up. Feeling tired and aching. Checked temperature, normal. We have to check our temperature daily to ensure we are fit to come to work during this pandemic. Meanwhile my husband made tea and brought it up to me in bed, so I could snatch a few more precious minutes. I'm a Christian but not really that good at it a lot of the time! But today I felt anxious and said my prayers!

Breakfast was toast and marmalade. My husband had fed the two cats so I just gave them a fuss. He had already left for work around 7.30. So I showered and got ready for work. My uniform is a tunic and trousers, dark blue with a white stripe along the collar and sleeves. I collected my belongings and lunch, ensuring I have my hand sanitiser and a notebook with me [. . .] Then set off for my first patient. There had been a frost and it was quite chilly but the sun was out so I didn't take a coat because I would have to wash that too if I did when I got home.

I obviously can't go into detail with my patients. However [. . .] I have seen COVID positive patients and patients with respiratory symptoms. Our personal protective equipment for this consists of surgical masks, plastic aprons and goggles. We have visors which we wipe and reuse that were donated by local companies and schools.

I stopped for lunch [. . .] at around 2pm [. . .] After that I undertook telephone consultations for the afternoon and spoke to my line manager by telephone. I checked emails. I answered a survey put out by our NHS Trust, asking if we had sufficient PPE and if we felt safe. My answer to this was 'No'. I left at around 4.40 for home.

When I got home [. . .] I stepped into the porch, used the wipes I had put in the porch to wipe down my car keys, lanyard, lunch bag and placed them on the stairs while still standing in the porch. Took off my shoes and left them on the rack in the porch. Then I took off my uniform and placed it in the waiting pillow case, and put on my dressing gown which I now leave in the porch. I then took the pillow case with my uniform and went through to the washing machine where I put it in straight away. Then straight upstairs for a shower before going to the rest of the house or greeting my husband. We are all afraid of bringing this virus home to our families.

Diarist 2035 (female, 50s, North West England, nurse)

Today I'm going to work for 2.30 – 8.30pm at the local community hospital as a staff nurse on the bank [. . .] Going in to work provides some normality in the strange times. Mixing with staff and patients is good. We all wear face masks and the usual gloves and aprons plus visor when providing personal care [. . .] Social isolating is almost impossible at work as most patients need two to help them. I suppose the masks do help. Some staff have recently tested positive and are off work. Like all hospital settings there are no visitors unless someone is terminally ill, and even then carefully monitored. This is hard for relatives and we help by organising FaceTime chats. Some patients with dementia can't remember why their relatives can't visit, and we have to remind them frequently. We have had family members waving through ward windows and this feels better than nothing.

Staff have been up and down throughout the last few weeks. Normally stoic staff, myself included, have been in tears about what is happening. Some scared for their families and themselves; going home after a shift, showering before hugging children and partners. We religiously take off our uniforms at work and change clothes. Donated uniform bags are good to take uniform home and can be put straight in the wash.

I have seen staff coping with the difficulties very well but then break down after 6 weeks – it has all got too much. Resilience is there in bucketfuls but every now and again it breaks down. We all support each other and I feel age and experience helps me and I try to support the younger and less experienced staff.

This shift was good [. . .] The camaraderie is good and the nurses and health care assistants do have a laugh at times. Someone has dropped off some cup cakes so we enjoy those on our break.

Diarist 2160 (female, 40s, South West England, mental health nurse)

I was working a night shift last night [. . .] At 7am I went to do handover to the morning team, like us, all in their scrubs and surgical masks. Usually we would be wearing our own clothes, but since the last couple of weeks we've been issued with scrubs which are washed on the ward overnight. We have to wear masks whenever we are within 2 metres of anyone else (i.e. most of the time!), and for physical contact with patients we have to also don plastic aprons and gloves. It has become less weird, but it's still odd.

Diarist 2261 (female, 60s, London, doctor)

Breakfast, dog walk, went to work. The team spirit at the hospital is fantastic. I feel very lucky to be able to go to work and feel this camaraderie. Today is the International Day of the Nurse and there seemed to be cake everywhere. One of my abiding memories of the pandemic will be the amount of food that kind people have given to the hospital staff.

Diarist 3062 (female, 30s, East of England, nurse)

I work [. . .] as a nurse in the recovery department at the [local] hospital. I am on a day off today. The shifts have changed due to the current pandemic from short days to 13 hour days and nights – which are total killers! But you do end up with more days off. Work is hard at the moment. My department has to help in Intensive Care, so I have been looking after COVID positive ventilated patients, which I do not feel competent to do, so this causes a lot of stress and anxiety. I am much happier in recovery! [. . .] [In recovery] we still have to wear all of the PPE, which is so hot! The worst part is the mask, it makes you feel so enclosed, and I've got so many spots and cold sores! My children say I'm Nanny McPhee in reverse!

Diarist 3569 (female, 50s, South West England, community health worker)

I work for an agency and visit clients in their own homes [. . .] I come downstairs to make a pot of coffee and spend a few minutes in the garden trying to get my head together for the coming day [. . .] My daughter gets up to spend a little time with me, she has been pretty anxious for my safety and scared I will die. Some days are better than others. She goes back to bed and I hop in the shower and get myself into Work Mode. Hair done, face on, uniform nicely ironed, hands washed and pick up my bag of PPE and food. I eat my breakfast later as it's a bit early yet. I get no breaks, so generally eat whilst driving between jobs. Terrible for the digestion [. . .] I drive 16 minutes to a village for my first call [. . .] I drive with my window down hoping the brisk air will perk me up as I am rather fatigued. Bit worrying at the start of the day!

My first client is a stroke victim with very limited mobility needing assistance with personal hygiene [. . .] We do all the necessaries [. . .] They always share their lives. I consider it an honour to be given windows into their worlds. These folk have lived amazing lives [. . .] I always try to get them outdoors for an airing and some sunshine. I place chairs on patios, balconies or gardens for those who have access to outdoor spaces. I open curtains and windows where allowed [. . .] For some ladies having perfume on or wearing makeup or their nails painted are part of who they are. It is important to remember who prefers what [. . .] Disinfected all door handles, disposed of soiled PPE, washed hands (for the third time in this visit) and off again.

A 7 minute drive through more chocolate box villages to lady with Dementia and limited mobility. She is a real character and laughs uproariously all of the time [. . .] All the necessities performed, then medication to administer [. . .] Whilst chatting and listening to clients I fill in quite a lot of paperwork, it's trickier than you think concentrating on both tasks simultaneously. More handwashing then off again.

A 10 min drive through more bucolic countryside [. . .] Arrived, washed hands, clocked on and rang in to log on so I get paid. Another client with slight dementia who suffered a stroke so has trouble moving and remembering. She is a jolly soul [. . .] We follow her daily routine for personal care in a swift manner as I only have 30 mins and there is a great deal to do. There is a hubby here too. He's always chipper and likes to be busy. He usually nips out to the shop while we're here but is worried it'll take too long because this Pandemic makes everything take twice as long. I reassure him I will wait for him to get back; the unspoken issue is we both know it's time I won't be paid for and will make me later than ever. But I genuinely don't mind. Ten minutes extra will mean they're all sorted for essentials and he will have had a change of scene and a chance to catch up with the neighbours [. . .] I trek out to my next client, 20 minutes' drive. I eat en route but also tricky as I have phone calls to make [. . .] The next client is my most challenging, extremely complex needs in a tiny cottage with stairs like a corkscrew [. . .] I arrived today to find she had dislocated her knee. I am a bit gobsmacked! Carers get fuck all in the way of training, you're supposed to pick it up as you go. Really??? Anyway I deal with the dislocated knee hoping the neighbours won't call the police because she's got a powerful set of lungs on her and is bellowing like a heifer. I somehow get a crocodile brace in place then we all take a breather. Tho I suspect that what she could do with is a Stiff Whisky.

After, I spend the next three hours sorting meds, equipment, talk to District Nurses team and various other departments and agencies organising essential ongoing treatment appointments as she is on about Level 7-8 on the pain threshold today [. . .] As well I try to blitz the wet rooms and get the kitchen ship shape. The laundry has become monstrous and I know she is upset at the state of her home. Her family usually support her brilliantly but she is under quarantine so that is cut off [. . .] More wash wash washing of the hands. (I'm up to about 20-25 times by this time of day) [. . .] I depart leaving them more comfortable than I found them. I am pleased with my input today.

This run is always challenging but easier by far than the calls where Loneliness is their only companion. Those calls make me weep, when I can only give half an hour to someone who will then sit alone all day with only the telly for company [. . .] If I could I would have them all live with me and my family.

Diarist 3797 (female, 40s, South East England, teacher)

I chat to my son, who has returned from work [at a local shop]. He told me that the click and collect service has been busy, so he hasn't had time to eat properly [. . .] He talks about opening up the store next week for customers, with social distancing in place. It is going to be difficult to control, as I've witnessed the people in the supermarkets not sticking to a one-way system, or just coming too close to people. He tells me that they will be allowing 45 people in the store at one time, which seems quite a lot of people. I am concerned that he won't get the proper face shields, like some stores have. People are often rude and aggressive, and it would only take someone with the virus to spit at him and he could die. It has happened already, so it is a worry.

Diarist 4671 (female, 20s, Yorkshire and Humber, carer)

6.50 Woke up by husband coming in from work [at a pharmaceutical plant] – first thing I ask 'how's work, how's his friend who is recovering from covid, has he made sure his hands are clean'.

7.40 must've drifted back off – [child] awake, time to get up, coffee, cig – obsession over news starts.

Turn on the news, watch in despair wondering whether this will ever end or will we just get used to the new normal.

Kids are running round, I feel like every day is just a battle for bedtime, they know what's going on but do they understand the implications for their futures?

It's hard being a carer [for elderly people with dementia] during this, it's hard knowing that the risk every day at work poses a threat to the health of your family. I've learnt to ignore that feeling for the most part though.

Husband's asleep. I am trying to keep the children quiet whilst struggling to maintain a normal family day.

Waves of despair, on and off throughout the morning [. . .] My thoughts often wander to work life. What if we get a case and I end up bringing it home. What if I lose one of my family members and I brought that home to them. For what? For a little over £8 an hour. You have to be slightly weird to be a carer anyway. Not your average job. I love my job I really do it's just hard battling the thoughts daily.

Diarist 4925 (female, 40s, South East England, midwife)

I walked into work at about 7.30am and the streets were very quiet. Just a few more people around as I approached the hospital itself.

Before covid19 the clinic was always horribly busy, the waiting room full of women who need to see a range of health professionals. Today many of the same people were reviewed over the phone so the waiting room was quieter. No partners are allowed in so very little chatting. It felt more edgy though. The women all feel vulnerable and may well be more susceptible to covid. I think almost every woman I saw today mentioned how they were feeling anxious – sometimes to the point of needing medication to manage it.

I was really pleased to see a friend who is also a midwife/nurse who had been redeployed to work in ITU [Intensive Therapy Unit] over the past few weeks. We have had relatively low numbers of covid patients so she was able to come back. I think her manager pleaded her case that her specialist work was important. She's just delighted to have got out of ITU. She said she finds it a lot harder now she's older and gets more affected emotionally by the sad things that happen.

LOCKDOWN PROJECTS

Those retired or furloughed had plenty of time to fill during lockdown. To make productive use of this time, or to keep anxiety and boredom at bay, they completed projects. They completed gardening projects and do-it-yourself projects, which had been on 'to-do' lists for years or which had been conceived once people started spending so much time at home. They completed administration projects, including the sorting of paperwork – the putting of affairs in order – in preparation for the event of serious illness or death, to which the context of the pandemic gave additional urgency. They completed creative projects: making photobooks, knitting, sewing, crafting, creative writing, learning to draw or paint, learning to cook, learning a musical instrument. They learned new skills, including new languages. They completed puzzles, learned new board games, mastered new computer games, read books they'd been meaning to read, watched films and boxsets they'd been meaning to watch, and kept diaries, including for Mass Observation. Many of these completed projects – these achievements – were displayed on social media. Of course, not everyone completed lockdown projects during this time. Some people couldn't find the motivation and found themselves distracted by news and social media, or personal illness or bereavement. Some people were not retired or furloughed. Their jobs were busier than ever. They now balanced work with childcare and home schooling responsibilities. To these people, displays of lockdown achievements on social media could seem insensitive. See also Anxiety; Furlough; Stay home; WhatsApp.

Diarist 46 (female, 40s, East of England, teacher)

Now that the working day is over, I have to try and keep myself busy. I would normally go for a run or run a cricket practice for junior members, all of which is currently prohibited. I am growing a lot more vegetables in my garden than I have done before and have spent many hours sorting family photographs into something like a chronological order.

Diarist 189 (female, 70s, North West England, nurse)

Recently completed 'Isolation Projects': An inventory of all our different, eclectic possessions inherited and collected from our travels abroad. I photographed, compiled and make comments about their provenance etc. into one document. This turned out to be more of a time consuming exercise than expected, but as someone who is better at starting projects than completing them, I was very pleased to have finished it. Pleasure strangely mingled with a sort of bereavement/sadness as it had prompted lots of happy memories, but now left a void about what I would 'DO' next!

Looking through my 'to do' list I realised that the two other big ones I have started (but not yet completed) concern **Remembering**:

1. My family history researches [...] Now, with so much time to spare, this seems to be the opportunity to finally complete my father's family story, and those of my grandmother and great grandmother [...] 2. The photo book of our 40 years of marriage. This was started last year with the intention of completing it before our Anniversary, but as usual it dropped down the list and I sit with an envelope beside me of final photos to add in, so the book can be finally edited before completion. *However again motivation lags.*

Diarist 221 (male, 20s, East of England, graphic designer)

To begin with, there was plenty to do in the garden, and I busied myself with painting the shed – now ready to be used as a pseudo summer house. But as the new reality set in, I found that motivation started eluding me. Days began to merge with less being achieved. A week or so ago I read a social media post asking what we'd tell our grandchildren about our time during lockdown, and it got me thinking – what *would* I tell them I'd been doing?

Diarist 286 (female, 60s, Scotland, retired building society cashier)

After tea, I finished writing cards and letters for the family, while Husband worked on indexing and captioning our photos from 1985. A few years ago we paid a teenager to scan all our 35mm colour slides so we have them digitally, but he'd never got round to indexing and captioning them all . . . until lockdown. He started with the 1960s ones, so is making steady progress.

Diarist 422 (male, 70s, South West England, garage forecourt worker)

After a pleasant salad lunch (some of which was home grown) I went back to trench digging at the back of my workshop. Having experienced repeated flooding of the workshop floor over the last three to four years I have finally got round to doing something about it. It's amazing how many major jobs that have been waiting some time are now being attended to. I have permanent back-ache but am getting fitter and have lost some weight!

Diarist 542 (female, 60s, East Midlands, retired accountant)

I am working on a jigsaw puzzle I started nearly 2 weeks ago. It's a 1000 piece puzzle. It's the 3rd one since the lockdown in March. I am at a difficult bit so it's taking a while to do. I usually take my cup of tea to the dining room and finish it while I put a few pieces in the jigsaw.

The jigsaw is a means of escape from what is going on in the world. The news can be so depressing. I can concentrate on the pieces and lose myself in what I am doing. My husband is reading a book on his kindle while I work on the jigsaw. I usually spend about an hour but so far today only manage about 20 minutes.

The days seem long. That's why it isn't much good being up too early [. . .] After lunch, we played a board game [. . .] We seldom play it except on holiday but we have taken it out and we play a few games every few days. Just for something to pass the time really. I won all 3 games today.

I have gone back to doing the jigsaw puzzle and managed to put a few more pieces in place. I might get it finished tomorrow [. . .] I am getting more annoyed at having to stay at home but there is nowhere to go. I can't visit or meet family or friends and there are no shops or cafes open. Trying to find things to do gets more difficult [. . .] I occasionally take a chair and sit on my driveway with a cup of tea and my next-door neighbour sits on her drive with a cup of tea and we chat for a while. We don't leave our home and we socially distance but at least we see another person. If I do it on the evening before garbage day you get to exchange greetings to the other neighbours putting out their bins. There are often people out for walks and they might stop and chat for a few minutes as they pass by. Something to do to pass the time.

Diarist 547 (male, 50s, South East England, consulting engineer)

Now it's 22:20, and I've failed to do the programming I should have done, nor undercoated the new woodwork in the soon-to-be-redecorated downstairs loo, nor planted out courgettes, or practised clarinet, nor emailed Aunt [. . .], or Skyped my little bro [. . .], or . . .

Diarist 858 (female, 40s, East Midlands, communications worker)

The extra time on my own has definitely magnified various previous interests. Suddenly, I have a heap of veg seeds on order [. . .] for which I need to take up some turf and do some digging, and a rapidly expanding houseplant collection [. . .] I've always knitted, and I think I'm currently standing at 3 pairs of socks and almost a cardigan since lockdown. I'm revisiting previous interests in dyeing fabric and yarn, and found myself ordering macrame stuff at 11PM the other day for something different to do that will also enable me to hang some of these plants suddenly festooning the house! I'm also thoughtfully eyeing the bathroom floor and wondering how easy it would be to replace. Amazing how extra time in our home not only gives us time to do things, but focuses our attention on our nests! [. . .] Haven't got around to that sanding-the-chest-of-drawers-down project that I've been vaguely meaning to get around to for the past five years, though. Oops. One day, maybe…

Diarist 1013 (female, 70s, Yorkshire and Humber, retired teacher)

My partner and I had coffee [...] I then used a shredder to dispose of past bank statements going back to 2015. These are uncertain times and I feel I need to get my papers in order unless I get the virus.

Diarist 1276 (male, 60s, London, retired physician)

During this lockdown I am learning how to cook. It could be argued that I have taken my time over this, being [in my 60s], and with a shape which strongly suggests that food and I have been good friends for some time. But, I decided that I should. Tonight's dish was Beef Bourguignon, done rather well, to a Mary Berry recipe. She does like her tipple – a lot of red wine, and brandy, but everyone agreed it was a success.

Diarist 1364 (female, 60s, East of England, solicitor)

I feel ashamed of the fact that I have not learnt a new language, or written a novel during this period of enforced idleness, some people are doing so much!

Diarist 1400 (male, 60s, South East England, retired accountant)

During the 'lockdown' period I have been trying to sort out many papers relating to my main hobbies and interests – folk music [...] church bell ringing, running and walking, and I have for many years (in fact since junior school!) had a great interest in buses (and also initially in trains – I was a 'spotter', collecting train numbers). These papers have built up over the years and have rather taken over one corner of our bedroom, so I am slowly sorting them, throwing away a lot that would now be of no use – out of date transport timetables, for instance.

Diarist 1423 (male, 30s, London, auditor)

This blog is the 58th day in a row I have written down my thoughts, starting with the Monday where the office said to work from home, which was 4 days before the country was told to go into full lockdown as part of the Coronavirus measures enacted by the UK government. In those 57 previous days I've written down some thoughts on the day, musings, and often a poem to commemorate how I feel. It's how I've been able to cope with the mental strain of living through a global pandemic.

Diarist 1456 (male, 50s, Wales, retired psychotherapist)

I have a perverse sense of my life becoming less structured than the current trend amongst Britons, who, it is reported daily, are sharing endlessly on Social Media about using Lockdown as a time to create more structure and thus more opportunity for self-improvement. Not me. I am loving the silence of my house and the stillness of my life, the sense of freedom that has become my new normal.

Diarist 1602 (female, 60s, South West England, school librarian and counsellor)

This afternoon I rang my daughter [. . .] She's started to create a photobook of her trip to Japan two years ago [. . .] Creating photobooks is one of the few things I've been able to concentrate on during lockdown; firstly I made one of our holiday [. . .] last year and I then made one of our trip to India [. . .] The biggest one I am working on now is of the family clan [. . .] It's comforting, joyful and sad in equal measure, to see all the happy times we've had together as a family.

Diarist 1691 (female, 20s, South East England, online shopper)

I spent the day updating my laptop, watching TV and finally reading *Silence of the Lambs*. I say finally because the bookmark in this book was a boarding pass from [. . .] 2017, the holiday on which I first attempted to read the book. If one good thing has come from lockdown it's that I can't use the excuse of 'I'm too busy' to read things that I enjoy.

Diarist 1710 (female, 60s, London, garden designer)

At the beginning of lockdown I decided that each day I would examine something in detail. When you are kept at home it is the small details that have to sustain you. So every day I write about an object and take a photo of it. Inevitably these can veer towards being nostalgic. This is not something that comes naturally to me but I've kept it going for more than 50 days now.

Diarist 1848 (male, 50s, Scotland, broadcast and telecommunications engineer)

A break for lunch [. . .] followed by a couple of games of chess. At the start of lockdown we'd dug out the chess set, and [wife] re-learned the rules, and we tend to play a game or two most days. Until now I've won fairly comfortable most times, although [wife] has had the odd win, but today I was outplayed TWICE! I must be more careful now, she's getting the hang of it and isn't the push-over she was 4 weeks ago! [. . .] Had a game of 'Wordfeud' (a mobile-phone app, based on Scrabble, but slightly different) with [wife] @ around 5pm. I lost this, too. [Wife] jubilant – chanting 'THREE-NIL! THREE -NIL!' after her 2 chess victories earlier, plus this 'scrabble' win.

Diarist 1866 (non-binary, 20s, South East England, student and proof-reader)

I've been marathoning the *Star Wars* films on DVD with my parents [. . .] We've been watching a film a night in chronological order of the narrative (rather than by order of release dates), starting with the prequel trilogy and including the *Solo* and *Rogue One* spin-offs [. . .] My mum is a half-hearted participant in all this. She keeps saying things like 'So when is Darth Vader going to get his face chopped off?' [. . .] I think we're going to try a Disney+ free trial to watch *The Mandalorian* once we're done with the films [. . .] Then, maybe the *Indiana Jones* films, which I've never seen but my dad likes a lot. I think it's important to establish and keep up little routines like this all the while the outside world is so uncertain.

Diarist 1940 (female, 30s, Scotland, assistant professor)

My oldest friend [. . .] is using the lockdown time to take a drawing class over Zoom and start learning Russian. I admire that. I initially planned to take up new things during lockdown, which now seems wildly naïve. I'm more concerned at this point about skill loss; my people skills must be atrophying with lack of human contact. Rather than attempting new things, I've been falling back on old coping mechanisms and soothing activities, like knitting, rewatching a favourite sitcom, and playing [old games] on my laptop.

Diarist 2070 (male, 70s, South West England, administrator)

Half an hour on the Duolingo Italian course that I started early in lockdown. It was encouraging to watch an Italian woman being interviewed this evening on [the TV news] and realise that I could understand almost all of what she was saying.

Diarist 2143 (female, 50s, North West England, secretary)

I'm finding that being at home a few days a week for the last however many weeks it is now, has left me, some days, not knowing what to do. The housework is up to date, the ironing is done, the garden is immaculate! And as I managed to get a delivery slot with Tesco, the shopping is organised for the week. It's now 9.30am and I'm wondering what to do for the rest of the day.

I used to do a lot of scrap booking/journal keeping and decided to start one about Covid-19. So far I have some paper, a few stickers and a rough idea of what to write. Apart from that I've drawn a blank. I keep staring at the pile hoping it will magically form itself into something amazing.

Diarist 2341 (female, 30s, Wales, librarian)

Back upstairs, sitting on my bed watching Castle on DVD – I'm on season seven of eight and have managed to watch the whole thing since lockdown began. Under normal circumstances, I'm very bad at binge-watching because I've always got work to do [. . .] These aren't normal circumstances though and I appreciate having the option to lose myself in someone else's imagination for a little while. I've clearly managed to develop my skills as I managed to cram the entire fifth season of Outlander into a single weekend.

Diarist 2070 (male, 70s, South West England, administrator)

I spent the remainder of the evening playing Animal Crossing on the [Nintendo] Switch I bought especially for lockdown. It arrived on Easter Friday (10th April) and I think I've already clocked up 70+ hours.

Diarist 2397 (female, 70s, South East England, retired secretary)

We have taken the opportunity during lock-down to undertake a long-overdue clear-out of files which resulted in much shredding of out-dated papers. We are making a list for my children so that in the event of our death they will have some idea of our financial affairs and know where to find things. I added a few important details to this list today.

Diarist 2473 (female, 60s, South West England, retired)

Continued to stick some photos into an album – they are of my younger daughter as a baby and toddler; I get very sentimental when I look at photos of my children when they were little. At the moment I sense a great urgency to finish things I have been meaning to do for a while. The thought that I might fall ill with Covid 19 is very much on my mind. So I want to feel that I have put my affairs in order as much as possible, in case I were not to survive. I am still trying to sort out my mother's belongings and papers, although it is more than two years since she died. (And cannot continue with this until travel is permitted again.) I want to spare my daughters this kind of overwhelming task.

Diarist 2627 (female, 40s, Northern Ireland, editor)

I have sentenced myself to dealing with all of the paper I have hoarded in boxes and bags for as long as I have been able to collect evidence of my existence in the world. On this diary day I opened a box of painful memories from the turn of the century, which doesn't seem as though it was 20 years ago. Some things I can't bear to keep, others I can't bear to throw away [. . .] After, I tried to scrub and rinse away the memories with the contents of the delivery of non-essentials I guiltily received from Boots.

Diarist 2721 (female, 40s, North West England, clinician)

Social media is full of friends and strangers making cakes, sourdough starters and bread, sewing, crafting. I have neither the time or inclination when I finish work. Evenings are for exercise, food, catching up with people and TV. Weekends are just a spread-out version of that (usually with some kind of cleaning or house fixing activity).

Diarist 2722 (female, 60s, East of England, museum educator)

I went to my emails [. . .] With [friend] I shared a moan about isolation [. . .] Fortunately we both very much enjoy reading and have extensive libraries. I really am going to read those 'great' political novels by Disraeli and Trollope which I have been putting off reading for the last fifty years.

Diarist 2788 (female, 60s, Scotland, retired teacher)

Beloved has eaten, taken his cycle ride and has started to remove skirting boards. A new kitchen will emerge from this lockdown.

Diarist 3051 (female, 70s, London, retired stage manager and personal assistant)

I started this lockdown almost glad to have the opportunity to finally get to grips with the domestic administration which overwhelms me. I'm a hoarder, and at last I could 'sort everything out'. After eight weeks [. . .] I've done very little of that. I envy those who've accomplished so much in these weeks but I also know of very many who, like me, seem to have no time [. . .] I spend a lot of time on texts, emails, phone calls, organising and cooking meals, and the day has disappeared before I think of taking down even one file [. . .] I have knitted a jacket for a nephew's new baby, which is something, and I restored and repaired my mother's old sewing machine which had been in the cupboard since she died [. . .] I've made two masks and will make more. There are a legion of films, theatre, museum tours offered online and I manage only a fraction of those. As for all the reading I thought I'd be able to do…

Diarist 3086 (female, 30s, London, archivist)

Read a chapter or two of Peter Ackroyd's *London*. I'm taking the opportunity to read as many of my large, heavy books as I can, as usually all my reading happens when commuting on the tube, which limits me to lighter volumes [. . .] I have dinner at 7:30 and watch an episode of *Life on Mars* on BBC iPlayer. Before lockdown, I was so socially busy I never had time to watch anything. Now I'm relishing the chance to catch up on all those series and films which have been recommended over the years. I have taken out subscriptions to three streaming services (Netflix, BFI, Now TV) and have a very long watch list!

Diarist 3134 (female, 60s, South East England, tour guide)

I go back to finish the last touches of my knitting which I have been doing on and off since lockdown. I sew the knitted flower on to the front of the little jumper for my grand-daughter and because it is finally complete and looking reasonable, I take a photo of it to send to my colleagues who have sent their 'creative' projects in to show what they have been doing.

Diarist 3284 (male, 20s, South East England, retailer)

I spent an hour working on a creative writing project. Furlough has freed up a lot of time for writing and editing. For passion projects, it's been the most productive period I've ever had.

Diarist 3899 (female, 50s, East Midlands, public health worker)

My afternoon consisted of drawing practice. I decided to do a self portrait every day, improve drawing skills and the virus made me a bit reflective on my own mortality. I've always hated looking at myself, really looking but this thing has made me think very differently about who we all are.

Diarist 3944 (female, 30s, London, event producer)

My husband clocks on to Netflix to watch a couple of episodes of Friends. When lockdown began, we decided to rewatch the whole series from the start. It's been very comforting, watching a programme we know so well.

Diarist 4001 (female, 40s, South East England, psychologist)

It has been 7 weeks since I have met up with anyone from outside our household and if I think too much about it then I feel as if I'm falling off a cliff, so I try to keep myself busy, literally at times by finding jobs to do around the house or garden, trying to work on some project or other to take my mind off what we've lost and what the future might possibly hold.

Diarist 4125 (male, 20s, North West England, music teacher)

I need to clean the kitchen. Actually I need to clean the entire house. I think I'd expected to do a lot of spring cleaning in quarantine and if anything I've done *less* than normal, which was already not very much. It's a little hard to feel motivated, what with… everything.

Diarist 4447 (female, 50s, London, art psychotherapist)

For the last week I have been doing a daily challenge on Facebook: 'to share MY LIFE for one week (take a new photo each day) no words, just pictures'. Each day I am meant to challenge someone else to do the exercise. These requests for people to share favourite album covers, book covers, movies etc. have become popular during the lockdown among social media 'friends' [. . .] I decided to add a twist to my interpretation as I have been using this quiet time to really concentrate on a new oil painting practice. So for a week I have been painting a new picture in oils each day that communicates some different aspects of my life [Figure 3] and then posting a photograph of the daily paintings on Facebook [. . .] I also posted the images on Instagram [. . .] I feel as if I have to an extent 'come out' as a painter during this pandemic and this feels liberating.

Diarist 4610 (female, 30s, South East England, maternity nurse)

On the way out of the house [wife] discovered a parcel in the porch (the number of home deliveries recently has been quite mad. Everything we need we have to buy online so there are deliveries being left in our porch every day, sometimes several times a day). She

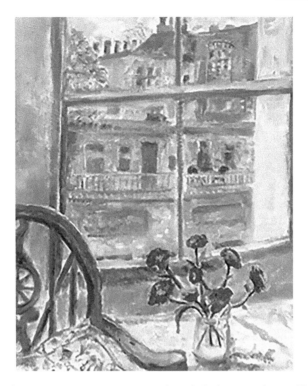

Figure 3 'I have been painting a new picture in oils each day.' Image submitted by Diarist 4447.

was curious as she hadn't ordered anything so she opened it immediately. It was a set of acrylic paints, brushes, a sponge and a mini trowel spreader. She hadn't ordered it, but instinctively knew it was sent by her dad. We've got a lockdown family art challenge with [wife's] side of the family – every week there is a theme and we all submit a piece of art via WhatsApp. Her dad is going to turn them all into a book at the end.

Diarist 4756 (female, 40s, Yorkshire and Humber, academic)

I'm getting sick of hearing about people starting new crafts, learning new languages and baking from dawn to dusk: I'm busier than ever, work is more challenging than before and doesn't show any sign of becoming easier, and [then there is] home schooling.

LUCK

Diarists wrote about their own lives but were keen to situate those lives for readers, to observe themselves and others, to record a range of experiences, in the tradition of Mass Observation. Many wrote about how they were lucky, fortunate, blessed, privileged – compared to others they knew or knew of via news and social media. What counted as lucky varied between diarists. Some felt lucky to have large houses, gardens, plenty of space, locations in the countryside. Others felt lucky to have their nice flat in the city they love. Some felt lucky to have company during lockdown. Others felt lucky to be locked down alone, without other people to deal with, and without responsibilities for others. Some felt lucky to have jobs they could do safely from home. Others felt lucky to be key workers, allowed to leave home for work and feel the camaraderie of face-to-face work situations. Many diarists felt lucky to be healthy and financially secure, with a roof over their head and food on the table. They acknowledged the difficulties faced by some during the pandemic, living with illness or poverty, in cramped conditions, perhaps with abusive partners. They wrote of people 'worse off' than me. They also noted how life in lockdown was hard for them in absolute terms – being separated from family and friends – despite their relative privilege. It is worth noting too how not a single diarist wrote of having good health, or a nice house, or financial security, or a supportive family because they had worked hard and deserved it. And no diarist wrote about undeserving people in difficult situations of their own making. 'I'm lucky to have . . .' is clearly a common, acceptable way that British people – especially middle-class British people – talk about themselves, but it is worth asking why this is and what it reveals about popular understandings of inequality and fairness and their political potential. See also Gratitude; Key workers.

Diarist 34 (female, 60s, North East England, retired teacher)

During the lock down I have been more fortunate than many, with a large house and garden. I am on my own and it is lonely at times, but I have kept in touch with friends and family over the last weeks. I have really felt for friends who have new grandchildren they have never held and for parents who can't ask for help with a new baby.

Diarist 99 (female, 50s, East of England, secretarial assistant)

I consider myself very lucky as I have kept healthy and had the benefit of going to work daily. This has meant I've been able to share my worries with other people and we've been able to support each other when we have had our down days.

Diarist 119 (male, 60s, South West England, retired teacher)

We are conscious of how fortunate we are to live in a beautiful part of the country with a large garden and miles of open space to exercise in from our front door. The contrast with the experience of, for instance, a wonderful father shown on the local news who lives on the 15th floor of a tower block in Bristol with his two sons is starkly poignant [. . .] The lockdown has provided us with the longest uninterrupted period together throughout our marriage, this has confirmed how lucky I have been to be married to such a wonderful person. I am only too aware that our fortune is not shared by everyone and that the incidence of domestic violence has risen steeply during the lockdown and that experiencing lockdown with an abusive partner or alone has for many been a very different and painful experience.

Diarist 139 (female, 15, West Midlands)

I'm lucky to live in [my village], surrounded by fields and countryside to walk through. Many aren't so lucky at this time, living in flats in cities with no outdoor space.

Diarist 250 (male, 30s, Yorkshire and Humber, researcher)

It's a beautiful sunny morning, and the light is catching the trees at the bottom of our garden and spilling in through the kitchen window. I feel lucky, as I have every day since the lockdown began, that we live in a house that has plenty of light, a garden where I can sit and read, and plenty of woodland nearby where I can walk [. . .] The lockdown has been easy for us, really – we have plenty of space, both still working, able to stay on good terms despite the confinement. I feel guilty about that too. My work often takes me into the lives of people who are experiencing severe poverty, but even so I've never been more aware of the privileges I have than now.

Diarist 522 (male, 40s, North East England, lecturer)

We are among the lucky few who are able to continue working through the lockdown, who are financially secure, and can look after themselves without further assistance. I am painfully aware that this is not the case for millions of others.

Diarist 530 (female, 20s, London, social media manager)

All in all, lockdown hasn't been too hard. I am very lucky to live in a stable location, in a safe and comfortable home with a lot of nature on my doorstep. My family has so far largely been unaffected [. . .] On a personal level my biggest challenge has been that my husband is in South Africa, and I haven't seen him since the end of February, so 2 and a half months now, with no idea of when we will be reunited. I am truly thankful for video chatting, but it will never replace physically being there.

Diarist 591 (female, 40s, Scotland, molecular biologist)

I am very conscious that my immediate family is coming at the current situation with a certain amount of luck and privilege. We live in a house that is big enough for all of us to have our own space when we need it, and a garden. We can walk from the house to lovely countryside. We have enough money and our jobs are not in danger at the moment. I feel for those with difficult family situations, lost jobs and who live in small flats. We have signed up to be on a list of community volunteers to offer help to any who need it but haven't been called on yet. We do the food shopping for our neighbour who is shielding with her husband who has severe dementia.

Diarist 622 (female, 40s, Scotland, sociologist)

Home and the space you inhabit has become so important. I feel so lucky to have a home all to myself and to not have to deal with the tensions that seem to be building in other households.

Diarist 884 (female, 50s, London, psychotherapist)

So far I have been lucky, no one close to me has been ill, I have enough money and I have work . . . I have a small flat and it's lovely, though I'd swap it for some modern glass minimal creation with a roof deck . . . so I am grateful and have donated money to various charities to help people, to combat my helplessness in the face of this.

Diarist 916 (female, 60s, South East England, retired teacher)

There has been a lot of talk about the difficulties faced by people in this lockdown. I have to say that, for me, it has not been too bad. I am blessed with a house, a garden, woods nearby to walk in, milk and other food deliveries from local suppliers – and being retired, I don't have to worry about losing my job.

Diarist 938 (female, 60s, Yorkshire and Humber, retired psychotherapist)

I and [wife] are in a privileged position, with adequate finance, space to live, and good health. It is such a strange time, as we know so much tragedy and trauma is going on all round us.

Diarist 1137 (female, 40s, Yorkshire and Humber, psychologist)

I know we are lucky. We have the space to be together when we want to, and apart when we don't, and both my husband and I have jobs we can do at home. We're healthy and well. I know that there are people so much worse off than us. But it doesn't feel easy.

Diarist 1248 (female, 20s, East Midlands, student support administrator)

It's almost time for bed, although I haven't been keeping consistent hours on this score. I feel very lucky that I'm able to work and get paid, not have any children or childcare duties, or have any major responsibility. I just work every day and do as I please in the evenings. It gets a bit lonely at times but the quizzes and whatnot are very helpful in curbing that problem.

That said, I cannot WAIT for all this to be over.

Diarist 1342 (female, 30s, North West England, actor and teacher)

It has been a slightly challenging day, with lockdown continuing and no guarantees of when we may get back to work but I feel lucky that I have all I need during this lockdown, some outside space and the beach at the end of the road.

Diarist 1352 (female, 50s, East of England, publican)

No telephone ringing, no hustle and bustle or voices raised in eagerness, no car doors or engine noises, live music extinguished, doors motionless in their frames, floorboards not creaking, how long since I heard the accidental smash of a glass ('HEADS!'). I clean the gents' floor.

I pour a small beer and take my dog out to the large pub garden. I sit on the trunk of our walnut tree, recently felled, oozing fermenting sap. And I am lucky because I am here, with a garden, a beer, freezers full of homemade meals and space in my house. The pub is dead! Long live the pub!

Diarist 1364 (female, 60s, East of England, solicitor)

We are ten – eleven? – weeks into lockdown. We (my husband and I) are blessed to have a lovely home with a garden and no money worries, though our needs are relatively modest. But it has been and is hard to be separated from our children, grandson and the rest of our family and friends.

Diarist 1490 (female, 50s, Yorkshire and Humber, nurse)

I am lucky compared to [husband] because I go to work so have face to face contact with colleagues there. But it must be odd for him and everyone else who has been in lockdown not allowed to see anyone they know in person.

Diarist 1751 (female, 30s, South West England, finance manager)

I set up the dining room for home schooling and get started at 9am with the kids [. . .] I think how lucky we are to have laptops, access to the Internet and a big dining room table to spread out on. Trying to focus on positives.

Diarist 2037 (female, 20s, East of England, PhD student)

I feel very lucky that during this pandemic we have not experienced any financial or health issues. We both continue to work and have not been furloughed (even though my fiancé wishes he had been so then he could play more video games!), so we continue to live reasonably normally, just at home.

Diarist 2044 (female, 30s, London, sociologist)

I feel weirdly calm about coronavirus right now because I can just work from home and read and write and live quite a small life which is relaxing. That is privilege.

Diarist 2290 (female, 30s, Scotland, historian)

We are very lucky to live in a tenement flat with a sunny, well-kept communal back garden, so there is a space for my son to run around, but he is asking to go out less and less.

Diarist 2386 (female, 60s, Scotland, coach and charity director)

I remind myself how lucky I am – not living alone, a lovely spacious and light home, a garden, beautiful walks close by, friends to keep in touch with. Still it feels tough.

Diarist 2390 (male, 60s, South East England, customs officer)

It's all a very uncertain time. However, I'm lucky. I'm healthy, I have an income, a roof over my head and enough to eat [. . .] The evening was closing in and my partner wanted to eat [. . .] I'm lucky to be with her, even more so in this situation. I feel for those who are isolated on their own.

Diarist 2394 (male, 50s, South East England, unemployed actor)

This lockdown life is basically my unemployed actor life writ large. Meaning that I feel very prepared for it all, it is all familiar to me – how to manage with limited resources, financially obviously but more significantly socially, how to maintain a healthy life on a tight budget from day to day, how to keep a sense of worth, to stay connected to colleagues and to a larger life, how to live a rich life in the moment while still holding onto a sense of myself as an actor despite having no job and no prospect of a job… so I feel lucky that this is not as disconcerting for me as for many many other people.

Diarist 2519 (male, 60s, East of England, retired teacher)

I consider myself lucky; although I have no garden, I have a large flat all to myself. Some large families must be very cramped.

Diarist 2723 (female, 50s, East Midlands, unemployed journalist)

I potter around in the kitchen, clearing up and then both of us sit down to watch the 10 o'clock news [. . .] But it brings the mood down and makes us feel tense. So many people are suffering [. . .] Economically, there are dire warnings of recession. And you can see why. To be honest, we went to bed feeling very fearful of the future [. . .] It's so worrying, it's almost laughable. But we have lots of compensations. None of us are ill, we live in a comfortable house, our children are surviving ok, we can afford food and we have some beautiful countryside around us. And we are not alone in the house, we have each other. That really is, to my mind, the greatest blessing.

Diarist 2891 (female, 20s, East Midlands, teacher)

What's next thoughts are mainly what goes through my head at some point in the day, every day of lockdown. When will this be over? How many more people will die? Will my baby be born in a pandemic? How long till I can let my baby meet his/her grandparents? When will my husband be called back to work? Will he be made redundant at the end of his contract? Then what?

146

Resolving to 'wait and see' is all I can do at the end of each day. I try and relax with yoga and a bath and sometimes this works really well and I feel so lucky to have such a cosy home, with a loving husband who always makes me laugh, a daft rescue dog curled up at my feet and a baby squirming around in my belly. So I haven't been out of the house in 8 weeks? At least we are all safe and well, fed and warm! If only it was the same for everyone else out there.

Diarist 2993 (female, 60s, South East England, retired GP)

I am very lucky to have a nice house and garden, a husband and dog and a pension. I really feel for people stuck in small flats trying to work from home and home school children at the same time.

Diarist 4479 (male, 70s, North East England, retired town planner)

[Friend] called me on FaceTime so we could chat over a cup of tea & catch up on how we are. That is always lovely, & much better than phone calls – we feel closer.

I'm lucky to have finances to afford modern technology & be able to use a smart phone & my iPad. Those without internet access, financial resources and ability to use such technology are really disadvantaged in the current situation. They cannot access online shopping or keep in touch with friends in as many different ways.

Diarist 4766 (female, 60s, East of England, family support specialist)

I've started going on an early morning walk in the local forest. I consider myself to be incredibly lucky because not only do I have a large garden, but within minutes I can access an amazing forest. I am aware that so many people are living in flats with no garden access, perhaps experiencing a job loss and huge financial concerns. Life can be unfair for so many hardworking people [. . .] Apart from physical distancing and not being able to participate in my usual activities, meet family and friends etc. I am living a fulfilling and contented life during the lock down. I also have the luxury of living in a very nice area with a kind and supportive husband. My aim is to make the best of the situation, but, I'm lucky as I have not experienced the death of someone close or work on the front line. I don't live in a violent and over-crowded household. Perhaps, then, my response to Covid-19 might be very different.

(NEW) NORMAL

The diarists were aware they were meant to describe everyday life for Mass Observation, but also that everyday life in the pandemic was not 'normal'. They wrote about how it was different from everyday life before the pandemic. They wrote of a 'new normal'. This could mean a number of things. It could mean the new routine followed by diarists in lockdown: getting up later, making Zoom calls, shopping online, going for daily walks and so on. It could mean the way of life developed in response to Covid-19 – locked down, socially distanced, anxious, fearful – which some expected to last for a long time, with no treatments or vaccines on the horizon. Or it could mean the way of life to come after the pandemic, once it had finally ended, which would be different to how things had been before – either because some things would not survive the pandemic (e.g. certain sectors of the economy) or because, having realized things could be different, a conscious effort would be made to develop an alternative future (less environmentally destructive, less unequal, and, at the micro level, less hectic, frantic, stressful). Of course, there were diarists who just wished for a return to how life had been before – to seeing family and friends, going to work, going to the pub, going on holiday. But they were the lucky ones. For some diarists, life before Covid-19 had not been great. Some people had felt isolated and lonely before any lockdown was imposed on them. Some people with disabilities had relied on deliveries and videoconferencing software before the pandemic, and they had benefited from the way the world had been reconfigured around them – had been made more accessible for them – during lockdown. For others, including those grieving loved ones lost to the virus, and the many thousands now suffering 'long Covid', it was unclear whether life would ever return to some prior normality. See also Birdsong; Cancellations; Hope; Stay home; Working from home.

Diarist 223 (female, 80s, East of England, retired medical secretary)

I look forward to the time when I can join in with the WI [Women's Institute] activities and holidays, long walks with the group I belong to and of course having my family around me [. . .] We must look forward and for me my holiday [. . .] postponed on 13th April 2020 has now been booked for 26th July 2021. Hopefully by that time a vaccine will be available and life will have returned to some normality!

Diarist 401 (female, 50s, Wales, manager of support line)

I have experienced the emotional rollercoaster that has affected almost everyone I know, with some serious bouts of stress and anxiety – counteracted by alcohol and chocolate, and some spontaneous weeping – now all firmly back under control, as I am now more immersed and better adjusted to the new 'normal' imposed by the restrictions on movement and physical proximity to people and things.

So, today, I woke up 715 after an undisturbed sleep.

Diarist 622 (female, 40s, Scotland, sociologist)

I have thought much about loneliness in light of COVID-19, where others are separated from each other and unable to participate in social life in normal ways. This is how I feel all the time! It is amazing how much of the world has suddenly opened up; that this was always possible so long as most people value these connections and make participation possible. I have felt able to participate in aspects of life that have felt blocked off to me for a very long time. I worry that things will revert back and it will all disappear when, or if, we go back to 'normal'.

Diarist 698 (female, 16, North East England)

I think that the most important thing I have learned during these unprecedented times is that we cannot go back to the world we had before. The canals in Venice are clear and clean for the first time in decades! There are fish swimming through them! Pollution is at an all time low and I am scared that when we are finally told that life is back to normal, all this environmental progress will be lost.

Diarist 884 (female, 50s, London, psychotherapist)

I long for normality . . . to see my friends in person, get a train to the countryside, plan a holiday . . . sit with my clients face to face…

Diarist 1088 (female, 40s, London, doctor)

For the past 7 weeks I had not travelled beyond the car park at the end of my road. Yet it feels comfortable and quite liberating to take a huge pause from the frantic pace of 'normal' life. I know I am not unusual in my view; everywhere I hear of people describe being able to hear birdsong now the traffic has lessened and enjoying views that had been obscured by pollution.

Diarist 1310 (female, 30s, South East England, business developer)

Life for me has been a series of lurching from one crisis to another and the one good thing about the Coronavirus crisis is that my life is relatively calm for once. I'm enjoying my own company [. . .] I'm enjoying my house and my garden and just relishing the simple things in life.

I'm not sure I'm ready for the world to get back to normal anytime soon.

Diarist 1346 (female, 60s, Scotland, retired doctor)

I think a lot about the virus that has called a full stop on life as we know it globally [. . .] Most of all I fear that after all this we will return to our relentless destruction of the planet and all this special time we have been given to reflect and live with so much less impact on the planet – will be in vain.

But I know many people are reflecting and I see the innovative ways some people are adapting their lives and businesses, I sense the clean air and loudness of birdsong. I am not too unhappy with this simpler life. I just hope we do not return to the old 'normal'.

Diarist 1423 (male, 30s, London, auditor)

Coronavirus has destroyed every semblance of normalcy here, with the notion of office work, and of frequent travel, seemingly smashed to pieces. The upshot of this is that locality now matters like never before. Having local groups to support one another, local businesses you can visit and rely on for goods [. . .] and finding more creative ways to connect and socialise. This is likely the new norm. I can't see commuting being standard at the end of this, which might reduce travel but also reduces stress of commuting and crowded bloody trains. I also think that it will mean we are now much better equipped for the greatest challenge facing us, climate change. This now has shown that there are ways to massively reduce greenhouse gas emissions and pollution, in a way I think before COVID we all thought was 'too big a sacrifice' and we felt we couldn't make the changes ourselves to make a sustainable go of it. This has shattered that perception. Flights for business should basically not be a thing anymore, neither should car journeys to client meetings. The fact that this has dented the issue and shown a brighter way forward gives me tremendous hope for the future.

Diarist 1428 (non-binary, 20s, North West England, fundraiser and consultant)

I can't wait for everything to go back to normal, but I also want a better normal than what we had before. Everyone deserves better than a world that is crippled by inequality and capitalist greed and environmental crisis. Everyone deserves a world where their needs are met and where their loved ones are safe and where they are accepted for who they are.

Diarist 1581 (male, 60s, London, office administrator)

This morning I woke at my normal time, 06.00am and followed my normal routine of a few simple exercises to help mobility, shower and breakfast. I think it is important to have as normal a schedule as possible, or I will find it very hard to return to work.

Diarist 1691 (female, 20s, South East England, online shopper)

During this very uncertain time it does make you reflect on the past and the life that you want back. I miss very normal things like seeing my mates, going to the pub and playing with my [. . .] niece. I hope that my future will be filled of the social contact that we are missing.

Diarist 1751 (female, 30s, South West England, finance manager)

Just after ten we go to bed and read until 11. A simple, uneventful day and tomorrow will be much the same and right now that's something to feel grateful for. Before lockdown, Tuesdays were incredibly hectic with multiple trips to school and after school clubs and evening activities for both me and my husband. I really don't miss that and will try not to go back to that pace of life if and when things return to normal.

Diarist 1874 (female, 40s, South East England, GP)

This episode of our lives has been strange. In many ways I have absolutely loved having my family around me all the time. We are very close and have had some really happy simple family times together. Daily dog walks, sitting in the garden and eating together have been simple but lovely events. The normal rush of school runs, after school clubs, mountains of homework, more clubs at the weekend – this has all vanished and none of us miss it much. We shall certainly think twice about what we add back when life eventually returns to normal.

Diarist 1920 (female, 40s, South West England, recruitment executive)

Very strange times. We so miss seeing friends and family properly. We miss being able to go out to do the things that a few weeks ago seemed so normal – going swimming, tennis lessons on a Saturday morning, going to the pub for a drink.

Diarist 1940 (female, 30s, Scotland, assistant professor)

Things I do not miss: Sports. Crowds. Lots of Traffic. Drunk people on the streets. Networking. Getting up early. People barging into my office with inane questions. Long train journeys.

Diarist 1942 (female, 40s, London, teaching assistant)

Today was a mix of normal activities like going out for a run, cooking meals and browsing Facebook, and activities that I've only done during lockdown such as meeting members of my running group online to discuss training and taking part in a Zoom 'strength and conditioning' class. I'm not too keen on Zoom chat. Actually even the running was a bit non-ordinary – pre-lockdown I'd meet with my running group on a Tuesday for a speed session. Today it was done alone but there were all sorts of people using the track at the same time who would not normally be there, such as children on bikes & scooters & families just having a stroll around.

Diarist 1966 (female, 50s, South East England, administrator)

How many days has it been now? Sometimes it feels like forever. When was life normal? When we went to work, saw friends, travelled and just lived!

Diarist 1979 (female, 60s, South East England, editor and retired nurse)

My biggest fear is that society doesn't learn from this and we return to the self-interested and grabbing lifestyles that were the norm. I am scared that having to close borders will lead to the wrong sort of nationalism, although I no longer feel a desire to leave the walkable space around me. I wonder how I will react when I am expected to resume more distant activities, and when the traffic outside my door starts to queue again.

Diarist 2341 (female, 30s, Wales, librarian)

They keep saying the virus is here to stay and that a vaccine may never come to fruition. There's a lot of talk about a new normal, a brand of normality that revolves around face masks and social distancing, elbow bumps and fear, where hugs are lethal, and whole countries can be locked down in minutes. I keep coming back to the proverb 'this too shall pass'. I hope it does. I really hope it does.

Diarist 2390 (male, 60s, South East England, customs officer)

I'm so looking forward to this terrible situation being over and getting back to a normal life. The older you get, the more precious your time becomes. I'm hoping we can get away on holiday.

Diarist 2425 (female, 50s, Yorkshire and Humber, researcher and editor)

I Skype my mother, as we have been doing every night since this started. She lives half a mile away, and in normal times we would be attending our place of worship together twice a week, sharing a meal at her home or mine after the Sunday services, and going for the occasional walk together in the local woods and parks.

Diarist 2471 (female, 30s, London, unemployed)

It's difficult to see an end to this at the moment. If I had a job I think I would be feeling much more positive about life returning to normal, at some point, but for my industry, even those with jobs are not secure. Even with the government's job retention scheme there will still be redundancies and companies that go into liquidation. Suddenly I'm looking at job adverts based on whether I think it's a 'safe' industry or not – is that a product that people need even during a pandemic? Is that a company which can operate remotely? [. . .] A few weeks back I thought we would look back on these 3-4 months as that strange isolated period in 2020 when the world stopped but I just read something about how the plague came and went for pretty much the whole of Shakespeare's life. Maybe this is the new normal and we just need to get used to it. Are the days of unlimited international travel, hopping on a plane for a hen do in Barcelona or popping to the pub for a few drinks after work gone forever?

Diarist 2637 (female, 60s, East of England, potter)

Shall I go and finish my homemade face masks? No, I am now sitting in the sun for a bit. I never normally sit down in the day but this is the new norm. Soon it will be time for some wine, is it too early? That and chocolate have kept me going. Better watch how much I eat and drink. So instead I start my grass weaving and water the plants. My husband joins me for a drink in the conservatory. The sun is going down nicely.

Diarist 2705 (female, 40s, Yorkshire and Humber, writer)

We began home learning with maths and quickly lost patience with it and with each other. Then we tried to look at some information about electric cars [. . .] We're seeing a resurgence of nature during this period and the pollution has cleared from the skies. It's been wonderful to have the roads clear of cars and there are even rumours that holes in the ozone layer are repairing. Speaking personally, I really don't want to go back to how things were but, at the same time, the economy is struggling and a recession is likely to follow. The government have been bailing people out but even I appreciate that they can't do that forever. But it seems so crazy that they have returned to chopping down woodland to build high speed railways when we've realised how easy it is for many of us to operate remotely.

Diarist 2709 (female, 50s, East of England, pharmacist)

Looking forward we have a week away booked [. . .] for 5 weeks' time with other members of our family including grandparents, which we are looking forward to. However it is looking more likely that we will not be able to go, or at least several people will not be able to join us. The uncertainty of whether we will be able to go is not nice. Other activities planned for the summer – having family to stay [. . .] my son's graduation and celebrating [. . .] birthdays and a [. . .] wedding anniversary in the family, are all on hold or cancelled which is very disappointing. We are hoping that we may be able to resume some sort of normal life in the coming months and visit family and friends again soon. The lockdown is beginning to be released but it looks as if it will take a long time for life to get back to normal for most people.

Diarist 2721 (female, 40s, North West England, clinician)

Work is a series of video calls [. . .] On one of my meetings we talk about how London traffic and tube travel has returned to normal so quickly and how it seems such a shame that we just went back to the same old when we could have seized this rare opportunity to change the way we do things.

Diarist 3150 (female, 50s, West Midlands, unemployed)

On the day the UK went into lockdown, I developed a fever, and over the course of the next week it became obvious I was suffering with Covid-19. My husband, son living at home and one daughter also caught it. As we are all healthy with no underlying medical conditions we had a good chance of surviving, but it was really worrying. At this time you couldn't get a test in the UK unless you were ill enough to be admitted to hospital, but the symptoms, and a link to a confirmed case, made us very sure that we had the virus. The rest of the family recovered within 1-2 weeks, but I didn't.

Evidence is only just emerging that for some people, Covid-19 causes a longer-lasting illness, with multiple relapses and very slow recovery. Today this is the reality of my life. I have now been ill for 7 weeks. I need frequent rest breaks or my breathing starts to deteriorate. I get very tired doing simple things like showering or walking round the house. Some days I struggle to sit upright for long. This diary reflects that – a life very different at the moment from usual, or from what I would have expected.

I woke at 8am [. . .] I stayed in bed for some time, saving my scant energy for later in the day [. . .] I showered (something that I am still finding very tiring) and then went down and had breakfast [. . .] I chatted a bit with my daughter, and helped her set up the Zoom call for her online saxophone lesson. While she was doing that, I came back to my bedroom, already tired although it was only 11am. I rested a bit [. . .] Around 12:00 my daughter came to find me, and I felt I had enough energy then to do some teaching with her [. . .] Since I have been ill I haven't been able to cook or do any household tasks, so the rest of the family have drawn up a rota. It was my daughter's turn to cook today, so I rested outside in the sun while she made lunch [. . .] I still had some energy after lunch so I spent some time preparing lessons for her [. . .] By 3pm however I was feeling very tired. With Covid I find that the first symptom that I am nearing the end of my energy is that I start coughing. If I don't rest then my whole body starts to feel heavy, like it will fall down if I don't lie down. Then I start to have difficulty breathing, getting very breathless even sitting still. The only cure is to go back to bed and rest totally [. . .] After about 20 minutes my breathing was improving, so I stayed in bed and started writing this, and responded to messages on my phone from friends, asking how I am doing. It's hard to keep having to say 'no real change' – I feel like they might think I'm a fraud, that Covid can't really be lasting that long, or I can't really be as ill as I say I am [. . .] The tiredness was starting to overwhelm me again, so I laid down for some more rest. Sometimes I fall asleep during the day, today I just lay still with my eyes closed. Just before 5pm I started to feel well enough to do things again, so still lying down I checked the latest news on my phone [. . .] Around 6pm I went down for our evening meal, cooked by my other daughter [. . .] We chatted for a while, but by 7.45pm I was feeling very tired and breathless so went to my bedroom [. . .] By 9pm I was feeling ill and tired, so I got ready for bed. There was still light in the sky – I would never normally go to bed at this sort of time, and it feels like I'm a child again having to draw the curtains and sleep when it's still light outside. But Covid has reduced me to this, and I don't have the strength to do any more today.

Diarist 3390 (male, 60s, South East England, retired NHS manager)

We had to cancel our planned holiday in the Lake District this month (we should have been there today) and have re-booked for next year. Hopefully this will be over by then, or at least we will be in a new normal. Will traditional local pubs ever re-open as they used to be? Will our local arthouse cinema re-open? When will I feel comfortable in a crowd of strangers, perhaps on a train or at a festival?

Diarist 4001 (female, 40s, South East England, psychologist)

In a strange way Covid 19 has brought us closer together as a family, and it has made me appreciate the small things in life. People always tell you to do that, but with no distractions now, it's finally possible to actually do. And there's a tiny part of me that is actually dreading having to release that pause button, and press play on life again. This morning I should have been driving over an hour to work [. . .] dropping my younger son off at his school on the way, and eventually arriving home around 7pm, shattered, just about making it through the boys' bedtime routine and our dinner before collapsing into bed, just to get up at 6.20am the following morning and do it all again.

Diarist 4125 (male, 20s, North West England, music teacher)

I wonder if, now most of the country is stuck at home, people will have a little more understanding of how it is to be disabled and housebound most of the time? I was leaving my house once a week for groceries *before* lockdown.

Diarist 4269 (female, 20s, South East England, editor)

Overall lockdown has been helpful for me, in that it's enforced a longer period of relative peace and quiet and a slower pace of life [. . .] Overall this period has made me realise how desperately I needed to slow down and how much I need to try to create some more peace and space in my 'normal' life when it resumes.

Diarist 4403 (female, 60s, South West England, community development consultant)

I am doing OK with lockdown [. . .] My life is generally calmer and I have more time to (attempt to) address the items on The List that I never get around to in my normal, overly busy life [. . .] There is a lot of talk about a 'new normal'. I am not so sure about what that will mean; but I know that for me, I want some things in my own life to be different.

PE (PHYSICAL EDUCATION)

In March 2020, children were sent home from school. Many adults started working from home. Gyms, pools and sports clubs were closed. Parkruns were stopped. Many people began living a more sedentary lifestyle. To counter this, to counter the treats people were baking and eating, to fill the time, to still the mind, to get fighting fit for any encounter with the virus, to connect with others in the same household or online, many people began doing some form of exercise. They counted their steps on daily walks. They ran or jogged round their neighbourhood. They lifted food items or books in makeshift garden gyms. They danced around their flats. Or they joined many others in classes on YouTube and other platforms: PE with Joe Wicks (viewed by almost one million people a day, mostly in the UK, in the early days of lockdown); or Yoga with Adriene (viewed by almost two million people a day worldwide in the early days of lockdown). Some people did get fit – the fittest they have been. Some adults enjoyed PE with Joe Wicks, initially aimed at children, more than their kids. For some people, such exercise was the highlight of their day. Others, of course, struggled for motivation, even hated every minute of these lockdown workouts. See also Anxiety; Cancellations; Home schooling; Lockdown projects; Stay home; (dog) Walking; Working from home; Zoom.

Diarist 390 (female, 20s, Yorkshire and Humber, furniture installations coordinator)

Woke up at 8.15 and joined Mum over WhatsApp video chat to do our morning 'Yoga with Adriene'. We have done this every morning for the last 6 weeks. It's wonderful for me to see her face every morning [. . .] After Yoga, met with [friends] on Houseparty for PE with Joe Wicks. We've done this every morning through lockdown and my mental health has definitely benefitted from it!

Diarist 635 (female, 13, North West England)

During the lockdown, I have done so much baking! Like at least twice a week [. . .] After all that baking it's important to do lots of the Joe Wicks workout.

Diarist 697 (female, 11, North East England)

Today I woke up at about six in the morning. The reason for that is that I got a visit from the tooth fairy! I put my hand under my pillow to find £5. I went back to sleep after that to be woken up by my dad saying nearly Joe Wicks time!

Diarist 1149 (female, 60s, Scotland, lecturer)

I'm slightly out of breath as I write this, because as it's raining outside I've just been 'jogging' round our tiny flat, waving two cans of tomatoes above my head [. . .] I've come to realise that physical activity is key to staying sane during the pandemic. If I sit still all day, I become grumpy. Dancing wildly around the sitting room for 10 minutes makes me feel much better, but I'm a bit self-conscious so try to do it when my partner is out or asleep. Having said that, some Friday nights we listen to music instead of watching TV and both dance around the room, and that makes us both happy.

Diarist 1284 (female, 50s, Wales, unemployed)

Went for a 6.5k jog. I aim to do this twice a week as part of my efforts to get fighting fit should I get Covid-19. I also took the dog for a 5000 step walk later, so I'm definitely getting my exercise in [. . .] As part of the health campaign I'm ensuring that the meals I cook for me and my parents are nutritious and varied. We all take Vitamin C and cod liver oil and I take a few more supplements. I've also given up coffee to calm my nerves.

Diarist 1331 (female, 30s, Scotland, restaurant worker)

Today is like every other day that has been since the lockdown. I wake up late (9.30-10am), feed the cat, make a coffee for me and my boyfriend and do some exercise. I am usually on my feet a lot at work – busy 12 hour shifts bustling around a restaurant but I have been aware that I probably am lucky to take 500 steps in a day if I do not make the concerted effort to do some exercise. So this morning I do a live yoga class on Zoom.

Diarist 1366 (male, 20s, South East England, student)

The past few days I have taken up indoor exercises each morning, when my girlfriend started up yoga, although I don't know how long it will last and I hate every second of it.

Diarist 1466 (female, 80s, East of England, retired teacher)

09.30am – Ready to start my usual exercise for the day – fifty-two laps of the garden which is approximately 2.5k. I've been doing this six days a week since week two of self-isolating.

Diarist 1473 (female, 50s, North East England, teacher)

At 8.30am it is soon time for the highlight of my day – 'PE with Joe Wicks' so I get my daughter up. She groans and complains as usual [...] I get really excited and my daughter pretends to be totally underwhelmed as Joe Wicks starts today's workout. He really is my hero! He is so full of energy, naturally funny and really motivating. He works us really hard today as he's increased the work time and reduced the rest time. The effort is worth it as both my daughter and I are getting unbelievably fit now.

 After 'Joe' I take a cold shower and get dressed.

Diarist 1557 (male, 40s, Wales, teacher)

I go straight into a 20 minute run [...] Exercise has been a vital component of my sanity – a 20 minute run every other day and Joe Wicks on the alternate days for 7 weeks now – and I'm probably physically fitter than I have ever been.

Diarist 1580 (female, 50s, Yorkshire and Humber, legal administrative assistant)

In between checking emails my husband and I did 'Joe Wicks' on YouTube – a fitness coach who is providing free ½ hour classes Monday to Friday. [Son] was initially enthusiastic, and now he sits on his tablet while we both do it the best we can.

Diarist 1757 (male, 40s, South East England, director of charity)

I woke at about 07:30 today, having slept quite well. I think my sleep is getting back to normal now after three weeks of worry about losing my job.

 Had a cup of tea and then did my usual quick run up the hill behind the school and along the Downs. Always so nice to get out into the countryside – especially first thing or at dusk when there aren't so many people about. Since we went into lockdown, to help prevent the spread of Covid 19, there are so many more people walking the Downs during the day! My wife also ran – a shorter route – and I caught her up on the main road and waved. My heart still jumps when she smiles at me – after 23 years.

Diarist 1813 (male, 30s, Yorkshire and Humber, researcher)

First, it's yoga. Like thousands of others around the world, I've used lockdown as an opportunity to practice daily yoga routines via 'Yoga with Adriene' on YouTube. Today is the end of my '30 day yoga journey', as she calls it, and I spend 40 mins stretching out my bones.

Diarist 1940 (female, 30s, Scotland, assistant professor)

I've been intending to do a little bit of yoga from a YouTube video each night before bed, however this habit has yet to be fully adopted. I haven't had the energy for it.

Diarist 1966 (female, 50s, South East England, administrator)

10.30 time for online Zumba. For years my great friend has been encouraging me to do it but I have always resisted. But now it is the highlight of my day. Love it. 10.30 am and I am there and ready to exercise. Do it with my daughter who thinks I am hilarious as a [woman in her 50s] dancing away to Beyoncé but it is uplifting and makes me feel good so I will keep on, even after this is over!

Diarist 1991 (female, 20s, East of England, student)

I'm going to go for a bit of a run because I think I need to get my heart rate up! My body has put on weight since lockdown and I'm not as fit as I was. I usually go to the gym once or twice a week, but I think the lack of movement, cycling to work and being on my feet in general is really taking a toll on me.

Diarist 2003 (female, 40s, South East England, housewife and artist/designer)

I worry that we are not getting enough exercise. We've been doing various online workouts and have been riding our bikes when the weather is nice, but the kids have become reluctant to go on walks as they are bored of the local area [. . .] I really miss swimming as we would usually go at least once a week and I just started the gym in January which I was really enjoying. I've tried working out with tins of beans, but it is hard to find the motivation especially when I've been busy all day with the kids.

Diarist 2172 (male, 40s, London, creative consultant)

I used to go to the gym every day. These days my gym is the back garden; weights are two canvas carrybags full of books.

Diarist 2517 (female, 50s, London, unemployed)

Did some exercise. Before lockdown I had begun a new successful exercise regime of going to my local swimming pool for water aerobics and swimming 3 times a week. It really helped with my pain and mobility. It was really good for me. I am devastated that the pools have had to be closed by the government.

Diarist 2627 (female, 40s, Northern Ireland, editor)

I ran, to [nearby town] and back. I stopped to take photos of the sea and sky to post on Instagram for a friend whose true love of nearly 40 years died with cancer and Covid-19 in the week before last [...] I'm so glad I can still run. I've been a long way, on the ground and in my head in the last 10 years, but still have – hope to have – many more miles to go. I miss the parkruns that saved my life [...] and made home a much better place to be. I worry about the people who stopped walking, jogging and running when parkrun stopped and an important connection with other people dropped away.

Diarist 3573 (female, 60s, East of England, humanist celebrant)

[Housemate] and I had our usual Badminton session, in the garden. We normally play in a local school hall, on Monday evenings, which we really miss [...] We have a ladder laid on the ground as a (very low) net and some dubious adaptations of the rules. We play five games, tallying wins with dry leaves slotted into the panels on the back gate.

Diarist 4127 (female, 20s, London, sex worker)

9am – got out of bed to get laptop, booked into online yoga class
    9:30am – failed to get ready for yoga and instead just spaced out on social media for some time

SHIELDING

In the first months of the pandemic, the UK Government identified those 'clinically extremely vulnerable' and at high risk of severe illness from Covid-19 – roughly two million people in total – and sent them letters advising them to 'shield' at home until further notice. It also advised those 'clinically vulnerable', including anyone over the age of seventy, to stay home and apart from other people as much as possible. It also advised care homes to isolate residents from visitors, though many care homes had already closed their doors to visitors before receiving this advice (sent April 2020). How did those categorized as 'vulnerable' and those close to them respond to such advice? Some, fearful of the virus and wishing to be a good citizen, or wishing to be a good partner or parent to loved ones fearful on their behalf, followed the advice to the letter. This was not easy. It required other household members to practise especially strict hygiene routines and to stay home and apart from others as much as possible. It made those categorized as vulnerable dependent on others – family, friends, neighbours – when previously they had been proudly independent. It made them dependent on infrastructure too, such as supermarket delivery systems, which worked for some – when their status as vulnerable secured them priority status for limited delivery slots – but not all. Isolation was tough, physically and mentally. People faced difficulties coming to terms with their own vulnerability. Advised to isolate, for longer and to a greater degree than others around them, people could feel outcast, forgotten, trapped. Because of these challenges, some people categorized as vulnerable interpreted the advice more loosely. They sought to balance the health risks of Covid-19 against the health risks of isolation. They took walks or went shopping, choosing quieter times to do so. Some felt guilty as they did this. Rather than guilt, some felt patronized by their categorization as vulnerable, against which they pushed back, arguing they were fitter than many people under seventy, for example, and that advice for the over seventies was ageist. See also Deliveries; Fear; Guilt; Shops; Stay alert; Stay apart; Stay home; (dog) Walking.

Diarist 46 (female, 40s, East of England, teacher)

It is 8 weeks since I left my house. I am following government guidance issued to protect people during the Corona Virus pandemic. The guidance states that people with some underlying health conditions, like the leukaemia I suffer from, are at risk of severe illness if I become infected with the virus and therefore, I am 'shielding' to protect myself.

This is stressful for me and places a lot of challenges on my family as well. My wife runs a nursery for pre-school children and has remained open throughout the pandemic to support key workers being able to stay at work – she has to follow a strict hygiene routine when she returns home to reduce the risk of infection, as does my [. . .] son who works as a delivery driver.

Diarist 401 (female, 50s, Wales, manager of support line)

[Dad] continues to follow shielding advice like most other older relatives and friends I know; unlike my mother who decided early on that her emotional well-being would suffer considerably if she could not get out of the flat, and this was a risk worth taking.

Diarist 404 (female, 60s, South West England, teacher)

I'm shielding until the end of June as my immune system is compromised after chemotherapy.

I woke early on Tuesday to a sunny but cold day. I needed to post a birthday card to my brother [. . .] This was the first time since March 18th that I've left my house to do something other than go to medical appointments. I feel like I'm doing something naughty as I walk up the street to the postbox. I hope no-one sees me. My neighbours have been so kind shopping and generally caring for me that I'd rather not be seen out and about. I see [. . .] the postman looking happy. He says he's enjoying the near empty streets of people and traffic. I get home without being spotted . . . as far as I know.

Diarist 486 (female, 80s, Midlands, retired)

I began to wonder when the osteopath who treats my back regularly would be able to open again, as my back is suffering from no treatment. Phoning her rooms I discovered that she had in fact opened, which left me disappointed she hadn't let me know. She explained that their professional organisation had advised discouraging older patients from coming. This really upset me, as from the outset the government's attitude to the over 70's – all lumped together regardless of general health and fitness, and labelled 'vulnerable' and not to go out at all, even for food – has felt very patronising to me, as if I am a child again and cannot be trusted to make sensible decisions regarding risk. Perhaps this is because they have been so poor at giving us information we can use, and is well meant, however the effect on me, and I know other over 70's, has been to make us feel rebellious rather than sensible! Fortunately my osteopath, knowing me well, agreed to see me the next afternoon, which was a great relief.

Diarist 1580 (female, 50s, Yorkshire and Humber, legal administrative assistant)

8 weeks ago, I was sent home from work due to having high blood pressure and a previous lung problem and as such was classed as being in a 'vulnerable group' by the government.

To be honest, I got home and cried. I did feel like it was the end of the world. Each day after that was just trying to get through this as best as you could.

Diarist 2030 (female, 70s, South West England, retired teacher)

A couple of neighbours have done small amounts of shopping for me, but a couple of times I've found it necessary to venture out to the supermarket to stock up on most things. I don't like to ask others (who should also be self-isolating) to do my shopping on top of their own. After visiting the supermarket at the quietest time, Sunday afternoon just before closing, I still feel anxious that I may have been infected. My children are adamant that I should not go out at all, anywhere, apart from my daily exercise of a quiet walk between the fields behind my house. I do not tell them about my shopping trips.

Diarist 2069 (female, 30s, East Midlands, scientist)

My activity is severely restricted due to my partner being highly vulnerable to the virus. We have been in full isolation since the 10th of March. We disinfect every parcel and every food item that gets delivered, and avoid going out even for daily exercise. We can't risk it [. . .] My partner left for his workshop around 10. I know he is fully isolated there, and he's very careful, but I still worry constantly about his catching the virus, as he really wouldn't stand a chance against it with his health condition [. . .] Other than to take out the rubbish I have only left the house four times since March 10th. Twice to mow the lawn, twice to check and drive my car for twenty minutes to keep it working, since I can't afford to replace it. The weather today was cool and cloudy, which I love. I miss hiking, just being outside.

Diarist 2341 (female, 30s, Wales, librarian)

As someone who is at high risk of contracting the Coronavirus, I qualify for priority delivery slots for groceries. Since in all other respects I feel like a total liability, I am more than happy to help my family where I can by adding things to my online shop [. . .] My sister has been to collect her groceries; she messaged when she was outside, and I took the bags to the end of the garden path. She waited for me to back away to the front door before she approached. It was nice to see her, and she looks well [. . .] I'm not supposed to leave my house at all as a person who is on the shielding list, but I've had to make a judgement call because the condition I have causes my joints to seize, so it's really important that I keep moving. I try to get out for a short walk each day, but I stick to wide open spaces and time the exercise so I'm not likely to meet many people. Mid-afternoon works really well [. . .] My housemate has just left to visit her boyfriend. They made the decision to break the lockdown last week and this is the second time she's gone to stay the night with him. I worry that their actions will increase my risk of catching the virus but at the same time, that makes me feel really selfish.

Diarist 3248 (male, 70s, London, retired engineer)

It was my turn to collect the paper from the local shop at about 09.00. It is lockdown. I am not supposed to go out until June but our delivery service was too unreliable.

Diarist 3524 (male, 70s, Scotland, retired IT specialist)

My morning walk pre-COVID-19 used to encompass a visit to the local Tesco to collect newspapers and other essentials but this is now verboten by elder daughter who insists that I – we – are at risk. She is of course right. So we get the papers delivered now and unbelievably efficient they are too.

Diarist 3647 (female, 60s, East of England, retired teacher)

I dozed until 6, then decided to get up and go for my early-morning walk [. . .] I quickly and quietly got dressed so as not to disturb my husband, had a drink of water and sneaked out of the house. I try to walk most mornings but feel slightly guilty doing so. Having had treatment for breast cancer, which finished just before Covid-19 arrived, I've had letters from the NHS and the government telling me that I'm classed as 'extremely vulnerable' and must stay indoors. Staying in for days on end makes me quite depressed so I decided to walk very early in the morning when there's minimal risk of encountering people. The few people I encounter generally respect the '2 metre rule' and I feel safe. Occasionally a jogger will pass me quite closely and I do wonder how easy it may be to catch the virus from one of them, as they are breathing so heavily. I also wonder if they are leaving a trail of virus-laden air behind and how long it takes to dissipate. Questions I shall never know the answer to. It doesn't stop me going out though; the exercise is great and I love to be out in the weather, wind, rain or shine. I usually say 'good morning' to each person I pass.

Diarist 3808 (female, 70s, North East England, retired school inspector)

5.30am I woke to find that husband [. . .] was already trawling the internet for the latest news on Covid 19. As usual he brought me a cup of tea to accompany a summary of his finds. I am getting used to this rather grim start to each day as we are settling with resignation to the life of self isolation recommended for those over 70. I turn over and snooze [. . .] 1200 noon Lunch – poached egg on toast and a proper read of the paper. There is much comment on the Government plans for easing the lockdown. I can't see it making much difference to [husband] and me – the over 70s are still being urged to be extra vigilant. Some people believe that singling out the old folk for especially punitive lockdown measures is 'ageist' – they claim that many older people are far fitter than some younger ones. I don't see it like that. It doesn't matter how fit someone is, it is a scientific certainty that as we age our immune system becomes less effective and statistics show that the vast majority of deaths due to Covid19 are in the 70+ age range. Whilst it has taken me some time to come to terms with the notion of being classified as 'old and vulnerable' I welcome the attention given to my protection, however difficult that proves.

Diarist 4054 (female, 70s, North West England, retired teacher)

In [. . .] 2018, my husband suffered a severe stroke which left him disabled and since then he has had to live in a nursing home. I have not been able to visit him for over 2 months which is hard for both of us [. . .] I used to see him and talk to him every day and spend most of my mealtimes with him. Since then I have only been able to speak on the phone, or an occasional FaceTime, except on his [. . .] birthday when they wheeled him out into the garden in the pouring rain so we could give him his cards and sing Happy Birthday. The staff made him a cake and did their best to make it a celebration.

The last few weeks have been worse than ever as the virus has reached the home. Several key staff are off sick and no doubt the residents will get it. All residents are being isolated in their rooms. The only good thing is that [husband's] room is on the ground floor at the front of the building so by climbing up a steep grassy bank and squeezing myself into a bush I can see him through the window. Sometimes if staff come into the room they will open the window a crack and I can shout to him through the gap. Today was one of the bad days. I stood outside the window for about 20 minutes and no one appeared. He was sitting in his special wheelchair and I could tell that he was in pain [. . .] He has not been able to have his essential physiotherapy since the lockdown began, and his leg is bent and stiff. I banged on the window and he saw me and waved and gestured to me to come in, but I had to gesture that I could not come in, although I longed to be with him. He had not had his lunch though it was past the dinner hour. I felt so helpless just waving through the window so I went away and walked to the beach.

It was a fine day with a strong, cold wind. The distant sea had white horses on it. I walked along the grass covered path by the beach and then down onto a sandy track. There were skylarks singing and swooping from sky to earth. It was very peaceful there with no other walkers on the lower path. I was enjoying the fresh air and the beauty of the world and the exercise but I was crying inside for my beloved [. . .] Of all the horrible things about the corona virus the way people are cut off from the people they love when they need them most is the cruellest.

Diarist 4149 (male, 80s, South East England, retired lecturer)

I have chronic heart and lung diseases and am on the government's list of the especially vulnerable to Covid-19 infection: supposed to be confined to the house and garden.

Partly overcome the restriction by going for walks just after dawn, which seems safe enough. There's the general problem of weighing up the pros and cons – I could easily die any day without the help of Covid-19.

Diarist 4217 (male, 70s, South West England, retired IT worker)

We are both coping well with the isolation but that's not to say that we're content with the current life style. Naturally there are things we long for – to have proper contact with our family rather than rely on electronic communication (yes – Skype is preferable to simple phone calls, but . . .), to resume social contact with our neighbours rather than hold whatever conversation you can reasonably conduct at two metres' separation, or to leave the grounds and head for a break in another part of the country (overseas holidays seem but a distant prospect). I have greatly missed watching [local football club] who were pushing strongly for promotion [. . .] when the season was suspended, and I am very sad that the [local cricket festival], due to begin in late June, surely cannot now take place. Furthermore, we have found having to rely on online shopping for food supplies frustrating and extremely tedious, rarely able to get all we want or even a slot for delivery. The weekly food shopping was never my favourite moment of the week, so surprisingly I am strangely longing for the day when I will again be able to go to a supermarket, find the shelves fully stocked and walk around at leisure choosing what I want rather than having to settle for what the online shops are prepared to offer.

Tomorrow, lockdown restrictions will be eased [. . .] But those like us who are defined as highly vulnerable must remain under lockdown, conceivably for many more months. The last seven weeks have been frustrating but tolerable while restrictions have applied across the board but as the majority gain their greater freedoms progressively over the next months, isolation for us will become harder and harder to take. Just when will it end?

Diarist 4479 (male, 70s, North East England, retired town planner)

I received an NHS letter dated 27th March stating that I should not leave my house because I am extremely vulnerable if I get COVID 19. I am being 'shielded' (i.e. advised not to leave my home for 12 weeks) because of Bronchiectasis, which has been well controlled for many years. I am otherwise a slim, fit active man with no other underlying health conditions, a non smoker, rare drinker & eat a healthy diet. I rarely use my car and stay fit by walking locally [. . .] I acknowledge that my bronchiectasis places me at high risk of serious illness if I contract the virus, but I cannot stay locked in the house without risking my physical health and mental wellbeing. I choose to walk briskly along in my quiet neighbourhood for an hour most days. I don't want to rely on my close friend [. . .] for my shopping any more than necessary, in order to minimise her risks from infection. I have managed to 'click and collect' groceries from local supermarkets for the last two weeks [. . .] I feel that the Government's partial relaxation of the lockdown measures [see Stay Alert] are making me feel trapped as a 'shielded' person. I'm concerned about the long term physical & mental health consequences on myself and others [. . .] 2.30. I started my walk around the local area & did 2.5 miles by my return at 3.30. I'm not supposed to leave my house – being a 'shielded' person – but it's a matter to me of balancing risks and benefits. I'd go crazy if I couldn't get out every day or two. I'm not ready for daytime TV and afternoon naps.

SHOPS

People stayed home and got deliveries if they could. But if they couldn't get a delivery slot, or if they decided to leave the available delivery slots for those more vulnerable than themselves, people went to the shops. They did this as infrequently as possible, using up food in cupboards and freezers first, and only after carefully making a list of items needed. A few people enjoyed visiting the shops. It was an excuse to get out of the house, something different to do, the highlight of their week. But most people shopped reluctantly. It was the most risky activity they did. They 'braved' the shops on behalf of higher risk family, friends and neighbours. They found shopping stressful. The atmosphere was tense, anxious, fearful. They chose what they thought would be quiet shops and times of day. They noticed the closed shops on the High Street and wondered if they would ever reopen. And they noticed all the new rules, guidelines, etiquette and rituals of supermarket shopping in a pandemic. Only a certain number of people were allowed in shops at the same time. Others had to queue outside. Some people wore gloves and face coverings. They sanitized their trolleys. Shops had one-way systems, indicated by arrows on the floor. Markings on the floor also encouraged people to keep 2 metres apart, as did signs and announcements over the PA system. Signs and announcements also encouraged people to keep moving – to avoid leisurely browsing. Shelves were generally well stocked by 12 May, after an initial period of panic-buying in March and early April, but some high-demand items were still rationed by some shops. Checkout assistants were protected behind Perspex screens. Payment was by contactless methods. On leaving shops, people sanitized their hands. On returning home, they sanitized individual purchases before putting them away. Then they washed their hands and sometimes their clothes too. See also Anxiety; Deliveries; Fear; Key workers; Stay apart.

Diarist 284 (female, 50s, East of England, retired nurse)

I got up at 8.45am and walked to the local newsagents [. . .] where one person is allowed in the shop at any one time. I paid my weekly newspaper bill, my parents' bill [. . .] and left a neighbour's newspapers voucher. The owner told me it was her mother's funeral that afternoon, only 10 people were attending, it was at the local crematorium and no wake. I was relieved to hear she had not died of coronavirus.

I walked down the High Street and went into the Butcher's on the market square [. . .] where 2 people are allowed at any one time. I bought sausages, eggs and a sausage roll.

I then walked to Boots the Chemist, where 5 people are allowed in at any one time. I had not been to Boots for 7 weeks. I bought a bandage, ibuprofen gel and tablets, hand gel, liquid soap and 2 pairs of cotton gloves [. . .] I then went home, where I unloaded my purchases, thoroughly washed my hands and cleaned the tops in the kitchen where the bags had been placed.

I do not like going to the shops and since lock down rarely go out.

Diarist 286 (female, 60s, Scotland, retired building society cashier)

I had my daily allowed walk, taking in the two beaches near our home [. . .] This walk also took me along the High Street. I got straight in at the Post Office for stamps (2 people only in the shop at any one time, and the assistants behind Perspex screens) but had to queue a while to be allowed into the chemist, where they have reduced their opening hours, and only let customers in one at a time. You have to knock on the door and wait for someone to come and unlock it and let you in. Again, a one-way system round the shop, and Perspex screens at the till. I paid by credit card (wearing gloves) at both places, to avoid handling cash.

Diarist 401 (female, 50s, Wales, manager of support line)

Forwarded weekly shopping list to daughter . . . supermarket shopping very stressful now . . . happy to abdicate responsibility and pass on; she finds it welcome respite from confinement to house with 2 little ones.

Diarist 414 (male, 60s, South West England, retired teacher)

Went to Lidl to buy some provisions. We chose Lidl, rather than Tesco which we also use, because we get impatient with the one-way system and fussing at Tesco in these times of plague.

Diarist 470 (female, 50s, East Midlands, child psychiatrist)

I have a daily walk – today through the park to Sainsbury's. I join a 'socially distanced' queue to be let into the shop. Announcements remind customers to stay 2m apart and use the automated checkouts. It's more relaxed than it was a few weeks ago when shopping was tense, with empty shelves [. . .] Supplies are back to normal and you can buy eggs and paracetamol but the baking shelves remain half empty. Furloughed staff and families out of school must be doing a lot of baking.

It's a dull day but there are ducklings in the park which is always cheering, although the swings are closed off to prevent kids getting the virus from surfaces. Lots of people out walking and cycling – many more than usual. On the way home I walk past shops all closed – estate agents and takeaways. Even McDonald's is closed.

Diarist 479 (female, 40s, South West England, clinical pharmacist)

I hate going to the supermarket. It takes so long to get through the shop. I try to distance myself from others but not everyone respects this when shopping. Some wear masks, some wear gloves. I wonder how robust their infection control attempts are. I see them touching their masks: touching everything with their gloves including their phones. I don't cover up. I wash my hands. I try to stay away from others. Some people even wash down their groceries before putting them away. I don't do this. To be honest I can't be bothered. I don't really believe that it reduces your risk of infection by such a significant amount that it is worth the effort.

Diarist 564 (female, 13, Scotland)

I went to the shop today with my Mum [. . .] We arrived at our local store and lined up outside. Usually, we would just walk straight in. There are signs everywhere reminding us of the rules and precautions. 'Always remain 2 metres apart', 'follow the one-way system' and, of course, 'If you have any symptoms, stay at home, protect the NHS, save lives'. Nobody talks to each other. We all stand divided. 2 metres apart. It is a one in, one out system, and everyone waits their turn. We reach the front of the queue, until a man tells us we can go inside.

The shop is unusually normal. Mum has told me that the shelves are usually empty but today they must have just re-stacked the shelves. We are in luck.

It's a one-way system, so Mum and I follow the arrows taped to the floor around the shop, avoiding people. Mum refuses to let me touch anything, so I tuck my hands in my pockets and they don't come out. I can't get over how unreal this is. It feels as if I am in some apocalyptic book. I never believed anything like this would happen to me. I thought where I lived was safe. I was wrong.

Diarist 591 (female, 40s, Scotland, molecular biologist)

We are trying to use up food that is in the freezer so that we reduce the trips we need to make to the supermarket. Some of the food is years old. I make a rather dubious salmon in pastry, which doesn't taste very fresh, but hopefully won't kill anyone.

Diarist 635 (female, 13, North West England)

The shops are quite scary as there isn't always enough food. That's why food shops [. . .] have put rules in place like anyone over 70 can shop between 9-11am Monday, Wednesday, Friday, Sunday. This is so that there is enough food for them. Shops also have tape around the floor as you need to keep two metres away from people. They also clean your trolleys and you can wear gloves. My mum does the shopping and it takes her so much longer than you would think because you can't go very quick and there is a one way system.

Diarist 989 (female, 60s, retired)

Every Tuesday I go shopping for us, my mother and one of our neighbours – if they need anything. I put on my virustastic snood and drive to the nearest small supermarket. Reducing exposure, keeping my mother safe – and my husband – men are more at risk.

Shops here still do not have some of the basics on my visits. It was nearly a month before I saw pasta or rice or tinned tomatoes. Flour is very difficult to get. There is no dried yeast but I have mastered sourdough starter and now make all of our bread when I can get flour. I have been able to get some home deliveries from our local butcher and a market garden and we are growing our own. The back garden is an allotment. We are eating our own salad now. I notice I am very careful with food. There is less waste – even though I was brought up to be frugal by the war generation. The dog is good for recycling odds and ends. Everything seems more precious; food, community, friends and family and most especially our lives.

Diarist 1005 (female, 19, West Midlands, student)

At lunch, I headed down to the shop at the bottom of the hill for milk and stuff for lunch; I made sure to keep my distance from everyone I came across, including heading off the pavement on the narrower parts of the street. Surprisingly, there wasn't a queue for the Co-Op like there usually is these days. I was in and out because I didn't want to risk passing anything on.

Diarist 1035 (female, 30s, East Midlands, manager for manufacturer)

7:05 – Mini shredded wheat for breakfast for the first time. We've avoided the big supermarket since lockdown due to the queues, one-way systems and increased likelihood of infection due to the numbers of people visiting the large store. We have got the majority of what we would usually buy from either our local small convenience store or from online delivery, and have also discovered some excellent local farm shops. However, one thing we haven't been able to get is my normal supermarket own-brand fruit-filled wholewheat cereal.

Diarist 1122 (female, 50s, London, service manager)

I clock off work early because yesterday was such a long day and suggest a car ride and possible shop to my daughter. I try and think of slight variations to each day to gee her up. It is hard to be an only child when you haven't seen your friends for seven weeks. On Saturday we agreed to one of them coming over and sitting by our gate. This seemed to satisfy both of them [. . .] We try one Tesco but turn round in the car park and head for the exit after seeing the queue. These masked queues are the bleakest aspect of daily Corona life for me; I don't want to be in them if I don't have to. We find a Morrisons and hey presto, no queue – just a helpful youth who sprays our trolley before we go in! We are over excited and buy far too much. I regret this when I get home and have to wipe down £100 worth of groceries. I have no idea if sponging down my Shreddies packet is necessary but having started this ritual a few weeks ago I feel I can't abandon it now or this will be our undoing.

Diarist 1153 (male, 20s, South East England, student)

I went on my weekly grocery run to Waitrose. I felt sad or disturbed in some way as I left the shop. People are very tense in the supermarkets and I think I often leave the shop with that feeling having permeated (not to say infected) me.

Diarist 1235 (female, 40s, Yorkshire and Humber, tutor and carer)

Between us, we had fish fingers, beef burgers, chips, beans and veg for dinner. Our meals are a bit haphazard at the minute, we do a lot of 'using up', combining foods that we wouldn't normally – it's because we are trying not to waste food at the minute. It's not really because of money, we are just trying to avoid going to the shops.

Diarist 1287 (female, 60s, London, retired teacher)

This morning I woke up later than usual, at eight thirty, and we were in Tesco Express soon after nine. I read a newspaper report that said this time, on a Tuesday, is the quietest time to shop, and it's proved to be true for us over a couple of weeks. We dressed up in our masks, and I also wore disposable rubber gloves. We took four bags-for-life to fill with enough main meals for a week [. . .] The bill came to £59.15. Because it was over £30 I had to tap the pin into the machine, which made me nervous [. . .] The supermarket floor was marked into two metre squares, with a one-way system, and there was a three in three out rule. The manager enforces the circulation when required. The cashiers wore gloves and worked from behind a screen. Floor staff were working stoically, filling the shelves. Most of them are young Asian men, but there's one white-haired woman of about my age who sits on a low stool and works without pausing. I imagine they're all vulnerable.

Diarist 1375 (male, 50s, Scotland, consultant engineer)

Lunch [. . .] – quiche and new potatoes. Fairly unusual for us, but it was cheap when my wife did the weekly shop. Up until recently, we were pretty disorganised and tended to shop for food every day. Now we are trying to avoid contact. My wife shops once a week. In theory, I am marginally more vulnerable to the virus (male with mild asthma), so she insists on shopping. Minimising the virus spread has become an exercise in probabilities for us.

Diarist 1473 (female, 50s, North East England, teacher)

Get dressed ready for what has become the highpoint of our week… food shopping [. . .] Under normal circumstances, grocery shopping is mundane and the drive tiresome. However, since 'Lockdown', we only get to see the house, the garden, fields and hills around our house (really I know that I am so lucky to live in such a beautiful place) so it is really exciting for my teenage daughter and I to go to a town and see different things [. . .] When I get to Morrisons' carpark I leave my daughter in the car listening to music and socialising with her friends on Snapchat and Instagram [. . .] The queue for Morrisons (which safeguards 2 metre social distancing) has grown considerably. I wiped down the trolley with an antibacterial floor-wipe that I brought with me and then I am allowed in the shop after waiting for 20 minutes. I am pleased to see that most things that I need are there [. . .] When I get back to the car, I get diesel and my daughter and I get something for lunch from Morrisons' garage. And therein lay one of the biggest treats of the day . . . a Costa coffee machine. Oh! how I miss my visits to Costa for a Cappuccino. You have no idea what little luxuries are important until you can't get them anymore [. . .] We make a quick pitstop on the, almost deserted, high street to pick up some bird food and chocolate rations [. . .] Before returning home, we drive to drop some shopping off at a friend's house who is isolating for medical reasons. It is great to see her, even if it is with her in her doorway and me in the garden, and we can't hug each other. My daughter stays in the car while we chat for a bit and then we drive home – our jaunty outing complete.

Diarist 1494 (female, 20s, South East England, student)

It's now nearly 4pm and I told myself I'd go grocery shopping today [. . .] The first time I went into the centre of town during lockdown I cried a little bit at seeing the streets so empty and devoid of life. I would have been embarrassed but there was literally no one around [. . .] I manage to get almost everything I want in the shops, which is a small miracle. Apart from baking supplies – everyone's been doing so much baking to pass the time you can't even find chocolate chips. I literally ordered flour online the other day. I rip my mask off as I leave the last shop – I hate wearing them, you get so hot and feel so claustrophobic. I also keep forgetting that my warm smiles at the supermarket workers are going unreceived, so I'm making a point to thank them out loud.

Diarist 1547 (female, 30s, East of England, innovation consultant)

It is our weekly shopping day, so [partner] is off to Asda with a list. It always makes me a bit nervous when he does this, although I know he'll take precautions with hand sanitiser and a mask and proper social distancing. He goes out about 8:30pm, which means it is quiet, but that we don't always get everything.

Diarist 1557 (male, 40s, Wales, teacher)

In the afternoon I undertake the weekly household supermarket shop, the only time any of us leave the house and its immediate surroundings. My wife and I have established a careful routine involving me taking latex gloves (mainly to deter my normal habit of constantly touching my face), bags kept separate for shopping trips and wiping down every product with dilute bleach on my return. I go straight into a 20 minute run outdoors and then undress completely into the washing machine and shower when I return [. . .] We are lucky to have a second fridge in a separate room with access from outside to use as a 'dirty' space, from which items will be released for eating over the next 3 days before anything left is considered safe enough to move to our kitchen. No-one in our family could be considered 'high risk' but my wife is very risk averse in general whilst I enjoy the planning, execution and evaluation of the operation. I'm pleased to have reduced the risk by pushing out this visit to 9 days since the last one but the interval since venturing out only heightens the sense of disconnection, even confusion, when I get in the car.

Diarist 1574 (female, 40s, Wales, public health practitioner)

On Tuesdays I do our weekly shop and also shop for my dad [. . .] and some local neighbours in their 90's who can't get to the supermarkets because they are all advised to avoid social contact as much as possible due to the Covid 19 pandemic. I go to the earliest slot I can so that the supermarket is quiet and safer for me. Because I work for the NHS I can go 30 minutes earlier than the public. So, every Tuesday I get up and go shopping at 7.30AM [. . .] When I go to the supermarket I put on a face mask before entering. I have only just started to do this, it feels strange and I am self-conscious. Being a public health professional I know that evidence is mixed about wearing face masks, but as going shopping is the most risky thing I do, I think I should protect myself, my family and others. It's a challenge shopping for 3 separate households at once and my trolley is always overflowing!

Diarist 1580 (female, 50s, Yorkshire and Humber, legal administrative assistant)

Phone my mum. We haven't seen both mums for any length of time for 8 weeks. I ring her in the morning and evening to check she is still ok [...] Luckily, I can do her shopping with ours once a week and drop it off at her door. She then wipes it down and puts it away and washes her hands. I think she misses her friends whom she used to meet on the community bus once a week to travel to the local supermarket but as they are of a similar age, that has been stopped.

Diarist 1582 (female, 50s, West Midlands, office manager)

I could really do with going out to get some shopping but I can't face the thought of queueing just to get a basket of stuff – I've been amazed at how much food I actually had in the house. Still working my way through the freezer and have got a ton of lentils!

Diarist 1692 (female, 60s, North of England, retired teacher)

I do a weekly shop which always feels dangerous. I feel anxious before I go and always relieved when I return, which is irrational as if I've picked up coronavirus it won't show for two weeks! I find men shopping on their own the worst for not keeping to social distance rules and can feel very cross with them.

Diarist 1739 (male, 20s, South East England, student)

12:00 – Went to the shop to get this week's shopping for the whole house since my boyfriend's mum is a key worker as a carer, and his dad is on the shielding list, so shouldn't leave the house. My boyfriend and I alternate weeks that we do the shopping. It wasn't busy today, but it is impossible to social distance when in the aisles. Shop was pretty much fully stocked, but still had no flour to buy.

Diarist 1940 (female, 30s, Scotland, assistant professor)

At 11:30 I got dressed then went out to do my grocery shopping. I wore a face covering for this for the first time. It's a tie-on fabric mask that a friend who is good at sewing made for me. The fit is good, so I didn't have to adjust it once I was outside. However, it felt a bit stifling, which at first put me on edge [. . .] Once I got used to it, the only problem with the mask was that my breathing kept fogging up my glasses. I realised that breathing through my nose reduced this, so tried to do that as much as possible. I also wore leather gloves while out shopping, although I had to remove them when using the touch screen automated checkout.

There's a large Sainsbury's only five or ten minutes' walk from my flat, so I went there. They have changed the store's entry and exit to enable social distancing, as well as having security people limiting how many can enter. I didn't have to wait to go in, as it was pretty quiet. I found all the foods on my grocery list except eggs, of which there were none whatsoever. This is the third week running that I've been unable to buy eggs and I'm starting to miss them. I'm a vegetarian, so they are my main protein source other than cheese.

Grocery shopping feels so very different to before the pandemic. I used to drop into one or two supermarkets (there are three different ones nearby) on the way home from work, three or four times a week. Now I buy groceries only once a week and carefully prepare a list of what I'll need. While I think this has on balance improved my diet (more vegetables) and certainly forced me to try and cook more, it's also stressful. Grocery shopping is now the most threatening part of the week. It's the only time I enter a building other than my home. I think less than half of the people shopping in Sainsbury's were wearing masks. Mostly it was older people covering their faces. The employees still don't have masks or gloves, I see. As the store is a large one and fairly quiet, keeping my distance from others was mostly easy.

I dragged my heavy bag of shopping home, went indoors, removed my gloves, washed my hands, removed my mask, put away my groceries, and washed my hands again. It's annoying that the halloumi I bought instead of eggs turns out to be the low fat kind. I must have misread the packaging due to fogged up glasses!

Diarist 1966 (female, 50s, South East England, administrator)

My theory is the optimum time to go to the supermarket is between 3-4pm as the queue is not too bad. And was right. Only took ten mins to get in.

Diarist 2100 (female, 40s, Yorkshire and Humber, nursery worker)

Drive to the nearest large supermarket with a massive list, a weekly shop has replaced little and often shopping since lock down. The queue outside is pretty small, only 5 minutes wait. Inside I'm pretty pleased to see caster sugar after not being able to find it for weeks.

Diarist 2147 (female, 40s, South East England, teacher)

I called mum. I have called her every day since this began because I can't bear the thought that she might not have spoken to anyone all day [. . .] She was fine – we spoke for about

40 mins – and had gone out to Tesco for the first time in seven weeks that morning. Glad I sent her the hand sanitiser.

Diarist 2408 (female, 40s, London, theatre worker)

As lunchtime approaches I realise I need some bread. I walk around to my local petrol station for this. It has a small co-op store attached and is the only largish food shop nearby that you don't have to queue outside to get in. 'Social distancing' is a bit haphazard as you dodge people in the aisles! I buy bread, a carton of juice and a bunch of flowers. I try to have a bunch in the house at all times to help cheer me up!

Diarist 2638 (male, 80s, North West England, retired teacher)

Today, May 12th 2020 I have experienced for the first time the queues at the local Post Office. Only one person is allowed in at a time [. . .] The members of the queue observed the two metre social distancing rule. The post office worker at the desk was obliged to wear rubber gloves throughout the day and admitted to me that it irritated the skin. I was lucky to get inside the post office in time to avoid the rain. Others were stranded there.

Diarist 2705 (female, 40s, Yorkshire and Humber, writer)

My son and I had porridge for breakfast. We ate the last of the bananas yesterday and will have to wait for a new shopping delivery before we have them again. I avoid the shops as much as possible. We're supposed to be keeping two metres apart at all times but it's so hard in supermarkets as it only takes one or two careless people to break the rules and it doesn't feel safe if people are reaching for the same vegetables or picking things up and putting them down again. They say the virus can exist on surfaces for several hours or days so we try to disinfect them when we get home and have to be careful not to touch our faces which is tricky for me as I'm a fidget.

Diarist 2869 (female, 60s, East of England, retired teacher)

To the shops. I needed to get top up for the electricity and a few groceries. My husband didn't come in the shop. I had to queue for a bit as it is one in and one out. There were two unaccompanied children who didn't have a clue about social distancing rules. They were walking backwards, going back and forth up each aisle, and when it came to the checkout, they stood very close to me. I had my mask on and sanitised my hands. When we both got home we washed our hands for 20 seconds.

Diarist 3573 (female, 60s, East of England, humanist celebrant)

Managed to sleep until 6am. Put Radio 1 on (I know it's meant for the youth but I still enjoy it). Made my Lady Grey tea and took it up to bed for my morning Facebook and E-mail catch-up, on my phone. I usually have my tea with Koko milk but shopping has become stressful and we try to go out as infrequently as possible, so I've switched to powdered whitener [. . .] The only protein left in the freezer is Quorn nuggets, so one of us will need to brave a supermarket soon. We have tinned beans, dry lentils, nuts and [. . .] plenty of eggs, so could probably survive another week [. . .] I've been obsessively editing the recently created spreadsheet shopping list.

Diarist 3739 (female, 60s, South West England, social worker)

Shopping is no longer any joy. Put on a mask, look outside, coast clear, set off, queue – sometimes people chat, sometimes not – don't browse because people are waiting, play aisle Jenga trying not to breach social distance – pay by contactless card at a machine, walk home, coast clear or cross the road.

Diarist 3761 (female, 30s, South West England, lawyer)

I prepare us a dinner of Thai green curry with chickpeas (an unusual combination but beggars can't be choosers when you're limited to buying 3 tins of legumes at a time from the supermarket to ensure there is enough for everyone!).

Diarist 3944 (female, 30s, London, event producer)

We finally left our house for our daily exercise after 3pm [. . .] We walked to the park and after a short mooch around the park, ended up heading to a nearby Homebase. It has only just reopened and as we were close, we thought we'd pop in and buy a few things for the garden – gardening is one of my main hobbies during lockdown. We queued up, 2 metres apart from those in front and behind us. There were probably 15-20 people ahead of us in the queue, but it moved quickly. I still find queuing to enter shops a very alien process and yearn for a time when I could enter and exit freely. Little things have come to mean so much more – a visit to Homebase became a much more enjoyable experience because it was something different to the day to day of lockdown. Signs advised that we were allowed to browse for 20 minutes only, in order to allow a regular flow of customers in and out of the store. We left a while later with a hose, some new terracotta pots, grass seed, a peony and a lavender plant. Exciting!

Diarist 4403 (female, 60s, South West England, community development consultant)

I decided, with some excitement, that I felt well enough and confident enough to go to [a nearby food store].

But I hadn't bargained on the 'new normal' in places like this. Apart from trips to the Co-op, I've hardly been out of my neighbourhood since before lockdown. The first thing that confronted me was the queue outside the shop. Socially distanced, and fearful. People no longer seem to chat in the queues outside shops. There is a sense of fear, distrust and resentment because it all takes so much longer and maybe the person in front will get the last of whatever it is that I want. It's not a pleasant atmosphere. The queue moved surprisingly quickly, and soon I was in the store. But . . . part of the enjoyment for me is to look, to appraise the food, to choose carefully what I want, to select carefully from the stock that's always on display outside the shop, to think about what to buy and what to prepare with it. Slow shopping. I didn't want to be slow, as I was mindful of people waiting outside as I had been [. . .] There's a one-way system in the shop so if I forgot something, I can't go back to get it. And, what are the 'rules' or at least the etiquette: am I 'allowed' to buy more than one dozen eggs? And when another customer came the wrong way down the aisle I was in, or the shop staff were re-filling shelves, should I be worried? And the produce was not as fresh as usual, no doubt because of the much lower turnover. And I was behind a mask which put a further barrier between me and the person at the checkout behind their screen.

I made my purchases and was pleased and relieved to get back home.

STAY ALERT

12 May came two days after a press conference from Prime Minister Boris Johnson, in which he announced a change of message – from the original 'Stay home, protect the NHS, save lives' to a new 'Stay alert, control the virus, save lives' – and a new set of rules and guidelines. Starting on 13 May, people should work from home if they can, but go to work if they can't work from home. If they do go to work, they should avoid public transport if possible. They would be allowed an unlimited amount of outdoor exercise. They would be allowed to travel for outdoor exercise or to meet one member of another household outdoors, so long as a distance of 2 metres was maintained. Starting in June, it was hoped that some shops would reopen and some children would return to school. Starting in July, it was hoped that some hospitality settings would reopen. How did the diarists receive these new rules and guidelines and this change of message? They noted how the general reception, on both news and social media, seemed to be confusion. They admitted to being confused themselves. Beyond confusion, they commonly interpreted the changes as a lifting, or easing, or loosening of lockdown – a new phase of the pandemic. This in turn was interpreted differently by different diarists. Some were relieved and excited. They began planning walks with family and friends they had not seen in person for months. They reemployed their housecleaner. Tradespeople happily went back to work. The roads and parks became busier. It would be good to get the economy up and running again. It would be especially good for those who'd struggled with loneliness in lockdown. Others were unsettled by the change and concerned by its potential effects. They worried it was too soon, when no treatment or vaccine was yet available. They worried it would lead to a second wave of infections, hospitalizations and deaths. They feared for their own safety and that of their loved ones – especially if they were dependent on public transport, or lived in the kinds of places people would now travel to visit, or were categorized as 'vulnerable' and 'high risk'. They worried they would be pressured to go to work or visit people – to take risks they weren't yet ready to take. They didn't trust the government to prioritize safety (over economy) and they didn't trust the public to make 'common sense' decisions. They argued among themselves about what now constituted a common sense decision. Some of those shielding or isolating felt particularly aggrieved. They were being advised to continue shielding or isolating. It had been relatively easy to stay home when everyone was mostly staying home. Now, as things changed, their situation would become relatively more difficult. Still, some of those concerned about the change would continue to stay home anyway, sticking to the original rules, guidelines and message, at least for now. See also Anxiety; Fear; Shielding; Stay apart; Stay home; Working from home.

Diarist 34 (female, 60s, North East England, retired teacher)

Now that restrictions are lifting, my concerns are for my family. How can my son go back into school safely, using public transport to get there? Will it be safe for my grandson at nursery? How can you stop little children from giving each other or their carers a hug?

Diarist 37 (male, 18, London)

I miss gathering with friends the most. Some have been doing it illegally, but most are trying just to wait it out. Today however, this 12th May, due to the new government advice we can now meet with one person from outside our household outside, as long as we social distance. This afternoon I am therefore going on a long bike ride with one of my closest mates where we will remain two metres but still have the opportunity to catch up and tease each other, which I am looking forward to.

Diarist 114 (male, 20s, South East England, student)

The government has loosened their restrictions for exercise from once a day to unlimited exercise, as if we were all training for the Olympics.

Diarist 119 (male, 60s, South West England, retired teacher)

The government's communications have become increasingly confused and confusing, moving from an initial message of Stay Home, Protect the NHS and Save Lives to a second stage of Stay Alert, Control the Virus and Save Lives. The PM, who boasted (before becoming infected with Covid-19 and nearly losing his life) of shaking hands with everybody despite scientific warnings that we should not be shaking hands, has advised the British public to use 'good solid British common sense' in interpreting new lockdown rules. The constant use of British this and British that speaks to a worrying sense of exceptionalism amongst some political leaders, ignoring the fact that other countries also have common sense and access to scientific advice.

Having updated the strapline to Stay Alert, Control the Virus and Save Lives, the government issued a 173-word explanation/clarification suggesting that the message wasn't clear. The BBC's Ten News on 11 May was totally devoted to the fact that nobody understands what the government thinks it is doing [. . .] The UK government's approach is leading to some interesting anomalies. From 13 May we will be able to meet with one person from another household in a public space at a distance of two metres. So, our daughters can only meet with one of their parents at a time. Yet, should we be employed as their cleaner we can meet with them in their house.

Diarist 175 (female, 70s, London, retired medical secretary)

I have 3 grown-up children and 5 grand-children [. . .] I miss seeing them daily as I would normally and Zoom or FaceTime is just not the same because you can't feel and cuddle them [. . .] On Thursday I am looking forward to meeting up with my daughter and grand-children for the first time in 7 weeks for a long walk. Am hoping for weather that is 'just right for walking'.

Diarist 189 (female, 70s, North West England, nurse)

While cooking I listened to the news and tried to decide what the implications and implementation of the government's 'Be vigilant' guidelines will mean. At a purely selfish and local level, it will mean that the golf course is re-opening on Wednesday. Being able to walk there has been a joy: a pond with a heron; green parrots as well as open spaces, mature trees and an ancient 'moat'. Walking there has been very therapeutic for my husband who has chronic fatigue syndrome. What will he do now? I'm contemplating getting him a crash helmet.

Diarist 250 (male, 30s, Yorkshire and Humber, researcher)

In the last days my partner and I have both felt a change in our mood, getting angry and frustrated at the changes the government has announced to the lockdown. The messages have been so inconsistent and confusing, and the priorities so wrong (all about forcing people back to work before it's safe) that we've struggled to feel good about what's coming. Today I'm going to make a conscious effort not to skim social media, as I know reading others' commentary on it won't do me any good.

Diarist 404 (female, 60s, South West England, teacher)

The prime minister announced an easing of lockdown restrictions on Sunday. I think this was interpreted as putting more of the responsibility of 'social distancing' (which should be called physical not social distancing in my view) on the individual. As a result, this 12th May turned into a really busy day. [The window cleaner] knocked on my door and I cleared a path for him to take his ladder through the house into the back garden and clean the windows for the first time this year. He told me they were filthy. Devon looks beautiful through clean windows!

   A quick bite of lunch (last night's leftovers, mustn't waste anything) and there was another knock on the door. This time it was [the handy woman] who had come to fix the downpipe before the next rainstorm breaks it again. Both my visitors kept 2 metres away from me at least. Today is turning into a very different day.

Diarist 472 (female, 40s, London, interior designer)

Today has been an exciting day [. . .] Last night Boris told us we could meet up outside with 1 friend so daughter & son have been walking with a chosen friend around the local park – first time they've spent time with their friends in the real (not virtual) world for 8 weeks. It's been a happy day!

Diarist 479 (female, 40s, South West England, clinical pharmacist)

There has been a new announcement over the weekend regarding the current lockdown situation. The Government's handling of this has been a shambles. There is currently so much confusion surrounding what we are allowed and not allowed to do that I have made a mental note not to get into a discussion with any patients about this today.

Diarist 529 (female, 50s, Yorkshire and Humber, company director)

We are in another period of change. 6 weeks ago we entered the 'lockdown' period but now we are coming out of it. I am finding the change unsettling. When we entered lockdown, I felt very scared of what might happen. My husband is in a high risk/shielded group so remember looking at him in the garden whilst I was washing up and crying at the thought of the suffering he might go through if the virus got into his lungs. Now it is deemed safe for me (although not him) to start to leave the isolated pod we have created for ourselves, but I feel scared. I do not trust the government; they have been so blasé about the impact on people's lives. If I had known back on 23rd March that over 30,000 people would die, I think I would have been inconsolable [. . .] Today my husband and I are arguing about whether he can play golf or not. The government advice is that they can play in pairs but he has also been told he is still shielding. He is counting the 12 weeks of shielding in his diary and reckons he has done 8 weeks already. Yet he knows that the 12 weeks is just an arbitrary period of time set by a government who are not really sure what to do. He does not feel that going to play golf on his own and having no contact with anyone is going to increase his risk – although he has been in the shielded group he has been out for a daily walk. I want him to be able to enjoy his sport but I feel worried about the risks. It felt easier when no-one could play golf or travel or work. Now there is so much to navigate and so much to decide.

My mum is already talking about me visiting them again. But it is 200 miles by train [. . .] and that exposes me to a whole lot of risk. 'But what is our exit plan?' my husband asks. I am somehow expected to know, to somehow be the grown up in all of this. He seems to expect me to set the rules for him and yet he doesn't really want that. I no longer know what to say to him about it all. 'Yes it is unfair that you cannot go out' and yes it is unfair that your asthma means you may not recover if you get the virus and yes I would feel very guilty if I was to bring the virus home.

At some point I will have to go out to work – so far I have been working from home [. . .] and then I will have the challenge of how do I safely travel when I do not drive [. . .] It is easier when no one can travel or work outside the home to keep safe but now it is about taking risks.

Diarist 542 (female, 60s, East Midlands, retired accountant)

I often read the news on my phone at breakfast but today I decided it could wait. I am a bit fed up of all the announcements and lack of clarity [. . .] The Stay Home, Protect the NHS, Save Lives was an easy message to understand. But I must admit by the middle of April I was truly tired of hearing about saving the NHS.

On Sunday I listened to our Prime Minister and I was confused about the new message. What does 'Stay Alert' mean? I am also disappointed that I can't yet see my children and grandchildren because of the lockdown restrictions.

Outside the weather has turned grey and dull. It looks like it might rain.

Diarist 1108 (male, 50s, West Midlands, teacher)

The 5pm briefing from Number 10 was something I was glued to at the start of all this, before it became repetitive and uninformative. Today, though, I watched. Over the weekend, the government made a mess of the change to a new stage of the lockdown and I wanted to see how they handled that today. Not well.

Diarist 1147 (male, 30s, East Midlands, psychiatrist)

I drove to work just after seven in the morning. The roads seemed a little busier today than they have been lately, as if the 'lockdown' for the coronavirus pandemic is beginning to sleep. The Government advice has become so woolly that it seems inevitable now that people will start to go back to normal. I am gravely concerned about what it will mean. The reality is that until we have either a solid vaccine, a reliable treatment or a better understanding of why some people are more susceptible than others, the risks of allowing further spread seem unacceptable to me at least.

Diarist 1480 (female, 20s, London, bar worker and sales assistant)

I decided to go for a jog [. . .] I jogged through the park which was lovely, but it was considerably busy for a Tuesday evening. The PM announced that people could visit the park and meet with one person outside their household, and people seem to have grabbed the opportunity with both hands. Considering the fact that 100s of people are dying every day still, I find this bizarre. It's stupid for the government to encourage it, and stupid for people to think we're over the worst of it. A second wave is on the horizon and people seem to think everything will be fine.

Diarist 1491 (male, 20s, North West England, student)

The new slogan of the government has changed from 'stay at home, protect the NHS, save lives' to 'stay alert > control the virus > save lives', whatever the hell that means. The new slogan does not really give me a great deal of confidence so me and my family will stick to the old slogan, we will continue to stay at home, to protect the NHS and key workers, and hopefully save lives, I just hope the rest of the country do the same for as long as it takes.

Diarist 1581 (male, 60s, London, office administrator)

This week the government has outlined a 'roadmap' of sorts to amend the previous restrictions and allow a return to some form of normality. The guidance is far from clear though [. . .] The government is encouraging people to return to work, but not to use public transport, which is almost impossible in London.

Diarist 1585 (female, 60s, South East England, therapist and chaplain)

Because Boris Johnson (our PM) gave a very confusing public address on Sunday about the new advice, everyone is talking about it and no one seems to have a scoobydoo what it all means! Clear, direct advice is what is needed now and the old slogan of 'stay at home' has now been changed to 'stay alert'. What does that mean? I am so confused.

Diarist 1651 (male, 70s, West Midlands, marketing consultant)

We took the decision late yesterday to ask our house cleaner to come back after [. . .] 9 weeks in lockdown. And, happily, she agreed. We reviewed the Govt documents and it seems that's allowed, so back to a spotless house again!

Diarist 1711 (male, 50s, West Midlands, geologist)

We both try to stop work at 5 to watch the daily coronavirus briefing from the BBC. The government have introduced new lockdown rules which are very confusing and although there is always a spike after the weekend it appears that hospital admissions are up, so are deaths. Because of this my wife is getting more and more anxious because of our daughter [recovering from cancer]. It's a worrying time.

Diarist 1721 (female, 50s, Yorkshire and Humber, nurse and lecturer)

Today is a slightly different day. For the first time in weeks, my husband is out for the workday. He was excited about the prospect of leaving our hill-side. Also today is the first day my border collie is going out with her dog walker (or as we call it 'dog-club') for weeks [. . .] I am concerned about returning to work [. . .] I live over 25 miles from my work place and usually commute by rail. I am not keen to get back on a train.

Diarist 1767 (male, 50s, South East England, project manager)

7:00 Awoke, could see sun coming in which is always nice. Read the news on the phone until about 7:30. Confusion around the gradual easing of lock-down restrictions seems to be the order of the day.

Diarist 1867 (female, 20s, West Midlands, cabin crew)

Today is the last day before some of the lockdown measures are slightly relaxed, but to be honest don't think I'll be doing anything different when the rules change as I'm still worried about the virus. Apparently we're now going to be allowed to meet people from other households in a public space, and people are allowed to hang around in parks outside, not just for exercise. It all seems too soon but what do I know. I'm going to keep staying home as much as possible.

Diarist 1874 (female, 40s, South East England, GP)

Two days ago our Prime Minister, Boris Johnson [. . .] addressed the nation and tried to describe how the lockdown measures could start to be lifted slowly [. . .] This address was painful to watch. It was confusing 'Stay at home, work from home, but if you can't work from home go to work . . .' and described ways in which people could meet members from outside their family – only one family member meeting another family member from another family outside and 2m apart. This all feels like the material of some horror film.

Diarist 1927 (female, 50s, South East England, artist and musician)

I watched the daily briefing last night and some of the lunchtime news today and am dismayed at the new guidelines [. . .] The message is confusing, it is scary for those who are being expected to return to work not knowing if they can arrange childcare or how they will be able to get to work if they have to avoid public transport, and it leaves so many 'guidelines' open to interpretation that you know many will make up their own minds about how to twist the rules to fit themselves. The fear is there will be a second wave of infections.

Diarist 1942 (female, 40s, London, teaching assistant)

The rules of lockdown are going to ease a little tomorrow. It will be lovely to be able to arrange to meet a friend for a socially-distant walk in a park. Face to face conversations!! Woo hoo!

Diarist 1984 (female, 60s, North West England, unemployed)

There are builders in our house! [. . .] They are relieved and happy to be working again though reckon it will be awkward getting supplies [. . .] I think this loosening of lockdown is too soon. When I had my mastectomy, I was fine in hospital, even positive – when the consultant said 'You can go home today' I burst into tears of panic – and I think that is almost where I'm at. I'm fine at home, even positive, things to do, healthy meals planned. But going out – not ready. The country's not ready [. . .] On the other hand, there are builders in!

Diarist 2030 (female, 70s, South West England, retired teacher)

I have been self-isolating as instructed, but our Prime Minister has changed his message leaving us all uncertain as to what to do now. I have no plans to change what I've been doing. I have no intention of joining the throngs who are desperate to return to 'normal' life. I am afraid of catching this virus, and of being left at home to die.

Diarist 2143 (female, 50s, North West England, secretary)

We're not supposed to 'travel for exercise' until tomorrow but I really want to go for a walk along the prom. It's been such a long time since we did that walk. I'm not one for breaking the rules and can honestly say that we haven't seen friends and family since lockdown started, we've only exercised to somewhere we can walk to from home, we haven't had anyone round to the house and we have stayed away from the shops as much as we can. I'm thinking that in 5 hours' time, the rules will change so what's the problem in going a little early?

9pm. 4½ miles later and a quick drive home and we're done for the night. The prom was really busy. Most people stuck to social distancing, but it seems that some people just don't care. They can see you coming but make no attempt to move out of the way or they walk down the middle of the path so you can't get past safely. Maybe I'm too much of a stickler for the rules but it is annoying when others just don't give a damn.

Diarist 2257 (female, 20s, North East England, artistic director)

Made plans to meet a friend in a park tomorrow now it's legal, even though probably not sensible.

Diarist 2463 (female, 50s, North West England, retired police officer)

At 00:11 I am still awake and exchanging messages on Facebook messenger with my best friend [. . .] We comment on the recent announcements from the Prime Minister about Covid restrictions. My thought is that him stating we should rely on the common sense of the public is scary as I have seen many examples over the years demonstrating just how little common sense people have [. . .] We both agree we are keeping in and away from people until things are safer.

Diarist 2466 (female, 20s, South East England, unemployed)

As I look out of the window at the sunshine, I wonder what the new restrictions (or lifting of) will bring to our seaside town. You can now drive to beauty spots and take unlimited exercise. I don't mean to sound paranoid, but Coronavirus does worry me a little bit. Not for me, although I would like to avoid getting it, but for my mum mainly. She isn't old, and is relatively healthy, apart from smoking, but she is my only living parent since my dad passed [. . .] I can see why they lifted the restrictions a little bit, as they have to keep the economy going, and people have been getting lonely, which has affected their mental health. But I don't think they should lift them at all. I think it is too early, and I worry that people will start going to places like the beach, which then makes it unsafe for locals.

Diarist 2705 (female, 40s, Yorkshire and Humber, writer)

Today I feel a bit grumpy. We're in the midst of the coronavirus and the government recently released some very unclear guidance about how to move forward. I'm tired of trying to educate my [son] whilst working from home but I don't want him to go to school until it is safe to do so. I worry about his health and about mine too.

Diarist 2723 (female, 50s, East Midlands, unemployed journalist)

After breakfast we both decided to go on a bike ride [. . .] Definitely a difference in activity levels. Although the roads were still quiet lots of the houses had traders visiting – for the first time in weeks! We saw roofers putting scaffolding up, builders, plumbers and gardeners. The 'get back to work' message is definitely being heeded by those that can social distance.

Diarist 2891 (female, 20s, East Midlands, teacher)

Tomorrow, we move from 'Stay at Home' to 'Stay Alert' according to Boris Johnson. For us that means we can drive the dog somewhere else for a walk – after 8 weeks of walks from our front doorstep that is incredibly exciting! But for lots of people it means going back to work without proper safety guidelines. We wondered about going to see our parents in their gardens but have decided not to.

Diarist 3134 (female, 60s, South East England, tour guide)

I make a phone call to my brother in the evening to tell him I will be allowed to drive over tomorrow Wednesday to hand over some bags of essential food and shopping & see him briefly standing well away from each other outside his flat. He is very 'low' and anxious having been isolated alone for over two months [. . .] I am determined I can do it tomorrow despite not having driven very far for months [. . .] I look forward to tomorrow when I will see my brother and be able to bring him a little joy and comfort. It will make me feel much better too.

Diarist 3210 (female, 30s, North West England, design manager)

We have just entered a new phase of the lockdown and we were allowed to now see one member of another household, outside, in public and stood two metres apart. It's been 8 weeks since we have seen my mum who has been in isolation alone and out to the shops rarely as there is only one to buy for. We decided the risk level was low and bent the rule a little and she came across to our house. It was unbelievable to give her a hug [. . .] My daughter was bouncing with joy, just jumping up and down on the spot, too excited to express her happiness in any other way.

Diarist 3367 (female, 50s, South East England, priest and bookseller)

The planned relaxing of lockdown rules from tomorrow has in fact already started for some people. There are more cars on the road, more people out and about, maybe a little less care when passing people to keep the 2-metre distancing. I have a sense of expectation, but also some trepidation, about the next few weeks. Will people go overboard and start having people round (as some have been doing all through lockdown anyway) or will they still be careful? If we get to open the shop what will that be like? Will we have to wear gloves and masks? How many people can we have in at any one time? With the older staff members still having to self-isolate we will be lone working most of the time, so how do we control numbers, or ask people to leave if they are chatting, as our customers often do, but others want to come in? How do you deep clean books? So many questions.

Diarist 3390 (male, 60s, South East England, retired NHS manager)

We are still digesting the details of the government announcements on Sunday and yesterday about easing the lockdown – encouraging people who can to go back to work (but not use public transport), saying we can drive to parks and beauty spots as long as we keep to social isolation rules, but not drive to see other family members unless we see them one at a time, in the open. There is a lot of confusion and I worry about what will happen to our seafront and promenade this coming weekend if people decide to drive [here] for the day. Last weekend the police had roadblocks outside the city turning day trippers away. This weekend that will, I guess, not be possible as the guidelines have been relaxed. A place to avoid for me, I think.

Diarist 3404 (female, South West England, 60s, retired curator)

5.00 o'clockish, so listening to the coronavirus briefing courtesy of Radio 4. So confused now as to what people can do or should do. And by confused I mean the government as well as the people they are talking down to.

Diarist 3562 (female, 50s, South West England, garden designer)

I went for my daily walk [. . .] The rules change tomorrow but for now we are only allowed out for an hour. Interesting to see how many more people and cars are about today, anticipating more freedom.

Diarist 3808 (female, 70s, North East England, retired school inspector)

5.00pm We watch The Downing Street briefing [. . .] I fear that the relaxing of restrictions will cause the graphs to rise again.

Diarist 3890 (female, 40s, London, urban designer)

I'm definitely unsettled today. Bozo has started lifting the lockdown and tomorrow is the big day. How many will come out and go back to work? How will they get there? This is London – not many people have cars, so what will the tube be like? Where will they all get masks from all of a sudden? [. . .] I'm unsettled after a bad weekend. A bank holiday and sunny, it didn't go too well in my neighbourhood! Generally younger people gathering in tiny front gardens that bump up against the narrow pavements and others from other households standing on the edge of the pavement. Chatting, drinking, smoking, laughing together. Finally, celebrating the end before it's been announced. This is not quite social distancing: a sign people are now confident that nothing will happen, no one will say anything anymore. It's done. Lockdown is done. People are done.

Diarist 4012 (female, 90s, Yorkshire and Humber, retired teacher)

Turn on BBC news [. . .] Loosening of lockdown – pictures of busy commuter traffic, people moving too close together without masks. Worrying – it's too soon.

Diarist 4756 (female, 40s, Yorkshire and Humber, academic)

Today I woke up still struggling to understand the Prime Minister's message on Sunday, which told us all to 'Stay alert' instead of 'Stay at home'. All very confusing, and I am now feeling more stressed than before about this situation [. . .] My daughter is in Year 6, so may be among the first of the guinea pigs/pupils to go back to school, and that's nerve wracking too. I'm white, but my husband is BAME and has various minor, underlying health issues such as asthma, high blood pressure, high cholesterol – and he also had TB in his 30s – so I really want to make sure he stays safe, and avoids respiratory problems. Our concern about this has been particularly high since his cousin (similar age and health profile) caught the virus and died last month.

STAY APART

To reduce transmission, people were advised to stay 2 metres apart from others not in their household. These others tended to be encountered when shopping or walking/exercising – the main two legitimate reasons for most people to leave home during lockdown. Such encounters could be minimized by choosing quiet places and times, and especially places without narrow paths, where staying apart would be difficult. Such encounters involved a kind of dance. People would step aside. They might turn away or hold their breath too. Avoidance measures might involve crossing the road or stepping into the gutter or a hedge on the side of the path. Usually this was done with good humour. People would smile or laugh, greet each other and say thank you. That is, unless others didn't keep their distance. This was annoying. It was seen as disrespectful. Joggers were seen as particularly disrespectful, or at least risky, for getting too close while panting heavily and so potentially spreading the virus. For these reasons, some people found going out stressful. A zigzag path had to be navigated, skirting dangerous others. But there were good reasons to go out. Lonely family members needed waving to from the end of their drive. Kids with birthdays needed singing to from the gate. See also Shops; (dog) Walking.

Diarist 138 (female, 11, West Midlands)

I cycled to my Grandad's house with my dad and we stood at the end of the drive and said hello, then we went home again [. . .] Next year, I'm starting secondary school and I'm slightly nervous. I mean, how will I make proper friends if we have to social distance?

Diarist 189 (female, 70s, North West England, nurse)

Meanwhile back to this morning and our visit to the doctor's for our shingles vaccinations (as we are now old enough to qualify as being at risk). Walked up the main road and had to take avoiding action, as the queue for the bank stretched out along the pavement and necessitated walking out into the road. Although the risk of getting knocked down was probably a greater health risk than passing breaking the 2 metre distance recommendations. The Practice's pharmacy was using a different door at the front of the building, instead of having to go inside, and there were only a few people waiting. The surgery itself was a very different experience from when I had been there a couple of years ago. The chairs were well spaced out, and cleaned as soon as someone left. We did not have long to wait, and the nurse was wearing a mask, apron and gloves.

Diarist 269 (male, 16, West Midlands)

I decide to go for a run [. . .] I get a fair way along the road before I see that I'm approaching two distant shapes on the pavement. Soon I can make out the features of a leisurely dressed couple walking towards me. I go to pass them, and momentarily catch their eyes. They both throw me quick glances as they hastily shuffle onto the side of the pavement away from me, despite already having enough room to pass by. Then they are behind me, gone. I try to place my focus back onto my breathing as I continue forward but that image of those two pairs of judging eyes imprints itself onto my vision. 'Is what I'm doing wrong?' I think to myself [. . .] I encounter several more people along the way. After that first experience with the couple, I choose to distance myself from anyone by stepping out onto the empty road momentarily and circulating past them, rather than causing a fuss on the pavement. It doesn't stop one woman from clearly holding her breath as I run past her, or one man from nervously recoiling away when he looks and sees me, but it does assure their safety from me, but also (though I don't fully acknowledge this at first) my safety from them.

Diarist 529 (female, 50s, Yorkshire and Humber, company director)

I miss my cycling friends and I miss the experiences you have on a group ride. But I cannot see how that is going to be possible again soon. Already I look at the photos from our last group ride before lockdown and the behaviour seems reckless. We are so physically close to each other when we are riding, and in the café. We all use the toilet in quick succession at the café stop and no amount of handwashing will have stopped the virus spreading between us. All you can do is hope that the others with you are not carrying the virus, but it is a silent killer and that is what makes it so scary.

Diarist 924 (female, 30s, Scotland, midwife)

My partner called for his repeat prescription anti-depressants from the doctor's. It is weird at the minute. You go and collect them at a set time from a box outside the GP's underneath a dangling bottle of hand sanitizer.

Diarist 591 (female, 40s, Scotland, molecular biologist)

The roads are quiet, and it is pleasant to walk [. . .] A strange etiquette has developed when people pass each other. Most people will happily move aside to give the other space to pass by. Many people give a cheery greeting. Occasionally, someone will make no effort to move and it makes me cross.

Diarist 1177 (male, 60s, South West England, finance director)

At 4pm I walked through the village to the doctor's surgery to pick up a regular prescription. Even this simple task is influenced by Covid-19 as I cross roads or walk in the gutter to avoid people. 'Oh, this makes me laugh' said one old lady as we passed at a respectable distance to each other. When I got to the pharmacy which is located in the surgery, I was met by a notice saying 'Do not enter'. I was directed around the corner where I had to knock on the frosted window and my drugs were handed out to me by an anonymous hand. In more normal times I feel I might have been arrested for such nefarious doings!

Diarist 1287 (female, 60s, London, retired teacher)

I took the dog for a walk. I used to meet up with other dog owners, and we'd go round the woodland in a posse. Now, we wave from a distance, which is sad. There's a country park near us, with fruit trees and wide green spaces and paths through the woods. It used to be almost empty except for dog-walkers. Today it was full of runners, families on bikes and teenagers surreptitiously meeting up with their mates. In different circumstances, I'd be happy to see them in the park, but at present I'm finding it difficult to maintain social distance, especially as our dog is very friendly.

Diarist 1289 (female, 50s, South East England,
creative producer and artistic director)

Short interlude to call the doctor, cystitis alert. You can't actually see a doctor at the moment because of the virus. Been advised to put a 'sample' in a plastic tub, Sellotape it up & stick it through the post box to the right of the surgery door; sounds dangerous, hope they've already collected the mail!

Diarist 1369 (female, 40s, West Midlands, housewife)

I dress and get ready for a dog walk with [son]. It is sunny today so everywhere will be busier and the runners will be out.

It is very busy out with the dogs. People are playing football and picnicking in the park which makes picking a 2 metre route a bit tricky. As I am trying to shut the gate – using a dog poo bag as a glove – the dog, who has been on the extender lead since lockdown began forays a few centimetres into the road. [Son] spots him first and pulls him straight back. An old lady cyclist in an orange waterproof has to slow down – very slightly – I immediately shout 'Sorry', she replies with 'Stupid'.

Diarist 1423 (male, 30s, London, auditor)

It is my younger daughter's birthday. And if you think that celebrating a child's birthday is hard in normal times when you arrange play dates or a small birthday party (why not rent a bouncy castle, we've thought in the past, what's the worst that can happen . . . Crying children. That's what can happen) arranging to have a birthday in the times of Coronavirus is outright difficult and challenging as anything. The friends playing are replaced by FaceTime calls with family members and social distance hellos. Young kids are not fantastic at realising how important it is to engage in these sessions [. . .] We also managed the new 'normal' of socialising by social distancing. 3 of her friends came to our house, stood at the gate about 2.5m away to sing happy birthday and drop off some gifts. Which admittedly given that we don't spray things we get down when we get them or wipe them down with some kind of super-gel (anti-bac stuff has to be strong to kill the virus) might defeat the point. But still, we got visitors which raised my daughter's spirits a good deal. That's how birthdays have to be for now.

Diarist 1426 (female, 40s, North West England, doctor)

My sexual health clinic is running a reduced service – most consultations are by telephone (booked online by the patients) and we can post out [. . .] testing kits for chlamydia and gonorrhoea (plus trichomonas vaginalis if relevant) to the patients if necessary. They take swabs or urine samples themselves then post them back in a prepaid envelope, and we text or phone them with the results. If patients need contraception, they can collect a supply of contraceptive pills from our reception following the telephone consultation. However, if a patient is suspected of having gonorrhoea, syphilis or genital ulcers, has been sexually assaulted or is under 16, or if they require an emergency copper intrauterine device, they are invited to attend clinic where I (or another member of staff who has no underlying health conditions) see them face to face wearing a surgical mask with visor, an apron and gloves. We also provide a mask for the patient [. . .] I have been surprised that a minority of patients have ignored lockdown restrictions to continue to meet sexual partners (sometimes meeting online via apps) and therefore have acquired infection or put themselves at risk of unplanned pregnancy.

Diarist 1490 (female, 50s, Yorkshire and Humber, nurse)

Once I'd got up and ready and opened the [birthday] cards that had arrived [. . .] we were very daring and instead of doing our walk from home, drove to meet [sister] on the canal bank because she wanted to give me my birthday present. We parked separately then engineered to be both walking on the canal at the same time. She caught up with us and we walked 2m apart and sat on a grassy bank 3m apart to have a chat. She gave me a home-made carrot cake and some leggings.

Diarist 1521 (female, 60s, South East England, customer service agent)

I walked this afternoon [. . .] to see my Mum who is still stuck in her flat due to this virus. Rang her on the way and told her I would be coming. She was pleased as is not coping very well with doing video calls on her new phone – she keeps switching the internet off or pressing the wrong button and it all goes off. When I got there, two of the old chaps were sat in the front hall of the flats and waved at me through the glass – not sure if they were warning me to stay away, or being friendly! Mum came down with her stick and sat outside on the wall whilst I stood on the pavement having a chat for a while. She messaged me later to say my son had passed by on his bicycle and waved to her from the car park. That was a good day for her she said. I am looking forward to when we can all meet up properly together and have a cup of tea. I just hope she can get through this ok.

Diarist 1548 (male, 11, South East England)

Woke up this morning and I remember something. It is my birthday [. . .] At 10:30 all my friends drive past in their cars shouting happy birthday and throwing cards to me. Later on I had a Zoom party with my friends and we did a scavenger hunt. After we played on the Xbox. It was fun chatting and playing with friends.

Diarist 1574 (female, 40s, Wales, public health practitioner)

My dad comes by and speaks to us over the garden wall and drops some compost off in the front garden. It is so strange and awkward to not be able to invite close family into your home. We are all getting used to it, but I hate it and it keeps conversation short.

Diarist 1585 (female, 60s, South East England, therapist and chaplain)

This afternoon I take [dog] out for our long walk in the farmland near our home. I try to find different paths, away from the general routes, in order to avoid people which is difficult if you are all on a narrow track. Today I got a little lost and, in my attempt to get back to the main path, we had to walk round the perimeter of a ploughed rough field to find a way over a deep ditch that I could manage. [Dog] has no problem with this but I do and got caught up in some nasty brambles which ripped my sock and skin. A mild sort of panic did set in but eventually we made it back to the main pathway.

Diarist 1679 (female, 30s, London, software engineer)

I clock off at 5.10 and think about going outside. I haven't done so for the last few days as it's been too cold (too cold for May). I quickly put my shoes on and go out before I can change my mind. There are plenty of people out and about doing the same – I skirt around the outside of the small square-ish park near my house, and duck inside round the top edge further up the hill, where it's always quieter. I find myself getting annoyed by a group of 4 middle aged people who are taking up the width of the path, even though they're facing away from me and couldn't possibly know I was behind them. I leave the park and head home.

Diarist 1794 (female, 70s, East Midlands, retired teacher)

2.30pm Exercise of the day: we walked about three quarters of a mile to a friend's house as it's his birthday tomorrow and we wanted to drop off a card. He asked us to come in and witness his and his wife's Power of Attorney forms. We shouldn't really have done this but we are all quite well and have been self isolating for weeks. We were very careful, kept our distance, washed hands etc. Probably safer than going to Sainsbury's.

Diarist 1815 (female, 20s, Scotland, unemployed)

I ran in [the local park]; it was quieter today than it has been, with plenty of runners and dog-walkers but fewer household groups out for walks. I was pleased about that, because the mental geometry of trying to maximise distance from others at all times can be quite stressful for me when I'm out.

Diarist 1866 (non-binary, 20s, South East England, student and proof-reader)

Me and my mum are thinking of getting up when low tide [. . .] is at about 5am next week, so we can take one of our dogs (the other is [old] and only likes short walks these days) to the beach when fewer people should be around than later in the day. That's the really difficult thing – avoiding other people when it's necessary to go out.

Diarist 1971 (female, 60s, Wales, writer)

Got up at seven and dressed to go for our 'exercise', a walk of 1.2 miles along a back lane from our village [. . .] We try to get out early so we don't meet anyone as the lane is quite narrow in places with tall banks and hedges that don't leave very much room to stand aside, especially if a large vehicle passes by; though we are seeing less traffic currently.

Anyway, we made it there and back without meeting a soul.

Diarist 1984 (female, 60s, North West England, unemployed)

In order to keep social distancing, my daily exercise is that I walk the dog only once, in the morning when fewer people are around. Usually, I've been wandering the golf course – less than five minutes across the road, on wide pavements to pass people and then acres of space. Social distancing can be a hundred yards or more, never mind two metres. I shall miss this all-over wandering when the golfers are back and we have to stick to the official public footpaths. The dog will miss it too. We've found lovely badger holes and rabbit holes to explore, and gorgeous views [. . .] However, today it is cold and wet and I guess there'll be very few people out yet, and probably no children, so I walk through the housing estate to the woods; a bit of a change for the dog, and more of a change for me. I cross the road to avoid a shopper coming away from the convenience store, and he is the only person I see on the streets. A mooch through [the woods] [. . .] Wish 'Good morning' to another dog walker who moved to the side so we are far enough apart [. . .] Back across the golf course. Two more dog walkers and we skirt each other with a greeting – so five people this morning, probably safe.

Diarist 2100 (female, 40s, Yorkshire and Humber, nursery worker)

I took the dog on our usual walk around the field. We passed lots of familiar faces, human and dog. Had a quick chat with some friends, all stood well apart shouting at each other.

Diarist 2172 (male, 40s, London, creative consultant)

At 15.30 my boyfriend and I head out for our daily walk [. . .] My boyfriend has mild anxiety. Where we go is usually determined by how he's feeling: if he can face the mass of joggers at the park or not. There are more people in the park than on any sunny summer Saturday I can remember! Today we decide to go to the cemetery which is more quiet than the park, and try to avoid dog-walkers, families with kids, and a handful of people who will not move out of anyone's way despite the need to keep 2m apart.

Diarist 2425 (female, 50s, Yorkshire and Humber, researcher and editor)

Out for my daily 'exercise' [. . .] I change into the 'outside' jeans that live in a box in the hall, wash my hands, and set out. I see my next-door neighbour walking her dog in the adjacent car park and say hello from a distance. After that, it's a brisk walk down the road [. . .] I step into the road for one young man coming the other way and skirt the edge of the pavement for another, but it's quiet enough that social distancing isn't really a problem. Back in just under half an hour, I slip off my jeans, wash my hands again, and pull on my 'inside' pair.

Diarist 2589 (female, 30s, South East England, actress)

At 2pm [. . .] my mum shouted down that we had visitors. My younger brother's fiancé and their [. . .] daughter came to visit. They stood in the middle of the garden, I stayed at the end and mum and dad by the house. Maintaining our 2 metre distancing at all times! I chatted with my niece about her school work, what books we are reading. She loves lending me books and I love hearing about how much she enjoys reading. After she left I ordered her a sequel of a book she loved that will arrive by the end of the week. I said to her it was weird not to hug and she said that's what she wants to do too!

Diarist 2806 (female, 30s, Scotland, tour guide)

After lunch I headed out into [the local park] for a walk. I've been taking a lot of walks in the park the past couple of months, exploring all these corners of it I'd never been to before. It's busier than usual on the main paths these days because everyone's out taking their exercise, but people are being respectful and staying 2m apart wherever possible. My favourite places now are off the usual paths, where you scramble up rocks and find hidden places that feel secret [. . .] I like to roll a joint, tramp up to the top of a hill in the park where there's no one around, and smoke while I look out over the city and think.

Diarist 2869 (female, 60s, East of England, retired teacher)

My husband and I went for our daily exercise. We are living by the sea, but there are too many people walking along the prom, so we tend to walk on the grass or in the road. We walked up the hill and sat on a bench overlooking the sea. Here we are away from everyone.

Diarist 2957 (female, 50s, North West England, careers consultant)

Today is not a typical day in either my life or a typical birthday, given the physical, social and mobility restrictions we are experiencing. Normally I'd be seeing lots of friends and family members over the course of the day, with people dropping in for cuppas and cake or evening drinks. It has been however, a really lovely day, with loads of messages, flower and plant deliveries and phone calls/video calls. After a relaxing bath, and a dog walk, my best friend invited me to her garden for a socially distant present giving! So I drove to her home [. . .] where she'd placed a little table and a chair outside her back door, laid with a pretty cloth plus blankets for the chair. She stayed inside her kitchen. The day was very cold, which was odd after all the warm and sunny weather we've had, so I went prepared, wrapped up in a big coat, hat and scarf!! She'd made a delicious Victoria Sandwich cake with cream, served me tea and gave me my gifts [. . .] I stayed for about 2 and a half hours

[. . .] What I loved most was just the joy of seeing my dear friend in the flesh after so long; seeing each other in video calls is just not the same. Strange though not to be able to hug and embrace. But it was a very happy occasion, one I'll always remember.

Diarist 3051 (female, 70s, London, retired stage manager and personal assistant)

We've been scrupulous in self isolating and talk to people from our window, and zigzag round people during walks. We spend some time in the front of other people's gardens, or in shrubberies, as we dodge oncomers. Most people accommodate others but it's noticeable that many are beginning to relax and not bother so much. Joggers have become everyone's bête noire as they frequently come up from behind, panting, with no mask on, and make no effort of avoidance. And we had a disturbing event in March when two cyclists passing on the road very near to us, turned and very deliberately coughed/shouted in our faces. We had to assume they weren't infected and were just being aggressive but it was shocking. I reported it to the police special virus line, not for any hope of a result but simply to record it.

Diarist 3404 (female, 60s, South West England, retired curator)

We take [. . .] our state-sanctioned daily exercise [. . .] via narrow paths through the allotments and alongside the railway, so there is a dance as we meet others coming the other way and try to maintain social distance, squeezing into the hedge and nettles or turning away. All very polite, we thank each other for keeping well away.

Diarist 3567 (male, 60s, North West England, retired engineer)

I go for a walk [. . .] As I make my way to the woods I see a neighbour walking towards me with his daughter. We perform the new social dance, who will move out of the way to follow the 2 metre separation guidance?

I move away to the far side of the grass verge and we have a socially distanced chat for a few minutes. It is even stranger than usual as this neighbour has only just come out of isolation having contracted Covid-19 about three weeks ago. All my instincts are to stay as far away from him as possible but I didn't feel that I could just walk away – it would have hardly been a neighbourly thing to do.

Diarist 3808 (female, 70s, North East England, retired school inspector)

1.30pm Out for our daily walk. We go via a local cash machine. I use disposable gloves to insert my card, press the key pad and take the money. I always carry some hand wipes or sanitiser too. We keep our 2 metre distance from other walkers, sometimes using the main road to do so [. . .] We have had to abandon walking in a local steep sided, wooded, dene because narrow paths make social distancing almost impossible. It is a favourite spot of young, fit runners who pant alarmingly (virus spreaders?) as they flash by.

Diarist 3987 (female, 70s, South West England, milliner)

Tango has been an essential aspect of my life for many years now. It is my main social activity and my main source of exercise [. . .] Now there is no tango. I last danced at a milonga on 2nd February. I suspect it will be a long time until I feel safe enough to dance so closely with another person again.

STAY HOME

During spring 2020, if they weren't key workers, people were asked to stay home. What this meant for people depended on their situations, roles and preferences. Those living alone were at risk of suffering loneliness. Those living apart from partners had difficult decisions to make about whether to move in together at the beginning of lockdown or not. For those who did, they found their relationship put under intense pressure. For those who didn't, the temptation to break lockdown rules was particularly strong. As for roles, the 'Stay home' instruction had particular consequences for women. In many households, they were still expected to do more of the cooking, cleaning and washing. There was now more of all such things. Some women were also used to having a little space and time to themselves at home. There was now less of this, as well as the freedom it represented. Still, some women appreciated the reduced pressure to dress up, wear makeup and watch their diet during lockdown. As for preferences, people who enjoyed their own company and found the pace of life prior to the pandemic too busy and stressful – all that commuting, all those extra curricula activities – found lockdown relaxing. They appreciated the slower mornings, the time to cook, the quality time with family. Some people only discovered they had such preferences when forced to live differently for a period of time. Of course, there were others who missed going out, seeing friends, losing themselves in the crowd. See also Birdsong; Home schooling; Working from home.

Diarist 8 (female, 14, East of England)

I'm actually enjoying quarantine because I get to be really lazy. When it ends, I'll probably go out to eat or something (I've really missed eating good food).

Diarist 37 (male, 18, London)

I hope to start university in October, yet as I write this there is great uncertainty as to whether universities will teach students face to face on campus, or whether it will all be done virtually through Zoom. Discussing this with my friends, the universal opinion is one of absolute desperation to start university in the autumn and to spend time away from their families who they have been cooped up with for the last two months.

Diarist 81 (female, 15, North West England)

Today is the same as any other normal day. Normal lockdown day I should say. For the past few weeks, I've grown accustomed to my new routine. I will definitely be late back to school on the first day back. Lockdown isn't so bad. I get to lie in, do my work in my own time, and eat whenever I feel like it! I don't miss my friends as much as I should do. I'm not sure what this means.

Diarist P293 (female, 30s, London, hairdresser and account manager)

Around 9.30am, [daughter] and I walked round to my sister's house which is about a 10 minute walk away. Although not strictly allowed we do regularly visit each other's houses, ring the bell, then quickly stand at the end of the path [. . .] The main reason for our visit today was for me to use their bathroom scales – mine are unreliable. I need to weigh myself once a week and then report back to my Slimming World Consultant [. . .] The scales were handed over the gate so that I could weigh myself in the street. Something I never would have done before Corona!

We do our best when visiting to stay 2 metres apart. But it is very difficult with the children. You can see that they are desperate to play closely with one another. I can't wait to hug and kiss my 2 nieces and my gorgeous baby nephew who is 1 next week, but for now that's all strictly off limits.

Before lunch, [daughter] and I made a huge rainbow for our front window. We used lots of crayons, paints, stickers, scraps of paper, glitter etc. to decorate it. [Daughter] was quite engaged and I love doing things like this anyway. One good thing about Lock Down is spending lots of quality time with [family]. On the other hand, it has been hard at times keeping [daughter] occupied for 12 hours a day largely in the house. I try not to rely on TV too much, so we've done lots of crafts, outdoor play (in the garden), puzzles, snap etc.

[Partner] has just taken [daughter] out for some daily 'exercise'. Think they are walking to the local park for a bit of a run around. This means I can get some precious time alone.

Diarist 482 (male, 40s, South East England, fundraiser)

My friend in Berlin wrote a luxurious reply to an email and really caught the mood of what this whole thing is like for couples in lockdown – he suggested he and his boyfriend have become somewhat infantile and, this is not a direct quote, cutesy. And I agree. So have we. What we're like here and now in our home, we would not be like in public. It would be embarrassing if we were.

Diarist 486 (female, 80s, Midlands, retired).

I am a widow [. . .], my husband died nearly six years ago of the effects of post polio syndrome. I still miss him enormously [. . .] I found life a big challenge since my husband died [. . .] However, I have learned to adapt, in particular to be comfortable in my own company, whilst also finding a social life through volunteering at our local library, at a large National Trust property nearby and at our local civic society. I sing in a small community choir, and love going to classical symphony concerts with friends [. . .] All this changed radically and rapidly with the advance of the coronavirus Covid 19 pandemic. Since the government's requirement of a lockdown on 23 March, I have stayed mainly at home, only emerging for a walk of around half an hour a day. I am fortunate in having the support of a home help one morning a week, and a gardener ditto. We are all very careful to keep our distance (minimum 2M) and with handwashing etc. I can't think how I would manage without them, or indeed without my garden, which has been a marvellous place of escape and activity through the past seven weeks (which feels much longer). But what I struggle with most of all is the physical isolation: it's called social distancing, but it isn't, it is very much physical distancing, and I long for a hug with a good friend and my family. It feels as if this is going on for ever.

Diarist 564 (female, 13, Scotland)

I can no longer go to school and sitting at my desk in my bedroom is exhausting. I miss my friends so much, as I am no longer allowed to see them in person. Talking to them through a phone screen is not enough. I want to hug them and joke around. But I can't.

Diarist 635 (female, 13, North West England)

The start of lockdown for me was on the 20th of March 2020. This is when we finished [school] for I don't know how long. The last day was really sad but fun at the same time. We finished at 1pm. There was hardly anyone in, but we had fun anyway. We got lots of photos which I will treasure forever! During that day we watched a Netflix movie and ate a few too many sweets. Everyone was hugging each other, some were crying.

Diarist 746 (female, 40s, London, consultant)

I'm in my 9th week of social isolation and staying at home. The nearest previous experience in my life to this weird suspended animation has been those days between Christmas and New Year, not venturing far from the sofa or fridge and not knowing what day of the week it is. Only this is going on for far longer and my wine, gin and cheese consumption is, if anything, higher than Christmas.

Diarist 924 (female, 30s, Scotland, midwife)

Lockdown makes me feel so alone. Living rurally away from friends makes me feel so alone. Being a parent of two young children makes me feel so alone. I am worried. I am sad. I am angry. I want to be around people who can support and love me but I feel I can't. Lockdown has me trapped at home. Alone. That is so hard.

Diarist 1005 (female, 19, West Midlands, student)

The world outside feels like it's stopped. You'd think, with less cars on the road and our near-ghost towns, that we were living through the apocalypse like it's *The Walking Dead*. There's no guns, no riots in the street, no gore; our 'apocalypse' is sitting indoors with our hand sanitisers on a throne of loo rolls, arming ourselves with gloves and masks when we step outside, and sharing the best bread-making tips on Twitter.

Diarist 1033 (female, 40s, South West England, author)

I started dinner. I normally love cooking, but it's become more of a chore now everyone is at home for EVERY meal. Well, I started making what I thought would be one thing (a sort of chicken in white wine cream and tarragon sauce with mash) and then realised I was missing so many ingredients half way through (because shopping has just become so random, what you can get, when). So it morphed into a 'chicken with any herbs I could find and green peppers in tomato sauce (and chuck in some cream and cheese)' with rice.

Everyone ate it, though. Win.

Diarist 1060 (male, 20s, East of England, scientist)

Overall, I feel pretty content with how everything is. Whilst I miss being able to see my family as everything is in lockdown, I am enjoying that I can spend so much time with my new-born daughter at the start of her life.

Diarist 1088 (female, 40s, London, doctor)

Today we had another of the type of days that have become the norm for my family and I since lockdown. We don't worry much about clock time; we wake whenever is natural for us [. . .] I worked as a hospital doctor until my pregnancy with my second child [. . .] Before lockdown we had a busy life with clubs and activities and dashing around at weekends and holidays. But we can't go anywhere, so we enjoy the garden and the stillness and small pleasures and being together [. . .] (the only negative effect of the kids being home full time is the permanent state of apocalypse the house is in!).

Diarist 1157 (female, 40s, London, archivist)

My partner [. . .] is married and in lock down with his wife [. . .] We have broken the lock down rules to see each other once a week in these difficult times. We both miss each other dreadfully and have been writing to each other throughout the lockdown. These letters are a great source of joy to me.

Diarist 1289 (female, 50s, South East England, creative producer and artistic director)

I am in a long term relationship, though we live separately; we're finding the lockdown is unbearable.

Diarist 1366 (male, 20s, South East England, student)

I have not left the house today. This is probably a bad idea, but overall the lockdown is not hitting me as hard as some others. I am naturally isolationist, so the lack of human contact touches me but a little – sometimes I miss friends, but mostly I get by, with the comfort my girlfriend brings me. I really feel for those who are alone at this time. One of my best friends was meant to get married this summer (I was to be the best man), but he and his fiancé are separated by the lockdown. It must be hard on them.

Diarist 1443 (female, 60s, North West England, project manager)

I've been on 'lock-down' since March so haven't been doing an awful lot really. Prior to 'lock-down' I didn't do that much either really – as I work from home and am perfectly happy with my own company. In fact, I have probably been in training for 'lock-down' all my life.

Diarist 1451 (female, 60s, Northern Ireland, retired teacher)

There is a new community garden project near us to which we planned to give spare plants. But we ended up asking our friend who lives alone whether she would like them, and we arranged to hand them over like spies at a quiet drop spot, without breathing on each other. She wanted to return books I'd lent. We put the plants and books on the ground and stepped away to let the other pick things up. We had our first slightly illicit walk on the beach, illicit because we walked two metres apart from our friend and talked loudly across at each other. We met no other people. The long beach was empty. I was glad to see her, but the main reason for this distanced walk is that I know she is very lonely so I felt it was OK to stretch a rule a bit.

Diarist 1491 (male, 20s, North West England, student)

My family is a family of four [. . .] Luckily, we are all together and have been for the last 8 weeks in lockdown, which has occasionally been frustrating as we all like our own space. However, the experience has generally been quite nice as we have found comfort and reassurance through being with one another which has maintained our morale. If I may say so myself, my family and I have not put a foot wrong during the lockdown and have made sure we have followed the rules properly and we have tried to go for the necessary shop we are allowed as little as possible and usually just one family member goes for a big shop. We have all been really frustrated, angry and annoyed when we have heard or seen people on the news and social media breaking the lockdown rules! I do not think we have gone a day of the lockdown without having a little rant about the inconsiderate nature of some people who completely lack any common sense or care for the most vulnerable of our society [. . .] It is very frustrating seeing people break the rules and the government softening the restrictions, as although I am very fortunate that all four of my grandparents are still alive, two of them are over 80 and the other two are in their 70s so all four classed as vulnerable [. . .] As for my grandad who has dementia, he lives in the next village and is at a stage in his dementia where he is still able to drive and so keeps driving round to our house at least once a week despite us telling him not to because of Coronavirus but every ten to fifteen minutes he asks why the streets are so empty and he has to observe the 2 metre rule in his local shop. I know people will probably think that him coming around means he is breaking the rules and allowing it is also breaking the rules. However, there is literally nothing we can do to stop him from coming round.

It is usually my mum who, when he comes to the house, stays downstairs in the kitchen with him [. . .] whilst [the rest of us] run upstairs so that we distance ourselves to avoid possibly contracting the virus (he does not have the virus but we cannot [risk] it in case he does or in case the member of our family who has done the weekly shop has contracted it). It really is heart-breaking hearing him have a conversation with my mum downstairs, with him repeating himself and asking why the streets are empty, and I often have to overcome the urge to go downstairs and just give him a hug.

Diarist 1547 (female, 30s, East of England, innovation consultant)

I've always been a bit of a 'home body', in that my main hobbies are baking, reading and gardening. Which means this is the one type of apocalypse I might be suited to surviving!

Diarist 1574 (female, 40s, Wales, public health practitioner)

We finally get our daily exercise. We walk through the park to the beach and have a paddle [. . .] One positive aspect of the lockdown is that we spend much more time together as a family and go out for daily walks and bike rides all together. Before this, we would have only done this at the weekend and my husband and I would have spent more time commuting and taking the girls to various activities. We also have much more close contact with our neighbours – I set up a WhatsApp group as soon as the lockdown happened. We now have over 50 people on it.

Diarist 1582 (female, 50s, West Midlands, office manager)

Been congratulating myself on de limescaling the bathroom taps today. My life's so rock n roll. And I even managed to walk down to the post office in a pair of trainers rather than flip flops. Things are looking up [. . .] G&T at 4.30pm? Don't mind if I do [. . .] It's not like I have to drive anywhere.

Diarist 1591 (female, 80s, South East England, retired teacher and lecturer)

This morning breakfast at 7.30ish. Weetabix, flaked almonds, honey and coffee which I think is decaffeinated. Looking out my big window onto [the road], it's quiet and deserted except for one or two people walking to work. The Brighton train gets in at about 7.30 and the train from London [. . .] at 7.45 and 8.15. Hardly any passengers though. The double decker buses run past my window but there is never anyone on the top decks, and few on the lower.

Diarist 1700 (female, 50s, London, piano teacher)

There have been some amazing positives from this experience – time spent with my daughter, games evenings and quizzes with friends and family online, regular contact on the phone and mealplans for every day – homemade cakes and bread as we have the time to cook and bake [. . .] Time in the garden that is pollution free, birds singing and quiet skies as no aeroplanes fly over. The kindness of people taking food and prescription medicines to the vulnerable and clapping for the NHS on Thursday evenings with many from our street. No stresses of having to entertain or dress up, wear a bra, put on make-up etc. I have learnt to stop stressing about the small things like paint on my daughter's carpet or a disagreement with a friend or family member and hurrying to book tickets for the theatre [. . .] and to appreciate that we are alive and safe.

Diarist 1815 (female, 20s, Scotland, unemployed)

I usually live in a houseshare with five other people, but since a few days before lockdown began I have been staying with my lover in his one-bedroom flat. We decided quite intentionally that we would rather lockdown together for the duration than be separated indefinitely [. . .] I split an orange with him since I'd grated the zest off it. Ugh, sharing an orange, that's some codependent-8-weeks-of-lockdown shit, isn't it? I worry about how we'll cope when the circumstances of our relationship change again, and we spend more time doing things separately, and seeing other people. I worry about how I'll cope, moving back into the shared house. In some ways, this is the purest form of a relationship: only seeing each other, and seeing each other all the time, and knowing there's no easy way to spend more than a few hours apart. I like it more than I thought I would.

Diarist 1857 (male, 11, North East England)

This morning I had a sausage sandwich which was delicious and then I got ready for school but we had to stay two metres apart because we were in this pandemic called covid 19 and basically we had to stay home and the country was in lockdown and I personally hate that because that meant that we couldn't go anywhere we had to literally stay home and protect our NHS and save lives and then we couldn't go like out and one person had to go out to do the shopping and then I just had to sit in the car and just watch the queue go down and then that was hell because I liked shopping and we couldn't go in and then we couldn't go and see family because we were going to their house and yeah that is the coronavirus and that was hell because we couldn't go anywhere.

Diarist 1867 (female, 20s, West Midlands, cabin crew)

My dad [. . .] has to try and work from home because he has a heart condition and is deemed at risk of the virus, so we spend the day together at the kitchen table. Every day we listen to a music quiz called Popmaster on Radio 2 at 10:30. After Popmaster we do a CD to learn French. I am good at neither the quiz nor the French but I enjoy that I get to spend more time with my dad, one of the few good things to come of the virus. After this my dad does some gardening. He gives me an update on how many of the beans have sprouted because that kind of thing is the highlight of the day when you're in a national lockdown.

Diarist 1966 (female, 50s, South East England, administrator)

Dinner with the family. What do you talk about when you are the only people each of you have seen for the past weeks? Not been anywhere or done anything to tell them about.

Diarist 1991 (female, 20s, East of England, student)

I live in a shared house [. . .] I also have a boyfriend who lives round the corner from me. We decided that as we both lived in shared houses [. . .] of young people who aren't at risk we would still go and visit each other during the lockdown. Breaking the rules a bit! But we did agree between our two houses that we were happy about it and if we treated our two houses as 'one house' then it was sort of justified. We are making an effort to be particularly careful when we do go to the shops, to try and make up for the fact that we are going between two houses. Well, I know we are breaking the rules and I could have asked him to move in with me for this period of time, but I have a small room and we only started seeing each other a few months before. Felt a bit soon.

Diarist 2003 (female, 40s, South East England, housewife and artist/designer)

We've just had lunch of baked potatoes. The grown ups had some left over chilli from the freezer and the kids had beans and cheese. We've been having jacket potatoes every Tuesday. I think it's become my favourite day lunch wise cause then I don't have to think about what to feed everyone. Usually I meal plan for dinners but lunches the kids would be having school meals and [husband] would be at work [. . .] However, with everyone here and having to make a week's grocery shop last a week (no popping out if you run out of things) it is easier if I make lunches for everyone. It's hard trying to make food last and everyone has had to change their way of eating. For example, cheese, condiments and milk are being rationed.

Diarist 2044 (female, 30s, London, sociologist)

I'll voice chat with my partner later before bed [. . .] My partner and I are still going to see each other; he is going to walk 2 and a half hours from the other side of London to stay at mine this weekend and in two weeks' time I'll do the same and go to his. This is going to go on for a long time so we all have to find ways to mentally survive as well as being responsible.

Diarist 2056 (female, 50s, Scotland, communications manager)

I measured myself for a bra. Need a new one, even though only sat at home at all times. Underwires are for going out. And we are not. Am not even wearing earrings or the rings I used to wear all the time when going out or to work. Wearing the same clothes on rotation. Strange and makes me wonder when I will wear the other 'good' clothes again. It is going to be weird choosing different clothes for when we are released.

Diarist 2143 (female, 50s, North West England, secretary)

2.30pm. [Husband] is in from the shed and rummaging in the fridge. We seem to do this a lot whilst we're staying at home. It's a shame he leaves the fruit and eats the sweets.

Diarist 2290 (female, 30s, Scotland, historian)

After dinner we put on CBeebies bedtime shows and my husband and son play with Duplo. I disappear into the bedroom for 30 minutes – during lockdown this is the only time I will be in a room by myself for the entire day.

Diarist 2354 (female, 30s, South East England, lawyer)

We all had pasta for dinner [. . .] I love cooking, but three meals a day at home gets a bit much sometimes.

Diarist 2408 (female, 40s, London, theatre worker)

A call from my partner who I have not seen since lockdown began! He is on the other side of London. We are used to being apart as we live separately and his work keeps us apart during the week most of the time but this is the longest we have ever gone without seeing each other! We are contemplating him visiting this weekend in a slightly socially distanced way (he'll come in the house, but no physical contact!) – I know this is breaking the rules but we have been good so far!

Diarist 2627 (female, 40s, Northern Ireland, editor)

At the beginning I thought about my inner resources, my long yet varied experience of having to put up with things, and I thought I would be fine. But although I still see the freedom that there is in restriction, and for all the conscious delight I took in stations, airports, galleries and cafes, it's only now that I appreciate what rest I found in motion and what true solitude there was for me in a crowd.

I am fine. Mostly because routine helps me [. . .] So, on this diary day, I got up at 0500. Since the lockdown started, I have kept the blinds in my room open and when I see that it's morning, I'm glad to have made it through another night. The windows and the [BBC] World Service help me to feel part of the world.

Diarist 2709 (female, 50s, East of England, pharmacist)

Life is very different at the moment as my husband is working from home, in our kitchen-dining room so when I get home from work I cannot follow my normal routine of having the radio on in the kitchen and doing the tidying/preparing supper and things – what I call pottering. Having my adult sons at home means more washing, cleaning, shopping, and altered routines.

Diarist 2721 (female, 40s, North West England, clinician)

I pop down to see the friend I co-habited with for the first 4 weeks of lockdown. I know it is bending the rules but I square it in that I was living with her a couple of weeks back so I figure her house is an extension of mine. I'm sure others would judge but I think we all have our interpretation of the rules and as long as we're broadly following and not taking the piss . . .

Diarist 2880 (female, 60s, East Midlands, retired librarian)

Being retired and living on my own, in a nice house with a garden, in a pleasant area, has meant that I haven't been psychologically affected too much by C19. I enjoy my own company and have plenty to do.

However C19 affects everything I do (used to do!) outside the home. No trips to large supermarkets, visits to [local towns]; libraries, churches & coffee shops closed. No society meetings or seminars at the university. I haven't been on a bus since early March. Rarely use the car [. . .] Safe at home it seems utterly unbelievable that the virus is devastating the world.

Diarist 3245 (female, 30s, South West England, painter and decorator)

We are going for a walk with my cousin. I am taking her some weed; I have also taken some to my brother. Despite what the law says I believe it's an essential service, their normal dealers are reluctant to be out and about as it is much harder to be inconspicuous and you are much more likely to be pulled over by the police [. . .] A few of us in my family smoke, I think it really helps with the type of minds that we have. I didn't make any money from my cousin, so I'm not dealing just gifting, helping [. . .] Google maps takes us through a well-kept housing estate where people are out the front of their gardens staring at us . . .I begin to sweat. I get angry at being here and just want to fuck off back home now. The pub car park where my cousin wants to meet is filled with signs telling people not to park there and the owners are present moving old furniture out of the pub. More stern looks. I feel very naughty!

Diarist 3367 (female, 50s, South East England, priest and bookseller)

As I house share with my sister, we have divided our days into upstairs and downstairs time, so we don't get on each other's nerves or disturb each other. Luckily today is an upstairs day for me so I can be in the office.

Diarist 3404 (female, 60s, South West England, retired curator)

I am at home all day drinking tea all day. I am trying not to eat biscuits.

Diarist 3890 (female, 40s, London, urban designer)

I decide to [do some gardening in the back garden]. It doesn't take me long to find my anger. I return inside but I can't control or ignore it. [The neighbours had] done the same thing on Easter Sunday: but that time it was different people: an older couple. They sat together eating lunch outside, chatting happily [. . .] This time it's a younger family, sitting together with them on their patio relaxing and chatting in the sun. I think of the other neighbours who live in the upstairs flats that overlook theirs and my garden; the kids that don't have a garden to run into, the number of people squeezing themselves into 2 bedrooms, the precarious jobs and lives, the rent that might not be being paid, the paramedics that came one night to the family above me in masks and gloves and aprons, the people above us that clap every Thursday, stay at home, do things the right way despite the greater effect this will have for them [. . .] It's enough. I go out. I stand on my garden sofa and look them in the eye. I shout (and I swear). I say the words 'responsibility', 'r-number', 'risk'. They shout back. It's not my business. Anyway, they are being safe. I end 'but you don't know that, you don't know anything', and go back in shaking.

Diarist 3987 (female, 70s, South West England, milliner)

Staying at home each day means there is very little structure or variety to my time, beyond that which we create for ourselves. I try to maintain a balance around my usual routines of meal times and relaxation. I very much miss meeting my friends and tango dancing. Each day I try to introduce new music, a short dance, a little gardening.

Diarist 4336 (female, 60s, Scotland, retired social worker)

After my usual breakfast of cereal, fresh fruit and yoghurt I had a shower and got ready to meet my friend [. . .] to go for a walk on a Golf Course about two miles from where I live. This is not strictly abiding by the rules [. . .] as we're not meant to encounter other people not living in your household. But we both live alone and it's not always easy going out on solo long strolls.

Diarist 4447 (female, 50s, London, art psychotherapist)

I watched [the evening news] and made myself a light supper of toast and marmite and an improvised salad of a red pepper, carrot and garlic. I love raw garlic and another Covid Silver Lining is that I can eat this as much as I like at the moment and not bother anyone with my smelly breath.

Diarist 4610 (female, 30s, South East England, maternity nurse)

Never in my working life have I spent so much time to just 'be' at home. Or to spend so much time with my wife. I miss the rest of our family [. . .] That's been the hardest part for us. But there is so much of the lockdown lifestyle I would love to keep for ever. Less cars on the roads, more time just to be with family at home, no rushing, no appointments. The pace of life which allows for early nights, daily yoga sessions, proper unrushed mealtimes, gardening, knitting and reading. It is enough to make me wonder how life became so messy and busy. This stripped back version of life has a lot going for it.

Diarist 4671 (female, 20s, Yorkshire and Humber, carer)

Can't actually remember the last time we all got up, dressed and ate breakfast by 8am. Like one big school holiday without the outings and with added fear and despair.

On with my day, washing up is done, washer is on, I swear the lack of getting dressed has in no way decreased the washing pile.

Diarist 4755 (male, 8, Yorkshire and Humber)

I'm not going to school but I am still learning in homeschool. It feels very different. I can still see my friends but only in a screen. I can still play football but only in the garden. I don't really like it.

(DOG) WALKING

In the weeks prior to 12 May, people were allowed to leave the house for one form of exercise per day. This became the 'daily walk' for many people, especially those with dogs needing walks. It was a risk. People tried to stay 2 metres away from other walkers. They tried to avoid touching gates and stiles. But it was also a pleasure. People would get a break from their rooms and computer screens. They would get a chance to relax and chat. They would see neighbours (at a distance). They would nose around the local streets, exploring and checking out people's front gardens. Over time, the same paths could become boring, but not for those people who walked daily and noted how the paths changed with the seasons: new flowers bloomed, new birds arrived and new kinds of litter were dropped – most notably, as the pandemic took hold, facemasks and gloves. See also Birdsong; Stay apart.

Diarist P125 (female, 30s, South East England, nurse)

The three of us walked in the open field near our house. The baby and I didn't touch anything and my husband only touched our door – such strange times. We spoke with a couple of neighbours at 2m apart and the baby enjoyed seeing people other than us!

Diarist 422 (male, 70s, South West England, garage forecourt worker)

After various household tasks we went out for a 3 mile circular walk which turned out to be a celebration of spring time in Devon. Lambs, bluebells and fresh green trees and fields. Although we used popular local footpaths we met only half a dozen other people. Stopped to chat (at a safe distance) to a lady exercising a young German Shepherd dog she was looking after, prior to his entry into training to be a guide dog. Were we breaking the rules?

Diarist 445 (male, 60s, London, retired banker)

On our daily walks, signs are appearing sometimes on the pavement about keeping 2 metres apart. Very sensible, but I don't remember voting to use French measurements.

Diarist 699 (female, 40s, North East England, nurse)

Kids are starting to get ready to go on our daily walk as a family. It usually lasts about an hour and it's lovely being able to get outdoors into the fresh air. You see, we're only allowed out of our house once for exercise, to do essential shopping or to go to work. We usually walk past my parent's house to say hello through the window as we are unable to go into their house. It's another rule to keep everyone safe!

Diarist 1022 (female, 50s, Scotland, nurse/carer)

My break [. . .] so me and my mature mini-dachshund set off up the hill [. . .] We pass maybe half a dozen other walkers and their dogs during our hour out, all keeping our respectful 2m distance (or more like 10m in most cases) but also saying a few friendly words to each other. I've noticed a significant upturn in friendliness and mannerliness since lockdown. Smiles, eye contact, a desire to connect – it's universal.

Diarist 1072 (male, 30s, East of England, IT engineer)

After lunch we went out for our walk around the block. The roads seemed busier (although they have been getting busier for the last few weeks). Some people are wearing masks and gloves while others don't seem to care and will walk right past you, not keeping the two metre distance. I'm somewhere in between. I don't think a mask will be of any benefit but I still think we should keep the distance.

Diarist 1247 (female, 60s, West Midlands, NHS worker)

I and my husband take [dog] out for a walk. We chat about the virus and my day. My husband seems relaxed and happy. I think we are happy to be out together and enjoy our new park, doubled in size since the covid crisis as the golf course is open to us.

Diarist 1316 (female, 30s, Scotland, school counsellor)

Everyone is a bit irritable and the dawdling and indecisiveness lead to a snap decision to go out for a walk, though we have walked pretty much everywhere we can go locally. We head out for a walk, and observe our neighbour and two friends he doesn't live with all getting out of the same car, seemingly flouting the social distancing rules. Our walk is a variation on a circular walk through a field of rape we walked round the other day, and tensions mount as we are forced to cross the road several times to avoid pedestrians coming from the other direction.

We get home and all are tired.

Diarist 1341 (male, 60s, East of England, retired doctor)

After a cup of tea my wife and I have a walk together. It's a 5 km walk through trees and farmland right from our doorstep. We are really fortunate. The highlight was seeing a fledgling Goldfinch and its parent sitting in the tree above us. As we walked together we chatted and occasionally held hands.

Diarist 1612 (female, 17, Yorkshire and Humber)

I didn't manage to get out for a walk today but probably should tomorrow because I'm going to bed feeling stuffy and slightly stressed.

Diarist 2037 (female, 20s, East of England, PhD student)

Our [dog] begins to stir at around 5pm because he knows that my fiancé will be imminently coming down the stairs ready for our early evening dog walk [. . .] We walk around the development in several different routes being nosy at what other people have done with their front gardens.

Diarist 2164 (male, 40s, London, student)

On my walk the other day I saw a rubber glove, inflated and tied off at the wrist, lying in the grass [Figure 4] It had a tension within it which made me half-expect it to scuttle away.

Diarist 2205 (male, 70s, North West England, retired teacher)

As it's still cold this afternoon, I'm not sure whether to go for a walk. I need walks to maintain muscle strength, but sometimes can't be arsed.

Diarist 2466 (female, 20s, South East England, unemployed)

I went for a walk along the beach with my mum this evening. It was lovely and sunny, and we stopped at a café and got coffee and ice cream. Most places are still shut, but a few have opened to do takeaway service only. I think mum would go crazy otherwise as she

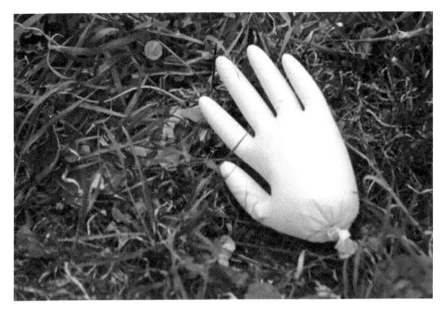

Figure 4 'On my walk the other day I saw a rubber glove.' Image submitted by Diarist 2164.

loves her cafes! It was nice to sit on the beach and watch the waves. The ice cream scoops were mint and chocolate, the combination tasted like After Eights.

Diarist 2471 (female, 30s, London, unemployed)

Walking down the residential streets, I noted that the roses have bloomed. We first had the blossom, then the Wisteria and now the roses are out – I've never noticed these changes before but it's lovely seeing the bursts of colour as I explore my local area.

Diarist 2519 (male, 60s, East of England, retired teacher)

In the afternoon, I went for a long walk (about 5km) in the country. I went with a friend although we are not supposed to do that until tomorrow. We kept social distancing. The walk made me feel better. Being outside, among trees and fields is better than any amount of anti-depressants!

Diarist 2880 (female, 60s, East Midlands, retired librarian)

Decided to forego yoga [. . .] and go for a walk as the forecast was for clouding over late morning. Wore a thick jumper and walking shoes, but with a thin wind-proof jacket. As

I live alone I texted my daughter to let her know my route and texted when I was home safely.

Diarist 2948 (male, 50s, Yorkshire and Humber, retired GP)

We ventured out for our evening's walk [. . .] It was a joy to be connecting with nature and not the laptop. The bluebells, may and horse chestnut blossom were something to behold and the crescendo of the birdsong was a delight as the sun began to set.

Diarist 3051 (female, 70s, London, retired stage manager and personal assistant)

We decided to go for our daily walk before lunch while it was still sunny. We walk every day and I feel almost superstitious about it now and would hate to miss a day [. . .] We've been discovering alleys, small lanes, and areas of green and woodland – parts that we haven't known before. Looking at houses that we've only driven past before is interesting too. We've hardly used the car at all.

Diarist 3426 (male, 70s, West Midlands, historian)

06.55 Left house, with dog, on a bright, still, frosty morning. Took with me my litter-picking 'grabber', because part of my entertainment on dog-walks is to pick up litter and take it to the nearest bin. BC (i.e. before the Covid-19 pandemic), I just used to pick up the odd can or bottle, but feel that these days it would not be sensible to handle such items any more. The litter-picker makes the task safe.

Diarist 4766 (female, 60s, East of England, family support specialist)

I decided years ago that while I was walking through the forest I might as well pick up the litter. I go armed with my litter picker and my husband kindly carries the bag. We probably walked for about 2 hours in the forest. We go off track and rarely see anyone. If we do, physical distancing is always maintained. It's become a natural response, although it continues to feel rude. I keep hoping I'll find some treasure, but, last week I did find a five pound note. The litter has changed from the usual poo bags, glass/plastic bottles etc. to face masks and rubber gloves.

WHATSAPP

Locked down, separated from family and friends, people connected via social media: WhatsApp groups (for family, friends and neighbours), but also Facebook, Messenger, Instagram, Twitter, e-mail and text. Groups were set up to provide mutual support. Information was shared, allowing people to keep in touch. Photos were shared, allowing people to display achievements and perhaps to compete. Funny memes and videos were shared to keep up morale. Under the guise of sharing jokes, people checked up on each other, making sure others were coping. Initially, there was much enthusiasm and a flurry of activity on such platforms. Over time, some people tired of receiving notifications and the demands often indicated by such notifications. Some wondered how to extricate themselves from new groups and associated obligations. See also Stay home, Zoom.

Diarist 39 (female, 40s, London, actuary)

At the start of Lockdown, the communications (WhatsApp, Facebook, FaceTime, Zoom, Skype, Houseparty) went into overdrive. There's one WhatsApp group that I have muted [. . .] I can't cope with the endless memes.

Diarist 119 (male, 60s, South West England, retired teacher)

One positive aspect of the crisis is the resurgence or rediscovery of community spirit. We are part of the village WhatsApp group providing support for everyone in the village, many of whom are elderly or vulnerable. We offer services such as shopping or collecting prescriptions or just someone to chat to on the phone.

Diarist 189 (female, 70s, North West England, nurse)

Our road's WhatsApp group has been bemoaning the late delivery of the post today and confirming just which rubbish bins are being collected. Oh the daily drum beat of trivia.

Diarist 1035 (female, 30s, East Midlands, manager for manufacturer)

Checked my phone messages again, as both our Facebook Messenger group with [. . .] friends from uni in it and my family WhatsApp group with extended family (cousins and aunts) have both been very active over lockdown. My family have been setting each other a challenge a week for something to do. This week's challenge is to make a zipwire for a cuddly toy, so I have a video to watch of one of my aunt's attempts in her garden.

Diarist 1097 (female, 20s, London, technology consultant)

It should be noted ahead of time that at continual intervals throughout the day I both sourced, sent and received excellent memes via Instagram from friends [. . .] Sometime in the afternoon my cousin group chat on WhatsApp kicked off about an image of a deer one of my cousins' dads collected as roadkill, and butchered for its meat. The vegetarians were outraged, it caused carnage [. . .] 7.30pm – start family quiz on WhatsApp. 3 teams made up of 3 families, my cousins. Each team provided 2 quiz rounds and sent all questions in the group chat. Everyone then had 10 mins to write down their answers. When the time is up, the person who wrote the round provides the answers and each team submits their scores. Our rounds were famous faces and music. Our team won this week by 4 points with 88 total!

Also throughout this time shared hilarious videos mocking Boris Johnson's Sunday address to the nation that just caused significant confusion.

Diarist 1270 (female, 30s, East Midlands, unemployed)

Having found a couple of funny animal videos on Twitter, I WhatsApped the links to a friend in York and one in Cancun and when the replies ('crying with laughter' emojis) come I feel a welcome sense of togetherness.

Diarist 1346 (female, 60s, Scotland, retired doctor)

Keeping in touch with friends and family and neighbours – I allow an hour every morning and more if other activities haven't taken over. This is so complicated and overwhelming. Texts, Facebook, email, WhatsApp, FaceTime, phone calls, Zoom . . . which could completely take over. Today I respond to our friend's email [...], speak to the grandchildren on FaceTime, check our son alone [. . .] is OK, find [funny videos] to send to our friend in Australia, fill in my COVID tracker app [. . .] send a comforting quote on the impossibility of home schooling primary school children while working from home to our daughter, WhatsApp friends – admiring their artwork and other distractions and check discretely if we have seen our very elderly neighbours out in their garden. Yet again I have not tackled my list of people I need, want or have promised contact. There is always tomorrow.

Diarist 1405 (male, 60s, London, lawyer)

The lockdown has really brought our local community together. My wife and a neighbour set up a WhatsApp group for mutual support and to maintain a feeling of togetherness. This has worked really well – almost everyone in our street and even around has joined, and is sharing supportive, witty, thoughtful comments, and sharing Ocado deliveries.

Diarist 1426 (female, 40s, North West England, doctor)

I did some tidying and vacuum cleaning, then spent some time (more than I planned, unfortunately) on social media (Facebook, WhatsApp) catching up with friends and work colleagues. At the beginning of the COVID19 crisis, one of my work colleagues set up a WhatsApp group for the team to share information. It has been a great source of support and also of humour – we often share funny 'memes' relating to the COVID situation (common themes include the frustrations of being relatively isolated in lockdown, the hygiene and social distancing recommendations, homeschooling children, and the weekly tradition of the public clapping for the NHS/carers at 8pm every Thursday).

Diarist 1604 (male, 20s, Yorkshire and Humber, graphic designer and communications officer)

Mum calls on WhatsApp at 5:45, as she has every day during the crisis. I don't mind as it's nice to have human contact, but I am slightly starting to fret about what the etiquette is for going back to our more usual schedule of chatting every week or so.

Diarist 1679 (female, 30s, London, software engineer)

At lunch I tried out a craft hack from a tweeted video, to make a mask out of a sock. I have a bunch of my partner's old socks lying around but they are not the best material for this. I catch up with my friends on WhatsApp – we have one chat for COVID related subjects and another chat for 'general'. I finally have sock mask success with one of my own (thinner) socks. I post a selfie to the COVID WhatsApp group, where my friends are showing off their own efforts.

Diarist 1794 (female, 70s, East Midlands, retired teacher)

Lockdown has meant a crash course in social media for many of us – we are Zooming tomorrow for a friend's birthday – but there is nothing quite like a phone call. We are also in several WhatsApp groups, mostly set up during lockdown, so the mobile pings all day with messages, photos, information, and rude videos about Donald Trump.

Diarist 1940 (female, 30s, Scotland, assistant professor)

During lockdown, I've become totally addicted to WhatsApp. Before the pandemic I'd never used it; now it's my main way of finding a sense of companionship during the day. I exchange daily messages with a least three friends and my Mum.

Diarist 1979 (female, 60s, South East England, editor and retired nurse)

Check Facebook and emails [. . .] A few family photos from the weekend on our 'Love and Support' WhatsApp group that I started at the beginning of all this. It's turned into a good natured 'my baby's cleverer than your baby' competition, but it brings us together. We've used it less this week as stamina is waning, but I'll keep it going for a time when one of us might really need another.

Diarist 2069 (female, 30s, East Midlands, scientist)

It has been hard being so far away from family during this situation, not being able to help and not knowing when (or if, in the case of my two elderly grandmothers) I will see them again. I am incredibly grateful for messaging services and social media. My mum, however, has been very demanding, keeping me on the phone for well over an hour every day. I love her, but for my sanity I decided not to call her today.

Diarist 2070 (male, 70s, South West England, administrator)

Checked email – nothing from friends. A flurry of exchanges at the start of lockdown with geographically-distant friends has tailed off.

Diarist 2390 (male, 60s, South East England, customs officer)

I got up late, had a lazy breakfast and spent too long on Twitter catching up with the news and seeing what those I follow have been up to. I also looked at all the jokes and short video clips that I've been getting on WhatsApp and forwarding many to friends and acquaintances. It's a good way of keeping in touch and for some it's been a great help, including one distant friend who, after a couple of weeks of exchanging messages, informed me that he's recovering from an operation for cancer. The poor chap is now going through chemotherapy. It was humbling to hear that the messages had in some way helped him.

Diarist 2476 (female, 50s, London, personal assistant)

Flicked through our WhatsApp group and more funny videos, especially re. PM's Corona virus address on Sunday! Forwarded them on to friends and family, we all need the laughs these days!

Diarist 2627 (female, 40s, Northern Ireland, editor)

I send off quick emails, saying *I hope you don't mind this message coming out of the blue . . . it's just . . . I had been thinking of you.* Covid-19 has made me bolder, in some ways [. . .] Replies when they come are like jewels and they remind me that I know the best, most brilliant people. It delights me to have their voices in my head.

WORKING FROM HOME

To control the virus, those who could were asked to work from home at various points during the pandemic. Such people recognized they were lucky, in that working from home generally meant less risk of catching the virus. There were other advantages to working from home. Not having to commute freed up money, but also time – for more relaxed morning routines, better meals, exercise, hobbies. Freed from the office, people could shower less, do their hair less, wear more casual clothes – even pyjamas, at least on the bottom half not visible on screen – listen to their own choice of music, get on with completing discrete work tasks and worry less about distractions from colleagues or surveillance from managers. There were also disadvantages. Some tasks where co-presence helps – e.g. training – were difficult to do well via videoconferencing software. Some people missed the camaraderie of the workplace and the energy they get from being with colleagues. Virtual coffee mornings could only partly replace their face-to-face equivalents. Back-to-back meetings on Zoom, Skype or Teams were found draining by many. Homes were full of distractions: housework, gardening, snacks, pets, children. People had trouble keeping work and home separate, since they now happened in the same spaces and, with many people juggling work and childcare or home schooling during the pandemic, at less predictable times. Certain rituals could help people keep work and home separate – changing clothes or computers at the end of the working day, or leaving the house for a walk after work – but only so much. Home workstations built from dining tables, sideboards, shelving units, chests of drawers, piles of books, ironing boards and so on could be uncomfortable and leave people with neck, back and shoulder pain. Working from home was especially difficult and disruptive for those living in small, crowded spaces, without access to spare rooms or garden offices. Quiet and privacy were lacking in such households. One homeworker's need for quiet and privacy had consequences for other household members, who had to adjust their usual activities accordingly. See also Guilt; Home schooling; Luck; Stay home; Zoom.

Diarist 14 (female, 30s, London, film producer)

I'm a film producer, so working during lockdown is a bit strange. We're developing lots of projects, so there's plenty to do, but I'm used to going to the office every day and used to the social aspects of work too. In truth, though, I rather like working from home. It's extremely quiet, as I live alone, but I find it fairly easy to concentrate (most of the time!). And I don't miss the 1.5 hour commute to work. The plus side of the pandemic is that I've got my mornings and evenings back. I love not having to get on the tube, squashed like sardines, and I love being able to go for a run before work and have the time in the evening to do things I enjoy (play the guitar, read a book, sew a quilt, cook, talk to friends/family on Zoom).

Diarist 250 (male, 30s, Yorkshire and Humber, researcher)

I'm writing this sitting in my kitchen, where I've been nosing around eating a hodge-podge breakfast – the end of a loaf of bread and a banana. I'm struggling to find any motivation to start on the day's work [. . .] Last week I was on holiday, which meant more time outside, but of course returning to the same rooms, eating the same food. It didn't exactly feel like a holiday, although I did feel rested by the end. Now I'm back 'in the office', so to speak, it doesn't really seem like anything has changed, except that I feel a returning sense of guilt for the work tasks I'm avoiding.

Diarist 390 (female, 20s, Yorkshire and Humber, furniture installations coordinator)

[Partner] is working from home at the moment. We only have a small flat and so it's difficult not to trip over each other and for me not to get in the way. He sticks to the spare

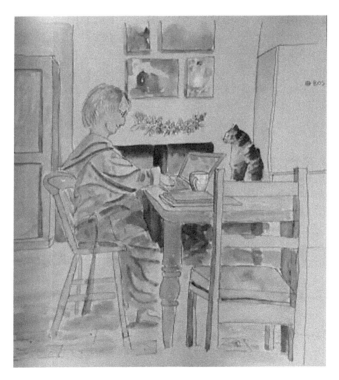

Figure 5 'I am enjoying not having to think about what to wear to go to work.' Image submitted by Diarist 484.

room and I stick to the living room/kitchen (it's one room) – sound does carry though so I don't have the telly on too loud! [. . .] [Partner] had his appraisal in the other room so put on Great British Menu – didn't want to overhear or seem to be earwigging!

Diarist 484 (female, 60s, Yorkshire and Humber, charity administrator)

I am enjoying not having to think about what to wear to go to work but it's very weird working in pyjamas and dressing gown [Figure 5] I could get used to this though! I only have to get dressed for a team meeting via Zoom at 11.00 am. The only downside to working from home is my cats who are wanting my attention and try to sit on my lap or on the laptop.

Diarist 602 (female, 50s, Wales, university tutor)

I love working from home, as a creative person, this suits me just fine. I can get more work done and even type when I am in meetings because I can't be seen. I love seeing people's ghastly wall decorations in the team meetings. I pretend to be the taste police; yesterday I saw someone's pyjamas on the back of the door; some people have bed hair!

Diarist 776 (male, 20s, South East England, journalist)

Since I am working from home, I don't shower as often as I did. Most days I wash myself in the sink basin with a bar of soap and a flannel. It sounds absolutely minging when I write it out like this.

Diarist 901 (female, 30s, London, unemployed)

My working housemate clears out the living room for a work call. After 8 weeks of living together, we've mostly worked out the kinks of our week-day dynamic. She tells me what to do and I do it quickly and quietly.

Diarist 1035 (female, 30s, East Midlands, manager for manufacturer)

6:30 – alarm goes off. Turned it off and stayed in bed 'til 7.

    7:00 – skipped shower today (hasn't seemed as important to have one every day in lockdown, and there's no need to do my hair for work as I would normally) [. . .]

    7:20 – Started work. My workstation is my work laptop set up on our card table (inherited from my Granny, so it's a proper old-fashioned fold-up square card table) in the corner of the spare bedroom. I have a beautiful view from here over the countryside. Logged in to the remote desktop at the second attempt today.

10:00 – today I have a scheduled training course to deliver. In the office I would be in a conference room face to face with around 15 people. For most meetings we are now very used to the multi-way conference calls [. . .] However, the training is still very hard work, as in a room I would be reading body language, checking people are following and not falling asleep, but with five voices on the end of the phone it's much more difficult and involves remembering to stop regularly with questions such as 'Does that make sense?', 'Any questions' – it's very tempting just to say 'Are you still listening to me?'!

Diarist 1072 (male, 30s, East of England, IT engineer)

After breakfast, I got washed and dressed [. . .] I then turned on my laptop that sits on what was a shelf in the corner of our dining room and connected to the company VPN [Virtual Private Network].

A couple of weekends ago I added some rails beneath the shelf and used a sheet of plywood to make a pull out drawer so that I have more room to work and I don't take up all the space on the dining table. It makes a good collapsible home office space and also allows me to keep work separate from 'home'.

Diarist 1122 (female, 50s, London, service manager)

I am waking and getting up later during lockdown than pre-Corona. This is one of the benefits and for me so far, there have been definite up-sides to this situation. As well as having more sleep, I am less stressed as I don't have to travel anywhere and I don't have to meet with my boss, other than via a Zoom call once or twice a week. Conveniently my camera glitches so I am only present as a still photograph most of the time. This also enables me to sneak away for short periods of time when boredom sets in during performance meetings.

Diarist 1149 (female, 60s, Scotland, lecturer)

I allowed myself to sleep until 8 this morning, so I feel quite human today. I'm not a morning person and hate getting up early [. . .] The more elastic working hours that people have adopted since lockdown began suit me in some ways, but have added to my stress in others. Previously, most colleagues sent emails only during normal work hours. Now I'm bombarded by emails and messages in Teams, WhatsApp and Messenger every evening and all weekend, as colleagues fit work around home schooling and so on. It means I can never forget about work.

Diarist 1212 (female, 16, Wales)

At 3.00 I did half an hour's violin practice in between my dad's work calls.

Diarist 1213 (female, 30s, London, IT consultant)

I got up at 6am and was ready to start work just after 7. I'm currently starting work at 7am 4/5 days because we're home-schooling our son during the COVID-19 lockdown [. . .] My partner and I are on a shift system. Today I was on 7am to 1pm. We are lucky enough to have a garden office – we had our shed converted a couple of years ago and we have never been more pleased at the decision! It means that whoever is on shift can work fairly undisturbed and the house itself doesn't look like an office [. . .] Finished my shift a bit late – [partner] was understanding today. He isn't always and we've had words about it over recent weeks.

Diarist 1248 (female, 20s, East Midlands, student support administrator)

Had a team meeting with my colleagues at 09:30. Had to drag myself out of bed on time to go to it. My punctuality is not great at the moment. We're discussing contingency plans for the university students and how we can best help them. Lots of assessment extension requests need dealing with and we are all very busy at the moment. My back is sore from the dining room chair I am using at my desk, and I am sitting down a lot more lately and for longer periods.

We are doing fun things in our weekly meetings though; today we did the first half of a quiz I wrote. We will do the second half on the next meeting [. . .] It's a way to brighten our days a little and have some non-work related social contact with the team.

I have been working from home now for about 8 weeks; I'm counting it by paydays, and I've had two since remote working began. I much prefer being away from the office as I have no commute, I can get up later and I don't have to worry about grubby work bathrooms or a messy office kitchen. The academic staff do so love to leave dirty cups and bowls and plates everywhere.

I get on well with the people in my team; we are a mixture of ages and nearly all women. They are a joy to work with. However, being away from the office removes a lot of the job stress; people bending over my desk to check on me or the worry of someone wandering into the office to spring more work on to you. That has all stopped since we started working from home which I love!

Diarist 1312 (female, 40s, Wales, research manager)

Since my daughter's school & nursery closed, we've been trying to manage one full-time job, one self-employed job and childcare, which has been challenging. I don't feel like

I've had a moment's peace in the last 7 weeks. I've either been working, looking after my daughter, or trying to keep up with life admin.

We've fallen into a bit of a pattern when it comes to childcare/work and Tuesday is one of the days I do a full day [. . .] I still dress for work even though now I'm working from home. It hadn't crossed my mind as being an unusual thing to do until I bumped into a friend during the state sanctioned hour of exercise in the park and I was wearing my work clothes and I suddenly felt really out of place. Anyway, the clothes give me a bit of a sense of purpose and help the week and weekends feel different.

Diarist 1405 (male, 60s, London, lawyer)

I have a shower and go off to work around 8.45 am. The commute, which used to take 35 minutes by tube into the City, now takes 35 seconds walking down the stairs to get behind my desk [. . .] With the lockdown, a conscious effort is made to stay in contact, with twice weekly practice group calls in the London office, a twice weekly partner's call to keep track of developments, and strategize. Add to that regular client calls, ongoing project management calls, individual calls with team members to check everyone is OK, and anywhere between 100 to 250 emails a day, and a day is quickly filled.

Diarist 1423 (male, 30s, London, auditor)

The day itself was surprisingly tiring. For me, as with many days, the issue with the new Work From Home (WFH) normal is that so much of what I do is now dependent on Skype meetings. Today was no exception, with meetings 10-12, 12:30-5 with one 30 minute break [. . .] Back to doing work 8PM-11PM [. . .] to try and get back on top of the work that I can't do during endless Skype sessions [. . .] Tomorrow is another hell-on-earth day. 2.5 hour committee session in the morning, followed by 3 hour session in the afternoon, with a couple of extra meetings sprinkled in for good measure. The WFH arrangements work really well in audit as everything can be done online, it's just surprising how drained you feel at the end of it all.

Diarist 1573 (female, 40s, North West England, analyst and programmer)

Started work at 730 in the spare room. It's a bit uncomfortable as the chair and desk aren't set right but I'm still better off here than at the dining room table, my normal space, with the children asking me questions about school work every few minutes.

Checked my tomato plants that are growing on the windowsill and looking good [. . .] Come back up for Zoom meeting at 1030 with my team. We have this daily to check up on everyone's workload/queries but it's also a coffee morning where we have a good chat/vent about our problems. Someone's kids were having a fight behind him, so he didn't want to come off the call [. . .] Finish work at 4 and go downstairs [. . .] Cook tea for everyone and we eat together at 5, which is the nice part of being at home more – normally we don't all get to eat together in the week [. . .] Lucky to be doing a job like this where working from home is pretty feasible really – I know people who have no income at the moment as they just can't work and have fallen through the cracks in the furlough system.

Diarist 1582 (female, 50s, West Midlands, office manager)

Working from home is OK really. I love not commuting and don't miss some of my colleagues certainly. I can just get on with things [. . .] Not commuting has saved me a fortune in petrol and the mileage on the car is considerably less scary than it would have been. It's been almost three months since I did a commute now.

Diarist 1604 (male, 20s, Yorkshire and Humber, graphic designer and communications officer)

I wake up to my phone alarm at 7am. We're seven weeks into lockdown so it's not as though I have much of a commute before work starts at 9:30 [. . .] Lockdown isn't too tough for my working patterns, since I'm used to working remotely already, and aside for a daily conference call with my colleagues, I mostly manage tasks over email [. . .] I sneak in a short walk before work, which usually means I'm far more productive since I trick my brain into feeling like I've had a commute. When you work remotely, exercise becomes a good way to keep yourself sane [. . .] The afternoon passes without incident, and I knock off at 4:45 because nobody is around to stop me (though I leave my emails open in case there are any emergencies).

Diarist 1711 (male, 50s, West Midlands, geologist)

Got up at 7 and fed both dogs and took my wife a coffee. This is a luxury as usually I am up at 5.30 to catch a train to the office and don't really see my wife and daughter until the evening. I must admit I am enjoying the lockdown. It suits me as I am an only one and don't get bored and don't need a lot of company. I had a quick bath and dressed ready for the day. Since lockdown my work attire has changed from white shirt, trousers and tie to shorts and a t-shirt [. . .] I work at the dining table as my wife occupies the study and we find it difficult to work in the same room [. . .] I made a point of contacting a colleague of mine who is on her own in a small flat to check in and make sure that she is OK. She is one of two colleagues who are completely alone during this and in our team we are making sure that they are contacted daily.

Diarist 1751 (female, 30s, South West England, finance manager)

Afternoon is taken up with work, the kids running into the office for various reasons and normal life distractions. I'm trying very hard not to think about the biscuit tin!

Diarist 1972 (female, 40s, East Midlands, communications manager)

I woke up at 7:15am – much later than on a 'normal' day as I am currently working from home due to the Coronavirus epidemic [. . .] I got showered. Didn't bother washing my hair today as I won't be seeing anyone, but I did put on a little bit of make up as it makes me feel more awake and ready for the day [. . .] I quickly popped some washing in the machine before getting to my desk that I have set up in the spare room, for around 9:30am. It's taken a bit of adjustment and I certainly don't like having my chunky old PC cluttering up the place, but I'm now quite enjoying working from home.

Diarist 1984 (female, 60s, North West England, unemployed)

Husband appears from his office in the spare bedroom – when he's working from home (barrister and mediator) I don't feel able to do what I normally do, not even have the radio on; it's a small cottage, very few doors. And I fear he has now discovered how little I actually do.

Diarist 1991 (female, 20s, East of England, student)

I set my alarm on my phone for 8:00am but I ended up snoozing until about 9:00am. It has been quite hard getting up every day during lockdown. I much prefer the days when I am up and about by 8:00am; it makes me feel so much more positive and productive, and motivation is hard when you're constantly at home! [. . .] I made a cup of Yorkshire tea and ate a banana. I went back upstairs and started to make my bed, wash my face, went to the loo and even dusted my desk. Because I am working at home and spending a lot of time in my room, I find I have to keep it really clean otherwise I'm going to go crazy! It's definitely part of my personality, maybe I have a mild form of OCD, but I really can't concentrate and have a clear mind if my workspace is cluttered or if my bed is unmade [. . .] I called my boyfriend [. . .] After that, about 10:00am, I cleaned up my room a bit more, shook out my feather duvet because my mum told me to do that. Cleaned the bathroom and sat down at my computer [. . .] I have an assignment to do [. . .] It is SO hard to motivate yourself at home! I have loads to do and I'm so lethargic [. . .] It's 11.16am now and I'm not quite sure how the last hour has passed! I think I was still on the phone at 10:00am, then after that did the cleaning and messaged my friends a bit more on WhatsApp [. . .] I'm going to sit down and try and write some of my assignment.

Diarist 2037 (female, 20s, East of England, PhD student)

Because of the lockdown in response to COVID-19, my fiancé and I are working from home so we have not had the need to wake up as early as we would normally to fit in our morning commutes. Instead, we find ourselves snoozing on longer and generally struggling as a result to get up.

When we do eventually get up my fiancé goes into the study to work and I head downstairs for breakfast and start my work. I am a [. . .] PhD student, and this lockdown has been challenging for me, workwise, because I should really be in the lab right now. The last few months have brought about a lot of uncertainty and anxiety, however for me this has not been financial, or health related like many during this time. Instead this has been just about moving my work to home and worrying about how I will progress my PhD without lab work.

PhDs generally involve a fixed period of funding, therefore not having access to the labs but that clock continuing to tick has caused me lots of stress. It took me about a month to get used to working from home and find something I can work on (computer modelling) that I could do from home and still helps me progress with my PhD [. . .] I have set up my workspace on the dining room table and our [dog] transfers between snoozing next to me or with my fiancé upstairs. I have found myself not being as productive at home as I might have been at work with the distractions of snacks, garden, the chickens and a dog. However, it has been much quieter, and I have managed to get longer periods of undisturbed working every now and then. I even worked outside for a bit but found that the sun glare was too much to see my laptop screen.

I have enjoyed having lunch with my fiancé every day, and saving money by not buying food at work, using the car as often and paying for public transport [. . .] Our [dog] begins to stir [. . .] Being at home constantly for many weeks has been great for him. We have taught him lots of tricks and he has enjoyed the company. However, we are worried that when we return to work he might struggle with us not being in the house. We have been intending to go out for runs in the morning to get him used to us leaving after breakfast, but we haven't managed to get up in time yet.

Diarist 2069 (female, 30s, East Midlands, scientist)

I had some cereal and milk for breakfast while checking work emails and my schedule for the day. Thankfully, I had no online meetings today! I had two long ones yesterday and struggled to concentrate in between. I have noticed that my productivity has been lower compared to what it was before the lockdown [. . .] I started working around 09:45, and stopped for lunch at 13:30 – an hour later than Before Covid. My cat was particularly demanding today. Unlike most cats she is indoors only, so I am her main source of entertainment. She is a great source of comfort, and I find it difficult to deny her.

Diarist 2147 (female, 40s, South East England, teacher)

We woke up at 8.30am [. . .] This was an hour later than 'usual' (although our usual alarm for normal school days is 6am). We're finding that the longer we stay off school, the later we sleep in [. . .] I got up, had coffee and enjoyed the quiet, slower start to the day. Although there are huge worries and challenges, these slower starts, actual breakfasts, time to *think* is so valuable. We're normally at our desks in school by 7.30am.

Diarist 2172 (male, 40s, London, creative consultant)

Work is an almost uninterrupted stream of calls from 08.00 – 13.00 on Zoom, Teams, and apps I've never even heard of since before COVID-19. I wear a clean t-shirt and sweat shorts. No one can see me below the shoulders [. . .] My 'office' is on the kitchen table. It's the one place in the flat that is sunny and also where I can have video chats without my boyfriend stumbling within camera range.

Diarist 2348 (female, 30s, London, project manager)

Working from home again today; had my standing desk (ironing board) set up and coffee good to go at 8:45am. I'd already dropped my other half at the tube station so he doesn't have to get the bus (he works at a hospital in town), jogged around the block and yoga'd at home which keeps some semblance of routine. The working day was boring – home alone with my cat [. . .] I'm an extrovert so usually thrive on conversations throughout the day. Listening to music I can sing and dance along to helps the time pass quicker. I also miss commuting. I used to spend train time learning German on Duolingo and reading. And looking out of the window over the Thames when I go over Blackfriars Bridge.

Diarist 2388 (female, 40s, South East England, clinical psychologist)

The day started at 7am with a cup of tea brought to me by my husband which I sat in bed and drank. This is one of the good things to come out of lockdown – no morning commute so a slower, nicer start to my working day! I flicked through Facebook – more habit than need – and listened to the morning news. This is an attempt to orient myself with the correct day of the week and try to separate one day from another. The danger of them all merging into each other is real and the blurry boundaries between work and home is one of the difficult things of lockdown. I noticed that I quickly log on and check my emails before I'm dressed and this is something I would never have done before.

Diarist 2390 (male, 60s, South East England, customs officer)

I've been working from home since the Covid-19 'lockdown' [. . .] I've found it very difficult working from home, I've not adapted well. Other than missing the camaraderie of my teammates, I've found it hard to concentrate, partially as it's such a boring process, but also because I'm easily distracted at home and I have poor self-discipline. We've had virtual team meetings via our lap-tops using Microsoft Teams. I've yet to use the camera as I just don't want to be seen. I've not had a haircut for weeks now.

Diarist 2589 (female, 30s, South East England, actress)

My alarm goes off at 8:04am. I am a trained actress but with no hope of theatre or film work I am glad I have a part-time remote admin job [. . .] Each morning all employees have to log in to an application called 'Slack', state where we plan to work from that day and in a few words state what we plan to do that day. I don't want to be the first person to post so I aim for a few minutes past 8. Usually I do this and go back to sleep for another 40 minutes or so.

Diarist 2721 (female, 40s, North West England, clinician)

I'm really enjoying working from home. I have lots to do, my surroundings are lovely – I've been buying bunches of tulips to have on my desk, I can get outside easily, I like being able to flex my day. After 6 weeks it hasn't really lost its novelty. I have a makeshift set up with my laptop sitting on a printer, so it is at the right height, separate keyboard and chair with various cushions to provide support. I also can use my sideboard as a standing desk for variety and so I can move.

Mid-morning coffee turns into hoovering as I discover a spider nest has hatched and there are loads of little spiders about to escape around my kitchen. I don't mind spiders but there are so many!

Diarist 3029 (male, 20s, North West England, editor)

Work was a little slow today, since I'm kind of in-between projects and so doing some 'filler' tasks. I listened to BBC Radio 1 through the whole workday. I only started listening to the radio during work last week – normally I wouldn't have any music on before lunch, then I'd play my own music from lunch on. I think I just got desperate enough for other voices that I decided to give the radio a try [. . .] I finished work at 4:30, turned off my second monitor, and disconnected my keyboard and mouse from my laptop, which is my little routine to signify that the workday is done – since my office is now my dining table, which is in my living room, I need to make a real effort to make sure that I establish a separation between work and free time.

Diarist 3086 (female, 30s, London, archivist)

This morning I did what I have often done since lockdown dispensed with my need for an alarm clock. I woke early to birdsong and sunshine streaming through my skylight but, instead of getting up, I went back to sleep and woke again after 9am, when I technically should have started work. However, time has relatively little meaning at the moment and I am making the most of not rushing around and worrying about being late. I am also not missing the usual 6am start and long commute across London [. . .] I spend most of the day as I usually do now during the week: lying propped up on cushions on my sofa, laptop on my knee and a cup of coffee beside me. Many of my friends and colleagues have created a desk space for themselves (some have even had money from their employers to buy fancy new ergonomic chairs), but I work best as I always do, mainly horizontal! I am lucky that I have plenty to keep me occupied at home. Even though my work usually relies on physically accessing archive and museum collections, there is still plenty I can do remotely, like improving online catalogue data, engaging with social media and answering enquiries from researchers. I actually love the freedom, flexibility and privacy of working from home, particularly being able to listen to music all day.

Diarist 3739 (female, 60s, South West England, social worker)

Up to my office to work [. . .] I work mostly on my laptop, talk to people on Zoom, or Teams. I miss being in a room with people, reading their body language, sensing the mood. I cannot do that remotely. I have been asked to deliver training using Teams. I use every aspect of myself to engage the audience in training, body language, off the cuff humour, relationship building in coffee breaks – how can I do that using a laptop? [. . .] In the afternoon back to work on the laptop again. I am determined to work whilst I can, but the garden beckons. I lack focus, and it takes me a long time to start, or finish, reports. I miss meetings, travelling and the energy that comes from contact with colleagues.

Diarist 3890 (female, 40s, London, urban designer)

The daily team 'touch down' starts in a few minutes at 9.30 [. . .] I look at the Teams window as the little white bubbles with initials pop up one by one, longing to speak to and see the people behind the bubbles. The ones I need don't speak much in these meetings, it's mainly the manager level that do that, telling us stuff we already know and making sure nothing has happened to anyone. In a kindly way they show their faces on video, in encouragement maybe, but not many others do the same. They also know there are a few isolating alone. I appreciate their good intention. Do I gather the little bubbles together after the 'touch-down' or do I just get into the work and on with another day? When we speak the cameras go on and sometimes, on bad days, that's magical.

Diarist 4459 (female, 30s, London, journalist)

[Daughter] started to get cabin feverish [. . .] As I kept one eye on my work email we built a den in the garden using a hammock as the roof and various cushions and blankets as the bedroom. I was hoping this might keep [daughter] entertained for a little while as I had to attend a virtual meeting but as I tried to escape she obviously followed me instantly to my work set up at the kitchen table [. . .] [Daughter] plays fairly well and independently for a three-year-old but on work days she knows that she doesn't have my attention fully and acts up until she gets a bit more. Frankly it is a disaster trying to work from home and look after her and I have had lots of ups and downs throughout lockdown about it. I have cut my days from three to two which helps, but I hate feeling like I am doing a bad job of work and parenting. It has been special having this intensive time with her [. . .] but we are all looking forward to nursery reopening.

Diarist 4669 (female, 40s, South East England, librarian)

Plugged in my laptop to start work. In my usual office I have a stand-up desk – an adjustable riser which sits on my standard desk, holds my workstation and allows me to stand rather than sit whilst working. I have found I have less back and shoulder pain since I began using it and being on my feet makes me feel more energised. I have tried to replicate it at home by building a tower of books on top of a chest of drawers in my spare room and placing my laptop on top with separate mouse and keyboard. So far so good!

As the weeks have progressed (I have been working from home for eight weeks now), I've found myself decorating my new 'office' (previously my spare bedroom). Last Friday (May 8th, 2020), the country celebrated seventy-five years since VE (Victory in Europe) Day. I hung some bunting in my window to mark the occasion and have decided to keep it up . . . until it falls down. Displaying a rainbow in your window as a symbol of support for NHS workers has become a popular trend, especially for children, during lockdown. I have created a mosaic rainbow to display and together with some Kalanchoe plants they brighten the room and help to lift my spirits.

Diarist 4722 (male, 40s, London, archivist)

Knocked off work a bit after 1730. Spent some time catching up on Twitter and other personal social media and then headed out for a walk [. . .] These walks have been really important during this strange time [. . .] They make a clear break between work and potentially sitting back down at the same desk to use my personal laptop later in the evening.

Diarist 4759 (male, 60s, Wales, CEO of a charity)

I am working from home [. . .] which consists of endless virtual meetings. I have a couple this afternoon. But now it's almost 10.00 am and I am still in my pyjamas – lockdown slobbery.

Diarist 4766 (female, 60s, East of England, family support specialist)

I woke early to check the laptop that has been provided by the hospital for working from home. For two weeks I have been trying, with little success, to access the specialist database that is used in my department. Failed again!

I listened to a meditation audio on Stoicism.

On Sunday I enrolled on a 4 week online Stoicism course. I have been observing my reactions in the hope that I will improve my ability to control my emotions and to live in accordance with my core values. This was particularly helpful this morning when I failed to access my database.

ZOOM

During the pandemic, much that would otherwise have been cancelled moved online. This included work meetings, but also meetings with family and friends (pub nights, cocktail nights, film nights, coffee mornings, birthday parties, quizzes, karaoke), meetings for clubs and groups (committee meetings, reading groups, music rehearsals, religious services), exercise classes, education webinars, theatre performances, music concerts, gallery tours. A variety of videoconferencing applications were used – FaceTime, Skype, Teams, WhatsApp – but the most common was Zoom, not least because it was free to download (in limited form, with limits on the number of participants and the length of meetings). Indeed, in a matter of weeks in spring 2020, Zoom went from being something most people had never heard of to something many people used daily. There were some teething problems to begin with as people learned how to set up and join calls, mute and unmute microphones, take turns and not talk over one another, turn cameras on and off, blur backgrounds, and so on. But most people adapted quickly. They looked forward to social Zoom calls in the evening, which filled up otherwise empty diaries – unless their work involved video calls, in which case fatigue from looking at screens all day could be a problem. There was so much now happening online. It was nice to see friendly faces. Indeed, many people had never seen family and friends so regularly – especially those living far away. Video calls were especially important for people living alone, or people isolating or shielding and so stuck at home even more than others during the pandemic, or people with disabilities meaning they had always been stuck at home more than others, even before the pandemic. Access to education, the arts and society in general had been improved for these people, who worried accessibility would slide back once restrictions were lifted and life returned to normal. This move back offline was a real threat, since many people found video meetings better than nothing, but still not quite the same as face-to-face meetings, remembered fondly for their energy and hugs. See also Cancellations; (new) Normal; PE (Physical Education); Shielding; Stay home; WhatsApp; Working from home.

Diarist 223 (female, 80s, East of England, retired medical secretary)

At just before 11am I get my iPad and log into Zoom and join up with my local exercise class. This is the third week and we all seem to have conquered the intricacies of this modern technology, turning the 'mute' button off when instructed. This took a bit of organising! It is lovely to see friends from our weekly exercise class on screen.

Diarist 286 (female, 60s, Scotland, retired building society cashier)

Daily family Zoom at 1630, which we started on Monday 23rd March, the first day of official lockdown. With 3 daughters in different parts of Scotland and England, and 5 children between them, it can be chaotic but is a lot of fun, and we have never seen so much of one another!

Diarist 529 (female, 50s, Yorkshire and Humber, company director)

Tonight I am joining my Tai Chi class via Zoom. It is nice to connect with people in this way. I run a virtual pub for my cycle club every Friday and it has been very successful. It seems strange to think how quickly we have adapted to these virtual formats for connection. But with both of these there will come a point where some people can socialise easily and others who are more at risk cannot. It will be really hard for people like my husband [categorised as vulnerable and advised to shield during the pandemic] but also people who have been socially isolated before Covid 19 because of their disability and feel more connected now than before. To have had a connection and then for it to disappear again will feel really painful for many people.

Diarist 542 (female, 60s, East Midlands, retired accountant)

Checking my phone after tea I see an e-mail with an invitation to a Zoom meeting on Thursday from the WI I belong to. That would be our usual meeting day. Never used Zoom. Not sure what I need to do. My husband downloaded Zoom onto the computer last week. Oh well have 2 days to read up what needs doing.

Diarist 622 (female, 40s, Scotland, sociologist)

I came back from my walk to enjoy a late lunch. I then caught up with a friend via an online meeting forum (Zoom), which has now become a bit of a life line [. . .] Later, I will be joining a virtual choir, with participants from all over the world [. . .] to sing this week's tune. We spend an hour singing a song and then there is an 'open mic' section where people perform songs, read poems, or share recipes. It is quite moving and beautiful.

Diarist 746 (female, 40s, London, consultant)

Podcasts and TV box sets, along with virtual video drinks with friends and family, are the great pleasures of lockdown. God knows how we would have managed before the internet.

Diarist 1089 (male, 40s, South East England, chaplain)

I've just got the invite to a shamanic medicine songs meeting on Zoom at 7pm [. . .] It's crazy how much stuff is happening on Zoom during the lockdown! [. . .] I've just noticed that the webinar I planned to attend at 5pm is hosted on Zoom [. . .] I'm going to Skype call [partner] in just over 20 minutes and see how her day has been [. . .] It's now almost half-past nine and I'm going to switch off my laptop by ten in the interests of good sleep hygiene.

Diarist 1108 (male, 50s, West Midlands, teacher)

Zoom meeting at 1pm with three colleagues. Nobody had even heard of Zoom a few weeks ago and yet now it is ubiquitous [. . .] On Wednesdays, I have two social Zoom meetings in the evening. The first of these is with a group of old school friends [. . .] And, ironically, this time has brought us closer. We're now spread across the country, having all started in London. And one is across the world [. . .] But every week, we laugh for 40 minutes. That's been an anchor.

Diarist 1153 (male, 20s, South East England, student)

Reading group was great. A lot looser and funnier than it's been in previous weeks. That's partly down to the group getting to know each other, but also because I think we're learning, collectively, how to create an etiquette in conference video calling where you can be funny or at ease whilst not talking over the top of one another, as we always do in reality. I kept changing my position around the room as the sun was setting, partly because some positions would cast me in absolute darkness, but truthfully more because I was trying to avoid unflattering lights. I hate having to look at my face all the time when I'm talking to someone, and I hope I don't re-emerge after lockdown with a new anxiety about how my face and teeth look when I'm speaking.

Diarist 1177 (male, 60s, South West England, Finance Director)

Microsoft Teams meeting at 11am. So much of my life now revolves around social interaction through a screen. The management meeting at 11 went on for two hours which, just like a face to face meeting with four colleagues, is far too long. Once it was over, I grabbed a sandwich and sat in the sun with my wife for 20 mins before getting back on the screen for a series of work based video calls through to 4pm. By then I was struggling to focus.

Diarist 1217 (female, 60s, North East England, vicar)

Got some coffee and joined a Zoom meeting (a system of which I'd not heard before March 23rd) for three of us from a charity I'm a trustee of to talk with a fundraising consultant. We were all hanging around and couldn't connect, then 3 of us did but the 4th couldn't – and then we agreed to try on Microsoft Teams. On this we all connected, but for some reason my picture was on its side! [. . .] I then looked at a few more emails and had a Zoom meeting of Slimming World – it is good to get together, though I much prefer being in a real group – and I was very aware I ate two 'Wagon Wheels' with my cuppa this afternoon [. . .] After that, it was time for a quick meal – a microwaved chicken noodle dish, and a zero fat coconut yoghurt before I needed to set up for the Christian Aid film night on Zoom. I was ready with my coffee about 15 minutes ahead, and that was good, as people came online early, and there was a bit of confusion about the code. In the end there were 19 households watching, many with two people [. . .] I had learnt last week how to share screen and put on the computer sound, and it all worked beautifully.

Diarist 1248 (female, 20s, East Midlands, student support administrator)

Hosting a quiz tomorrow on Zoom which will be fun! In a weird way, this distance has forced me into making a lot more effort with my friends, especially people I haven't been in touch with even for years. Despite the physical distance it's been a uniting experience for me personally.

Diarist 1380 (female, 40s, Northern Ireland, librarian)

My daughters are busily chatting in separate rooms on a group quiz with friends using the Zoom app. It's good to hear their animated voices.

Diarist 1547 (female, 30s, East of England, innovation consultant)

I put on bright red lipstick for my client call, but decide to rely on Zoom filter rather than bother with tinted moisturiser and concealer. The lipstick makes me feel more like the professional version of me, and I hope serves as a distracter from the rest of my make-up less face. I've noticed that most of our clients also seem to be wearing a bit less make-up in the case of women or being a little more casually dressed than usual. It has been odd, seeing the inside of people's housing, that odd blurring of personal and professional lives. I spent the first week worrying about whether it was possible to read the titles of the books in the bookcase behind me.

Diarist 1661 (female, 13, Wales)

Dad came in with a letter from a friend – we've been pen palling during the pandemic, as a more romantic way to keep in touch [. . .] I started writing back to my friend. We decorate our letters and put lots of little trinkets and drawings in – she's a very talented artist and I enjoy writing poetry, so it's a perfect match! In the envelope (which I hand made for the first time) I put the letter, a pressed flower, some origami, a little badge and a poem. I also made the same friend a birthday card, and put in a necklace I've been making for her, which has a little heart-shaped piece of slate on it that I sanded into shape.

Diarist 1676 (female, 50s, West Midlands, St John's Ambulance worker)

Well it's been a day similar to every other day in Lockdown. Being single I am missing not having my Daughter and Son-in-Law for Sunday dinner but hopefully we will be able to return to that soon, meantime using WhatsApp and Teams virtual get togethers is so important, so planning another Girls Virtual Cocktail Night with friends for Friday – something to look forward to.

Diarist 1700 (female, 50s, London, piano teacher)

I sat at the computer, looking at the beautiful paintings that my daughter did for me for Mother's Day and my birthday (thank goodness for Zoom and the ability to see friends and family online) [. . .] Then the doorbell rang, my friend was standing at the bottom of my driveway having come to collect a necklace that I fixed for him. I left him a letter to post for me on my doorstep (he was wearing gloves) and we had a lovely chat [. . .] So nice to socially-distance see a real person instead of one on a screen.

Diarist 1711 (male, 50s, West Midlands, geologist)

At six some friends of ours [. . .] have asked us to join them on Facebook. I'm not on Facebook so my wife gets it up on her tablet. They are doing a Car Pool Karaoke [. . .] and at the end name us to do it next. My wife and daughter are good singers but I can't sing at all and hate performing. I'm very anxious about this. I wish people would ask first.

Diarist 1822 (female, 10, North East England)

At 7:00 o'clock after I'd just had my dinner I went onto Zoom to do drama. It was quite fun to see lots of smiling faces around me because I had only seen my brother's and mum's smiling faces which you can get a bit tired of when you are stuck with them for 7 weeks.

Diarist 1848 (male, 50s, Scotland, broadcast and telecommunications engineer)

[Friend] popped up on Facebook Messenger at around 9:15am.

He wanted to know my thoughts on how to 'tactfully let [another friend] know that he needs to make his quiz questions a little less obscure' without upsetting him. We have been doing a weekly Friday night quiz using Zoom and one of our circle of friends seems to think it's an excuse for showing off his own esoteric knowledge by asking almost un-answerable questions. . . . Hopefully he's got the message now.

Diarist 1867 (female, 20s, West Midlands, cabin crew)

Today is Tuesday and every Tuesday evening at 8 I have an online quiz with my friends. We take it in turns to write the quiz. I come second place in the quiz and after that we spend a long while talking about everything we're worried about, talking about silly things, and trying to reassure and cheer each other up. Whilst I'm doing the quiz upstairs my mum does an online yoga class downstairs. We all use Zoom. It's a website where you can video chat with lots of people at once. Zoom and specifically quizzes are big things nowadays.

Diarist 1979 (female, 60s, South East England, editor and retired nurse)

We've all learned how to use Zoom, Skype, and FaceTime as if we were born to it. Watched the youngest baby eat her lunch on Sunday whilst I chatted with her parents – it's been hard for some grandparents, but I feel lucky to see the families this way. I probably wouldn't have seen them as much in normal times.

Diarist 2003 (female, 40s, South East England, housewife and artist/designer)

My youngest's birthday [. . .] We are organising a virtual party via Zoom on Saturday. This is all new technology to me and I'm worried it will all go tits up.

Diarist 2035 (female, 50s, North West England, nurse)

I have started doing Pilates via Zoom. Like most people I had not heard of Zoom before the lockdown. We all adapt.

Diarist 2070 (male, 70s, South West England, administrator)

There was a plan for a Zoom Trivial Pursuit session with our [son and his children] this evening, which has been postponed until tomorrow due, I think, to several of the children having other virtual engagements.

Diarist 2348 (female, 30s, London, project manager)

I sing in a barbershop chorus (and quartet) and we've had virtual rehearsals for nine weeks now. After trialling a few options we've found the best option is initial Zoom chats to say hi, then an online pre-recorded rehearsal video which is played to us all via SynchTube. We keep the Zoom running and it's nice knowing and seeing others are singing along at the same time, although we're all muted. Some of us send in videoed sections of our repertoire that are played during rehearsal so we can duet. I miss being able to harmonise with others, and really miss the people. Zoom chats only go so far, especially in a large group. I miss those side-conversations you can have when you're face to face. That chat finished at 8:30pm – I feel the energy dropping in them each week, like everyone is getting video call fatigue.

Diarist 2394 (male, 50s, South East England, unemployed actor)

A quick check of tomorrow's schedule.

An almost-complete blank. Which is exciting, or challenging, or depressing, depending on how you choose to take it. (I'll go for option one, please.)

Except that I do actually have one item on the calendar: my [Dad's birthday], so I will join my siblings & family members on a Zoom call and we will each bake a cake in our various homes and celebrate with him; this will replace the big family party we had planned before all this happened [. . .] So that's something to look forward to.

Diarist 2408 (female, 40s, London, theatre worker)

Time to have my regular daily WhatsApp video call with my mum [. . .] We have done this every day since lockdown started. When the virus and lockdown was first announced she went into a bit of a panic as she lives on her own and also convinced herself she was going to catch it and die, so to begin with my daily calls were to check in with her to make sure she was ok – But now she is fine it's just nice to see her face and talk to another adult every day! We fill each other in with the details of our quite boring days!

Diarist 2473 (female, 60s, South West England, retired)

Checked my emails; as almost every day, there were messages from museums and theatres, offering virtual tours of galleries and online theatre performances; it is nice to have this option, but I miss the real experience of going to an exhibition or to see a play and wonder when this will be possible again; I feel I have been spending too much time on my computer and watching television during lock down!

Diarist 2621 (male, 70s, North East England, retired lecturer)

It is hard not to see our son and daughter-in-law [. . .] We now meet as a family online via Zoom which is lovely in itself just to see each other via this video link but is hardly a substitute for hugs or playing on the floor with my grand-daughter.

Diarist 2627 (female, 40s, Northern Ireland, editor)

In the evening [. . .] I Skyped the last person I hugged. Her uncle was in hospital and her shower was blocked. I wanted to get up from my desk and go round to help her fix it and felt furious, and wretched, that I couldn't.

Diarist 2640 (female, 60s, Scotland, counsellor and therapist)

I joined The College of Medicine's free online Mindfulness session at 8am, it is brilliant! It is taught by one of the experts in the field. 200+ of us took part on Zoom. I hadn't heard of Zoom a month ago! I also did a yoga class late morning on Zoom [. . .] While we are all locked in there is such remarkable availability of free health and exercise classes and spiritual workshops, meditation teachings by the world's leading Buddhists and even the great and the good in the music business giving Instagram mini concerts from their homes [. . .] For people with mobility problems the stream of arts, crafts, courses, exercise classes and even online support groups is a very positive offering amidst a very terrifying reality.

Diarist 2707 (female, 40s, South East England, painter and decorator)

We were due visits [from family] this month but all that is now on hold due to the pandemic. I miss seeing them in person but we video chat and WhatsApp a whole lot more than we did before. In a strange way, I currently feel closer to them even though we're separated by 300 miles!

Diarist 2722 (female, 60s, East of England, museum educator)

I have a Parish Council meeting on Zoom this evening. I have registered with Zoom, printed off the Agendas [. . .] and the annual accounts so I am all ready [. . .] I switched on to [colleague's] email and pressed the link for the meeting. It told me that the meeting would start in a moment. I waited. The page changed and now I was being told to click on 'join a meeting'. I clicked. Nothing happened. Till not quite 7 o'clock so I waited. Still nothing. It reached about ten-past seven. I went back to the email and re-clicked on the link. Same result. This time I scrolled down below the 'Join a meeting' button. Tried 'Register for Zoom'. It told me that I was already registered and logged in. Phoned [colleague] to explain why I wasn't participating. Called to [nephew] for help which, after a few minutes of fruitless attempts, he found he was unable to give. Together and then on my own, spent the rest of the designated meeting time desperately pressing everything, going round and round in circles and becoming more and more frustrated. Sometime before 8 o'clock, I gave up and went to watch 'Midsomer Murders'.

Diarist 3390 (male, 60s, South East England, retired NHS manager)

Zoom is changing the way we live! I use it for a social friendship group (sitting with a glass of wine in front of the screen), for a music session I am part of (playing along to a lead musician with the rest of us on mute so that the internet latency does not create a cacophony). This week I will be on Zoom for four consecutive evenings.

Diarist 3562 (female, 50s, South West England, garden designer)

I haven't seen anyone face to face for two months. That is an unreal thought, something I never thought I'd say, but I speak to people every day. Today I had some FaceTime and Zoom calls with friends and family. It's not the same but it is the closest thing I can get to seeing people.

Diarist 3835 (female, 50s, South East England, social care worker)

11.30 Zoom meeting with colleagues and management.
    12.15 Meeting over. Colleague suggested by text to me that I get my breasts out for the next meeting to add to the interest a bit. I agreed that I would change my clothes and wear something more revealing.
    12.30 Zoom meeting hosted by me [. . .] Flirted in private chat with my colleague during the meeting. He made me laugh at one point which confused the rest of the team – not fair and will try not to do that again.

Diarist 4688 (female, 60s, Yorkshire and Humber, researcher)

Tonight is Zoom choir night – which is better than nothing but not that easy when not surrounded and cushioned by other singers [. . .] The head of the choir cannot hear us but we can hear her. Probably just as well no one can hear me!

Diarist 4768 (male, 9, South East England)

I have not been able to see my friends, apart from on Zoom. If we didn't have Zoom, then we wouldn't be seeing anyone.

CONCLUSION
PRESENTING EVERYDAY LIFE

How to bring the everyday into focus?

The introductory chapter situated this book in a tradition of experimental, non-linear writing on pandemics. In the spirit of Defoe, Camus, Grover and Spinney, I've sought to capture the Covid-19 pandemic's broad and shallow shape, to interpose the thinnest fabric between reader and event, to include a variety of testimonies and a mass of minor details, to include the compromises and ambiguities of the pandemic and to identify my own set of Covid keywords. This concluding chapter situates the book in another tradition of experimental, non-linear writing: everyday life studies.

My approach to everyday life studies is taken in part from Ben Highmore.[1] For him, such studies approach the everyday as a problematic to be brought into focus. The challenge, then, is how to register and represent everyday life? In *Everyday Life and Cultural Theory*, Highmore wrote: 'A significant concern for theorising the everyday is the problem of generating a suitable *form* for registering everyday modernity. In other words, all the projects dealt with here can be seen to contribute to the creation of an aesthetics of and for everyday modernity'.[2] In *The Everyday Life Reader*, he wrote: 'The "coherent narrative" and the "rigorous argument" have been the dominant forms encouraged by social science approaches, but whether these forms of presentation fit the material world of everyday life is, I would argue, in need of questioning'.[3] He continues:[4]

> I want to suggest here that the future of everyday life studies will necessitate a form of articulation built on the fault line that divides the social sciences and art. Or using another academic vernacular it will require an inventive 'blurring of genres' (Geertz 1993: 19–35): sociology and literature, for instance, but not the sociology of literature, rather a literary sociology.

The challenge is one of form and aesthetics. Highmore rejects coherent narrative and rigorous argument for literary sociology. He takes inspiration from nineteenth-century realist novels; twentieth-century modernist novels; Brecht's dramatic and artistic works; Manet's impressionism and theorists including Simmel, Benjamin, Lefebvre and de Certeau.

In the rest of this chapter, I situate the form and aesthetic of the present book in the tradition of everyday life studies, taking inspiration from my own selection of literature, sociology and theory: modernist literature of the 1920s; avant-garde social and cultural studies of the 1930s and 1940s; experimental literature of the 1970s and 1980s;

experimental history, geography and theory from around the turn of the twenty-first century; and recent attempts to extend and reflect on this tradition. In doing so, I take one caveat from Highmore: the secondary literature on some of these works is huge and this chapter is not meant to be a comprehensive discussion. Rather, I mine these works and some of the secondary literature for resources that helped in shaping, encouraging and justifying this book. And there is a second caveat: I focus on some writers and works in everyday life studies more than others. Certain key figures in the tradition are largely missing from this chapter (most notably, Simmel and de Certeau). Again, my primary aim in this chapter is to make clear my influences and inspirations for the book, not to provide an exhaustive survey of everyday life studies – and certainly not to claim a place in this tradition alongside those I view as intellectual heroes.

The next six sections introduce these influences and inspirations. The two sections after that reflect critically on the compositional decisions made in this book and encouraged by everyday life studies, and so reflect critically on the strengths and limitations of the book as an account of the Covid-19 pandemic. The final section calls for more experimental studies of the kind attempted here; for more humanizing, democratic representations of life in the twenty-first century and for a renewed science of the people, by the people, for the people, with a repoliticized Mass Observation at its centre.

Just one day

12 May 2020 was just one day in the Covid-19 pandemic. Books focused on just one day, though, can do a lot for our understanding – both of the broader period in which that day is located, and of more timeless phenomena. This was demonstrated by the original Mass-Observation's *May the Twelfth*, which we'll return to shortly. Before that, however, it was demonstrated by two novels from the 1920s: James Joyce's *Ulysses* and Virginia Woolf's *Mrs Dalloway*.[5]

Published in 1922, *Ulysses* takes place over just one day: 16 June 1904. Leopold Bloom and Stephen Dedalus wander the streets of Dublin, bump into each other and form a connection. Otherwise, nothing much happens. As Jeri Johnson puts it, 'nothing much happens on this day in Dublin and nothing much happens in *Ulysses* [. . .] Mostly in *Ulysses*, people talk, or think, or remember, or drink, or argue, or gossip. The rest of the time they walk, read, eat, bathe, defecate, urinate, fall asleep'.[6] Yet *Ulysses* is often seen as one of the great novels of the twentieth century. Why? It represents both the culmination of one tradition – the nineteenth-century realist novel of meticulously recreated characters, streets, shops, commodities, newspapers, current events and so on – and the birth of another tradition: the twentieth-century modernist novel of fragments, montage, open-ended narrative, multiple viewpoints, pastiche, parody and form for its own sake.[7] Ulysses exploded the conventions of the novel. Readers are thrown into the middle of the narrative from the first page. Depending on the page, readers are confronted by a novel, but also a drama, a catechism, a poem, an epic and an encyclopedia. Anne Enright notes how Bloom and Dedalus are 'porous to the world' (and so, we might add, is the day).[8]

Events from the past are remembered. Thoughts intrude and voices interrupt. The prose is fragmented. It is difficult to know always who is telling the story and what story is being told. For Enright, this difficulty is part of what makes reading Joyce so liberating: '*Ulysses* is about what happens in the reader's head. The style obliges us to choose a meaning, it is designed to make us feel uncertain. This makes it a profoundly democratic work. *Ulysses* is a living, shifting, deeply humane text that is also very funny. It makes the world bigger.'[9] I love this last phrase. A book focused on just one day when nothing much happens can, through its stylistic choices – its use of fragments, montage, open-ended narrative, multiple viewpoints – *make the world bigger*. In doing so, it can make us uncertain. And it can provide an account of a time and place, porous to other times and places, that is both humane and democratic.

Ulysses was read by Virginia Woolf, who published *Mrs Dalloway* in 1925.[10] The two novels are often contrasted: the elevated, mythical, masculine *Ulysses* versus the realistic, ordinary, feminine *Mrs Dalloway*.[11] However, there is much shared by the two novels. *Mrs Dalloway* also takes place on just one day: 13 June 1923. Perhaps a little more happens than in *Ulysses*. Clarissa Dalloway is organizing a large formal party. But again, the day is porous. The characters remember other days – other times and places. In particular, Dalloway repeatedly remembers the pivotal day when she was eighteen and decided not to marry Peter Walsh. Elaine Showalter has noted the influence of psychoanalysis on Woolf, whose publishing house (Hogarth Press) began publishing Freud in 1921. Woolf saw the self as multilayered and constructed by actions and thoughts, but also memories, fantasies and dreams. *Mrs Dalloway* makes 'brilliant use of flashbacks and fragments from childhood experience, images that have stayed in the character's consciousness, preserved and frozen like photographs or snapshots, and that come up in unexpected contexts'.[12] Showalter also notes the influence of cubism on Woolf. Like *Ulysses*, *Mrs Dalloway* provides views from multiple perspectives. For example, the novel opens with a motor car travelling up a London street. Woolf pans from observer to observer; from one set of thoughts and fantasies to another. Showalter describes this narrative technique as cinematic: 'Woolf makes use of such devices as montage, close-ups, flashbacks, tracking shots, and rapid cuts in constructing a three-dimensional story.'[13] Showalter also wrote:[14]

Woolf gives us a full range of portraits spanning the seven ages of woman. Elizabeth Dalloway is almost eighteen, just beginning her adult life. Rezia Smith is in her twenties. Milly Brush and Doris Kilman are past forty. Clarissa and Sally Seton are in their fifties. Millicent Bruton is sixty-two, but dreams of being a little girl in Devon, playing with her brothers in the clover. Miss Helena Parry, past eighty, lives in her memories of India, and the glorious triumph of her book about the orchids of Burma. Finally, there is the nameless old woman Clarissa sees from her window, putting out her light, and going to bed.

This full range of portraits is possible not least because *Mrs Dalloway* focuses on just one day. The day might be porous, but it still acts as a constraint, encouraging inclusion of multiple perspectives on the same events. *Mrs Dalloway* shares this and much else with

Ulysses. Both novels emerged from and helped to produce a modern context populated by psychoanalysis, cubism and also Surrealism.

Surrealism connects this modernist literature of the 1920s to the avant-garde social and cultural studies of the 1930s and 1940s – Mass-Observation, Jennings, Benjamin – discussed shortly. Joyce and Woolf combined fragments in montages. They incorporated dreams and fantasies. They used cinematic techniques: close-ups, flashbacks, tracking shots, rapid cuts. During the 1920s, people like Louis Aragon and Andre Breton articulated these techniques and objects as Surrealism. Ben Highmore is helpful again when approaching Surrealism.[15] He sees in Surrealism an art form, but also – in its 'journals', 'bureaus of research', 'laboratories' and 'investigations' – a form of social research into everyday life. The surrealists wished to defamiliarize and make visible the everyday. They imagined the everyday to be marvellous, if only it could be freed from capitalism, and if only people could be freed from rationalist consciousness. In pursuit of these wishes, the surrealists developed methods for attending to the social and recognizing the everyday:[16]

> Collage (or montage) provides a persistent methodology for attending to everyday life in Surrealism. In its juxtaposing of disparate elements (umbrellas, sewing machines etc.), it generates a defamiliarizing of the everyday. If everyday life is what continually threatens to drop below a level of visibility, collage practices allow the everyday to become vivid again by making the ordinary strange through transferring it to surprising contexts and placing it in unusual combinations.

Highmore adds: 'What is at stake here is the production of the "spark", generated by the juxtaposition of different materials.'[17] The spark 'jolts us out of the familiar'. Juxtapositions within collages would defamiliarize the everyday, making it strange, vivid, visible. They would shock people into recognizing the marvellous everyday. They would be taken up as methods by avant-garde social and cultural studies of the 1930s and 1940s, including the original Mass-Observation.

The whole rope

In the introductory chapter, I introduced M-O via its three main founders, two of whom were heavily influenced by Surrealism: Charles Madge and Humphrey Jennings. I also introduced *May the Twelfth*, one of M-O's first books, published in 1937.[18] Like *Ulysses* and *Mrs Dalloway*, *May the Twelfth* is focused on just one day: 12 May 1937, the day of the Coronation of George VI. Madge collected reports from observers around the country. Jennings edited these reports using surrealist techniques from his documentary film work: montage, collage, juxtaposition, close-ups and long shots, detail and ensemble. He allowed the material to speak for itself, 'which had the effect of putting the reader there'.[19] Instead of a single clear image or narrative whole, he provided fragments, partial perspectives, different points of focus, different voices (allowed to speak for themselves).[20]

The day-survey of 12 May 1937 was one of a number of day-surveys completed by M-O during its first couple of years.[21] Day-surveys, however, were not the only way M-O collected materials in these early years. While Madge organized the day-surveys (reports of a particular day, made by observers spread across the country), anthropologist Tom Harrisson organized research not of a particular day but of a particular place: 'Northtown' (Bolton, also known by M-O as 'Worktown').[22] M-O was influenced by Surrealism but also by anthropology. Harrisson was an anthropologist. M-O claimed to be doing an 'anthropology of our own people'.[23] A leading anthropologist of the day, Bronislaw Malinowski sat on the committee controlling M-O funds and wrote a chapter in *First Year's Work, 1937–1938*.[24] Some students of M-O have seen it as the coming together of Surrealism and anthropology: an experiment in 'surrealist ethnography'.[25] Others have seen M-O less as a coming together and more as two distinct projects (or even organizations):[26] Harrisson's Worktown Project, positivist in character, informed by his background in ornithology;[27] and Madge's National Panel, a collaboration with Jennings (more than Harrisson), until Jennings left M-O before the end of its first year.

M-O was a complex organization that evolved over time. It also had many influences: Surrealism, anthropology, the social survey tradition (think: Charles Booth), the Middletown studies of Robert and Helen Lynd (which influenced M-O's naming of 'Worktown').[28] For the purposes of this discussion, I've been interested in a particular version of M-O: the early years, when Jennings was involved, when day-surveys were prominent in M-O's repertoire and before Madge aligned himself more closely with Harrisson's vision for M-O. This particular version of M-O was influenced by Surrealism and also David Hume's radical empiricism, which encouraged observation as a means to producing imaginative, sensitive, full accounts of human life.[29] Furthermore, it was influenced by what Boris Jardine has termed the 'scientific humanism' of continental Europeans like Benjamin, Freud and Tarde, who took a particular approach to the individual/group problem of social research.[30] They sought to describe and explain without aggregating. They favoured record-keeping of concrete particulars over research method, theory, classification and statistical analysis. They aimed to give voice to the masses and not to speak for them. And they were oriented to both scientific and literary ways of knowing, to both science and aesthetics, to the scientific problem of representation and literary solutions to that problem (found in compositional techniques, e.g. juxtaposition of different perspectives, or treatment of the individual as a microcosm of society).

Benjamin's scientific humanism will be discussed shortly. It shared much with the M-O of Madge and Jennings: a horizontal focus on a particular period (if not a particular day); the influence of Surrealism (fragments, montage, juxtaposition) and an interest in quotation and letting people and materials speak for themselves. Before moving on, though, it is worth dwelling on what happened to Jennings after he left M-O in late 1937. He worked in journalism and film, ultimately producing another inspiration for this book: *Pandæmonium*.[31] The ideas behind *Pandæmonium* were developed in an essay on the machine Jennings wrote for the *London Bulletin* (1938) and a film Jennings made for the Crown Film Unit (*Listen to Britain*, 1945).[32] Jennings died in 1950, leaving an enormous, unfinished manuscript (the similarities to Benjamin are many). Roughly a third of that manuscript was published in 1985 as *Pandæmonium*, edited by Jennings's daughter, Marie-Louise, and Charles Madge. Indeed, Madge had to write up the introduction from extensive notes left by Jennings. This introduction is worth quoting at length:[33]

> In this book I present the imaginative history of the Industrial Revolution. Neither the political history, nor the mechanical history, nor the social history nor the economic history, but the imaginative history.
>
> I say 'present', not describe or analyse, because the Imagination is a function of man whose traces are more delicate to handle than the facts and events and ideas of which history is usually constructed. This function I believe is found active in the areas of the arts, of poetry and of religion – but is not necessarily confined to them or present in all their manifestations. I prefer not to try to define its limits at the moment but to leave the reader to agree or not with the evidence which I shall place before him. I present it by means of what I call Images.
>
> These are quotations from writings of the period in question, passages describing certain moments, events, clashes, ideas occurring between 1660 and 1886, which either in the writing or in the nature of the matter itself or both have revolutionary and symbolic and illuminatory quality. I mean that they contain in little a whole world – they are knots in a great net of tangled time and space – the moments at which the situation of humanity is clear – even if only for the flash time of the photographer or the lightning. And just as the usual history does not consist of isolated events, occurrences – so this 'imaginative history' does not consist of isolated images, but each is in a particular place in an unrolling film.
>
> And these images – what do they deal with? I do not claim that they represent truth – they are too varied, even contradictory, for that. But they represent human experience. They are the record of mental events. Events of the heart. They are facts (the historian's kind of facts) which have been passed through feelings and the mind of an individual and have forced him to write. And what he wrote is a picture – a coloured picture of them. His personality has coloured them and selected and altered and pruned and enlarged and minimised and exaggerated. Admitted. But he himself is part, was part of the period, even part of the event itself – he was an actor, a spectator in it. So his distortions are not so much distortions as one might suppose. The event had its effect on him. Undistorted him, opened his eyes.
>
> What have these extracts in common? They have no political or economic or social homogeneity. They are all *moments* in the history of the Industrial Revolution, at which clashes and conflicts suddenly show themselves with extra clearness, and which through that clearness can stand as symbols for the whole inexpressible uncapturable process. They are what later poets have called 'illuminations', 'Moments of Vision' – some obviously clearer than others – some intentional, others

unintentional – but all in some degree with this window-opening quality – it is this which differentiates these pieces of writing from purely economic or political, or social analyses. Theirs is a different method of tackling, of presenting the same material, the same conflicts, the method of poetry.

There is so much in this extract. Jennings was interested not in political, mechanical, social or economic history, but in 'imaginative history': 'mental events', 'events of the heart', 'facts passed through feelings and the minds of individuals'. He wished to *present* this history, not to describe or analyse it; to place evidence before the reader and leave them to make their own judgements. The evidence he presented took the form of quotations – from poets, novelists, scientists, philosophers, social critics, working people, capitalists, journalists – chosen for their 'illuminatory quality', their 'window-opening quality', the way they 'contain in little a whole world', the way they work as 'symbols for the whole'. And while this whole was large – the industrial revolution from 1660 to 1886 – Jennings viewed it horizontally as just one cross-section of history. This comes through in another part of the introduction:[34]

> The analytical historian's business is to disentangle shred by shred like plucking the strand out of a rope. The result is the length of the rope but only one strand's thickness, and although the strand may still be twisted from its position among the other strands it is presented nevertheless alone. The poet might be compared to a man who cuts a short section of the whole rope. The only thing is he must cut it where it will not fall to pieces.

Jennings saw himself more as a poet than a historian, or at least an analytical historian. He was interested more in the 'whole rope' at a particular moment in time – the industrial revolution in the case of *Pandæmonium*, the Coronation of George VI in the case of *May the Twelfth* – than one strand of the rope, followed over time. For Frank Cottrell-Boyce, who wrote the Forward to the 2012 edition of *Pandæmonium*, this cross-sectional view, and the techniques of Surrealism (montage and juxtaposition), may not have allowed Jennings to make an argument, but allowed him to communicate an experience: the *feel* of the industrial revolution; its heat and velocity, the clank of machinery, the roar of the furnaces, the shouts of protest, the thrill and the fear, the injustice and the excitement.[35]

Quotations constitute the main work

He was interested in a particular historical period. He was interested in poetry as much as analytical history. He wished to capture the feel of this period. He sought to do this by presenting quotations, viewed as illuminations. He developed his ideas in a published essay on the machine. He died in the middle of the twentieth century, leaving an enormous, unfinished manuscript that was eventually published closer to the end of that century. This could be Jennings or it could be Walter Benjamin. There are many similarities between them, and many differences too. Benjamin was influenced by Surrealism but also Marxism (to a greater extent than Jennings, who saw conflict in society, but hardly through a Marxist framework). Benjamin was particularly interested in Surrealism's revolutionary potential. He saw in Surrealism the potential to replace religious illumination with profane illumination (i.e. inspiration that is anthropological and materialistic). On Breton's *Nadja*, he wrote:[36]

> He [Breton] was the first to perceive the revolutionary energies that appear in the 'outmoded', in the first iron constructions, the first factory buildings, the earliest photos, the objects that have begun to be extinct, grand pianos, the dresses of five years ago, fashionable restaurants when the vogue has begun to ebb from them.

He continues:[37]

> Breton and Nadja are the lovers who convert everything that we have experienced on mournful railway journeys (railways are beginning to age), on Godforsaken Sunday afternoons in the proletarian quarters of the great cities, in the first glance through the rain-blurred window of a new apartment, into revolutionary experience, if not action. They bring the immense forces of 'atmosphere' concealed in these things to the point of explosion.

Surrealism located revolutionary energy in objects, moments and experiences. Taken by this view, Benjamin became a 'peculiar Marxist', interested more in superstructure than base, and particularly interested in the *spirit* of the nineteenth century, to be found in almost anything from poems to street scenes.[38]

Benjamin sought 'to document as concretely as possible, and thus lend a "heightened graphicness" to, the scene of revolutionary change that was the nineteenth century'.[39] He was interested in 'the image of the epoch'; not the great men and celebrated events of that century, but traces of daily life of the collective, to be found in refuse, detritus, trash – the outmoded materials of everyday life he'd learned to notice from Breton. It was in these ruins that history could be seen; that the process of modernization, with its incessant accumulation of debris, continual demand for the new, production of obsolescence and broken promises could be seen.[40] This last point is Highmore's, who makes a further point regarding Benjamin's purpose. For Benjamin, modernity produced a wealth of material goods and an intensification of sensation, but also a paucity of communicable experience. It produced *erlebnis*: experience that is immediate, inchoate, simply lived-through (think: bombardments on the battlefield, the sensory assault of the modern city, the shock of modern everyday life). But it didn't produce *erfahrung*: experience that is accumulated, reflected upon, examined, evaluated, communicated, made socially meaningful. Daily experience had been revolutionized, but forms of consciousness and communication had not kept pace.[41]

All this left Benjamin with methodological challenges. He collected drawings, photographs, quotations, reflections – often in black-covered notebooks he carried with him everywhere.[42] He arranged these items to produce 'dialectical images': montages of elements 'that, in combination, produce a "spark" that allows for recognition, for legibility, for communication and critique'.[43] As a collector, with a collector's attitude, he was careful to arrange these items in a way that allowed them to remain unique, original, untypical, unclassifiable.[44] He then made much of these individual items. His method of materialist physiognomics encouraged him to infer the interior (the signature of the nineteenth century or the essence of capitalist production) from the exterior (the tangible object or concrete historical form – the machine, product or building).[45] It encouraged him to infer the whole from the detail, the general from the particular; 'to assemble large-scale constructions out of the smallest and most precisely cut components. Indeed, to discover in the analysis of the small individual moment the crystal of the total event'.[46]

An early experiment in producing such a montage, in which illumination would be achieved by juxtaposition of details – and sometimes just the presentation of details themselves – was *One-Way Street* (written during 1925 and 1926).[47] Benjamin's ultimate experiment, though, was *The Arcades Project*, written between 1927 and 1940, unfinished, and published posthumously in 1982.[48] In the period before his death in 1940, Benjamin collected a huge volume of materials and notes on the nineteenth century, including the arcades of Paris, which he saw as that century's most important architectural form.[49] He then grouped these fragments, including thousands of quotations, into bundles or 'convolutes' – the term used by Adorno, who first sifted through Benjamin's papers after the Second World War – covering various topics: arcades, sales clerks, fashion, boredom, exhibitions, advertising, prostitution, gambling, mirrors, modes of lighting, railroads, the stock exchange, idleness, and so on. There has been some discussion as to whether these convolutes left by Benjamin reflect an earlier stage of the research (filing of materials) or a later stage (composition ready for publication). Hannah Arendt argues for the latter:[50]

When he was working on his study of German tragedy, [Benjamin] boasted of a collection of 'over 600 quotations very systematically and clearly arranged' (*Briefe* I, 339); like the later notebooks, this collection was not an accumulation of excerpts intended to facilitate the writing of the study but constituted the main work, with the writing as something secondary. The main work consisted of tearing fragments out of their context and arranging them afresh in such a way that they illustrated one another and were able to prove their *raison d'être* in a free-floating state, as it were. It was definitely a sort of surrealistic montage.

Arendt notes 'Benjamin's ideal of producing a work consisting entirely of quotations, one that was mounted so masterfully that it could dispense with any accompanying text'.[51] The fragments and juxtapositions constituted the main work. Eiland and McLaughlin, who translated *The Arcades Project* for Harvard University Press, also make the case:[52]

Many of the passages of reflection in the 'Convolutes' section represent revisions of earlier drafts, notes, or letters. Why revise for a notebook? The fact that Benjamin also transferred masses of quotations from actual notebooks to the manuscript of the convolutes, and the elaborate organisation of these materials in that manuscript [. . .] might likewise bespeak a compositional principle at work in the project, and not just an advanced stage of research. In fact, the montage form – with its philosophic place of distances, transitions, and intersections, its perpetually shifting contexts and ironic juxtapositions – had become a favourite device in Benjamin's later investigations.

The Arcades Project, however unfinished, was meant to be a montage of quotations. It was meant to describe the nineteenth century graphically, to document it concretely and to capture its feel or spirit by selecting fragments that illuminate its essence and composing these fragments to make sparks fly between them, encouraging further illumination and, ultimately, revolutionary consciousness.

Listening, preserving, exhausting

Quotations were central to Benjamin's works. He described them as 'robbers by the roadside who make an armed attack and relieve an idler of his convictions'.[53] Quotations work to shock readers out of the familiar (and perhaps into revolutionary consciousness). They allow authors to speak for themselves. They allow editors to accommodate multiple, diverse, unique, original, eccentric voices and perspectives. They can open windows on particular times and places, putting the reader there, illuminating events. All this appears to have been appreciated by authors of experimental literature during the 1970s and 1980s, especially Studs Terkel and Svetlana Alexievich. Terkel explained his oral history approach, developed over three decades and numerous books, in *Working* – one of his earliest experiments in publishing 'talk'.[54] He was 'prospecting' for the daily experiences of others, especially non-celebrities: people not often heard from, ordinary people. What such people said often shocked him, providing him with 'prospector's gold'. He sought to treat such people as unique persons and not statistics. Still, he trusted that many of the dreams and hurts felt by these unique persons were felt by others too – a trust seemingly confirmed by the wide readership Terkel found for his books.

Since the mid-1980s, Alexievich has published oral histories, or what she calls 'missing histories', of numerous historical moments: the Second World War (as experienced by Soviet women), the Soviet Union (as experienced by children), war in Afghanistan (as experienced by Soviet soldiers), post-Soviet life (as experienced by post-Soviet citizens). In *Chernobyl Prayer*, she describes her approach as follows:[55]

This is not a book on Chernobyl, but on the world of Chernobyl. Thousands of pages have already been written on the event itself, hundreds of thousands of metres of film devoted to it. What I'm concerned with is what I would call the 'missing history', the invisible imprint of our stay on earth and in time. I paint and collect mundane feelings, thoughts, and words. I am trying to capture the life of the soul. A day in the life of ordinary people.

Her interest is in *the world of the event*, not just the event itself. It is in everyday life: mundane feelings, thoughts and words. It is in the daily – 'a day in the life of ordinary people' – if not just a single day. Elsewhere in the book, she notes her interest in experiences of the disaster, the imprint of the disaster on the senses and emotional life, the meaning of what happened and the perspectives of ordinary people (not high-ranking officials and military men, but peasants, workers at the power plant, scientists, doctors, displaced people, clean-up workers). A part of her project is to collect the stories of such people, to tell those stories and to donate them to the future.

If Terkel and Alexievich use quotations to great effect in representing everyday life – or, better, *presenting* everyday life – then other experimental authors of the 1970s and 1980s introduced other devices to the repertoire of everyday life studies. Based in Paris during this period, Georges Perec is of interest here not for his connections to Lefebvre (and, by extension, Marxist everyday life studies),[56] but for his focus on method: methods of noticing everyday life and methods of depicting everyday life. In his writing for *Cause Commune*, a 1970s review of 'the anthropology of everyday life', he asked how we should 'take account of' the everyday:[57]

> The daily papers talk of everything except the daily. The papers annoy me, they teach me nothing. What they recount doesn't concern me, doesn't ask me questions and doesn't answer the questions I ask or would like to ask [. . .] How should we take account of, describe what happens every day and recurs every day: the banal, the quotidian, the obvious, the common, the ordinary, the infra-ordinary, the background noise, the habitual?

He called for 'our own anthropology': 'What's needed perhaps is finally to found our own anthropology, one that will speak about us, will look in ourselves for what for so long we've been pillaging from others. Not the exotic any more, but the endotic.'[58]

Perec was interested in what he termed the 'infra-ordinary': those parts of everyday life that we struggle to see and speak about. He developed exercises for noticing these things, some of which are reported in *Species of Spaces*:[59] a project to describe and classify all 200 or so places he's slept in; a project to rename the rooms of his apartment to fit different senses (the auditory, the smellery, etc.) or days of the week (the Mondayery, the Tuesdayery, etc.); a project to describe all the apartments of an apartment block, and all the rooms and activities in them (this project became *Life: A User's Manual*);[60] a project to cross town only taking streets beginning with one letter of the alphabet (making notes while walking, taking one's time, looking closely, asking questions). Another exercise is reported in *An Attempt at Exhausting a Place in Paris*.[61] For this project, he spent three days in cafes in place Saint-Sulpice. He wrote:[62]

> There are many things in place Saint-Sulpice [. . .] A great number, if not the majority, of these things have been described, inventoried, photographed, talked about, or registered. My intention in these pages that follow was to describe the rest instead: that which is generally not taken note of, that which is not noticed,

that which has no importance: what happens when nothing happens other than the weather, people, cars, and clouds.

Perec confined himself to just one place in the same way others have confined themselves to just one time (the single day). He sought to exhaust that place, describing all the items he saw and heard – from advertising slogans to overheard conversations, and from passing buses to the titles of books for sale. Indeed, for Perec, self-imposed constraints were important devices for directing attention to the infra-ordinary. In his work with OuLiPo (*Ouvroir de Litterature Potentielle*, or Workshop of Potential Literature), he experimented with various games and rules, including the use of mathematical formulae to shape his projects. Perec practised a 'literary sociology'[63] that sought to 'see flatly' – to see without the usual hierarchy of attention (using devices like inventories and meticulous description)[64] – and to 'write flatly': to communicate observations without the usual hierarchy (using devices like bullet points and lists).[65] He practised an 'extreme empiricism'[66] that was quite different to the project of, say, Alexievich. Still, these different means were oriented towards similar ends. As we have seen, a part of Alexievich's project is archival: to collect stories and preserve them for the future. Perec justified his writing in similar terms: 'To write: to try meticulously to retain something, to cause something to survive; to wrest a few precise scraps from the void as it grows'.[67]

The arbitrary factor of the alphabet

If the preservationist impulse connects Perec to Alexievich, then Perec's interest in classification and hierarchy – in seeing and writing flatly – connects him to another experimental author of this period (and the Paris of this period): Roland Barthes. I have in mind specifically Barthes's *A Lover's Discourse*.[68] For Barthes, the lover's mind races and so their discourse exists in bursts of language: 'adorable', 'agony', 'catastrophe', 'I am crazy', 'at fault', 'the heart', and so on. These fragments of language occur without order. They are not linked by logic. They are 'distributive', not 'integrative' – always existing on the same level. They are 'non-narrative'. Barthes structured his book to fit this 'horizontal discourse' – a collection of quotations and reflections – using the device of the encyclopedia. With encyclopedias, there is no classification and hierarchy. There are no firsts and lasts – beyond those determined by the arbitrary factor of the alphabet.

The device of the encyclopedia – or, rather, the devices of the encyclopedia (entries, cross-references, alphabetized sequencing) – can be added to the other devices for registering and presenting everyday life encountered so far in this chapter: the day-survey, the constraint of the single day (or period, or place) and the horizontal, cross-sectional view; the devices of Surrealism (fragments, montage, juxtaposition); the devices of (surrealist) cinema (close-ups and long shots, rapid cuts and flashbacks, tracking shots and panoramas); the methods of anthropology (fieldwork, observation, participation); quotations and convolutes; and Perec's devices for seeing and writing flatly (inventories, lists, meticulous description). The encyclopedic form was especially prominent in experimental history, geography and theory around the turn of the twenty-first century.

In History, Hans Ulrich Gumbrecht structured *In 1926* as an encyclopedia.[69] The book caters to a perceived desire for direct, immediate, first-hand experience of past worlds (their look, sound, smell, taste, touch); a perceived desire for 'historical reality' or 'history as environment' (not history as narrative). It aims to conjure the worlds of 1926, a random year; to re-present them or make them present again; and to produce for the reader the effect of feeling like they are in 1926. This aim would be achieved by aligning content with form:[70]

> [. . .] the primary, and perhaps crude, desire behind this book – the desire, that is, of coming as close as possible to making present a moment of the past, and of making it 'present' in the fullest possible sense of the word. Such effects of presence, I assume, are more likely to come through reference to concrete historical detail than through abstract, 'totalising' overviews.

Gumbrecht's chosen form, to which concrete historical details would be fitted, was the encyclopedia:[71]

> I have opted for the encyclopedic structure of multiple entries, using the word 'entry' to refer to the individual texts that constitute an encyclopedia or dictionary, but also using it as a way of stressing that everyday-worlds have neither symmetry nor centre and can therefore be entered from many different directions. Each entry leads towards an encounter with an element of concrete historical reality, and each of these elements is connected to other elements via myriad labyrinthine paths of contiguity, association, and implication. The arbitrariness of the alphabetical order in which the entries are presented and the encyclopedic device of cross-references mimic the nonsystematic character of our everyday experience and suggest that readers constitute the world of 1926 as an asymmetrical network.

The entries referred to here cover topics like airplanes, assembly lines, automobiles, bars, boxing, bullfighting, cremation, dancing, and so on. Readers are encouraged to find their own path among these topics, these elements of concrete historical reality, making their own connections between entries:[72]

> Do not try 'to start from the beginning', for this book has no beginning in the sense that narratives or arguments have beginnings. Start with any of the fifty-one entries in any of the three sections [. . .] (the alphabetic order of the subheadings shows that there isn't any hierarchy among them). Simply start with an entry that particularly interests you. From each entry a web of cross-references will take you to other, related entries. Read as far as your interest carries you (and as long as your schedule allows). You'll thus establish your individual reading path. Just as there is no obligatory beginning, there also is no obligatory or definitive end to the

reading process. Regardless of where you enter or exit, any reading sequence of some length should produce the effect to which the book's title alludes: you should feel 'in 1926'.

To achieve this effect, Gumbrecht used the encyclopedic form – entries, alphabetical ordering, cross-references – in combination with other literary devices. He wrote in a 'strictly descriptive' style and refrained, so far as possible, from expressing his own individual voice. He focused on surfaces, as opposed to depths (hermeneutic depth, interpretive depth, depth of meaning). He focused on simultaneity (a single year, if not a single day), as opposed to sequence, causality, subjectivity (Jennings's disentangled shred of rope – the length of the rope, but only one strand's thickness). He included multiple perspectives and favoured paradoxes and contradictions over logic and integration.

In Geography, Pile and Thrift also chose the encyclopedia, its form and devices, for their *City A-Z*.[73] This was their solution to the problem of how to bring the city to print (if the city is not a coherent system, but is rather a 'complex jumble of practices', a 'patchwork of intersecting fields', a 'discordant symphony of overlapping fragments'). The encyclopedic form allowed them to capture the city's multiple constituent parts: airports, amusement arcades, animals, art, beaches, benches, borders, building societies, buses, and so on. It allowed them to capture the city's serious, oppressive side and its vital, playful side; its dreads, violences and frustrations, and its jokes, dreams and delights; and also its sights, sounds and smells. With different authors writing the many entries, this form allowed Pile and Thrift to include a multiplicity of voices and perspectives. Like Gumbrecht, they encouraged readers to make associations between entries, to be disturbed by juxtapositions, to use the book for thinking differently – a 'modest [. . .] act of theorising'.[74]

Why such an interest in the encyclopedic form – and also fragments, connections, associations, experience, environment, re-presentation (over narrative) – around the turn of the twenty-first century? One answer is provided by Featherstone and Venn's introduction to *Theory, Culture and Society*'s 'New Encyclopedia Project'.[75] The project was prompted by two destabilizing processes. Globalization encourages a focus on alternative cultures, traditions and knowledges; and on variability, connectivity and intercommunication. Digitalization encourages a focus on how data are stored and retrieved, and how the world is structured and classified. In this context, the encyclopedic form would open a more dialogic space of engagement (compared to the journal or monograph form). It would accommodate counter-knowledges. It would allow for the constitution of an alternative corpus and the reconstitution of 'the global archive'. It would be appropriate to the 'de-classificatory mood' of the period. Featherstone and Venn are not naïve or romantic in their view of encyclopedias. They prefer Diderot's *Encyclopédie*, produced by a cosmopolitan association of individuals for a cosmopolitan public readership to stimulate discussion and dialogue, to the *Encyclopedia Britannica* (a servant of nationalism). What they take from encyclopedias are certain devices: the expandable list, because knowledge is always incomplete and unfinished; and the multiple, multiply-connected entry – because knowledge doesn't fit easily into just a few separate categories.

Everyday life studies: Intellectual tradition and popular repertoire

There have been numerous recent attempts to extend and reflect on this tradition of everyday life studies. Inspired by Perec, David Matless has tried to 'see flatly' the appropriately flat Broads of eastern England. He constructed *The Regional Book* as an encyclopedia of the region's geography.[76] Forty descriptions of marshes, nature reserves, riversides, seasides, towns, waterways and so on make up a 'cross-regional democracy' due to their non-hierarchical arrangement in the book. Inspired by Perec and Barthes, and more immediately the Austin Public Feelings group and the 100-Word Collective, Berlant and Stewart wrote *The Hundreds* as an exercise in using constraints – the constraint of hundred-word units or units of multiple hundreds – to shape attention.[77] They experiment with classification in the book, providing four different indexes from four different colleagues, and also some blank pages at the end so that readers can themselves experiment with indexing. Inspired by Benjamin, among others, Colin McFarlane structured *Fragments of the City* using vignettes juxtaposed in a 'discontinuous text'.[78] His purpose was to move urban studies beyond the utopian desire for wholeness and completeness; beyond modernity with its technologies for making the city appear coherent (maps and statistics) and for governing the coherent city (bureaucracies). The book emphasizes fragments, scraps, ruins: material fragments (bits of housing and infrastructure) and knowledge fragments (different ways of knowing, traces of historical memory, alternative mappings). Most recently, Karl Schlögel's *The Soviet Century* was also inspired by Benjamin and especially one particular line from *The Arcades Project*: 'Method of this project: literary montage. I needn't say anything. Merely show'.[79] Schlögel eschews commentary and focuses instead on providing evidence. This takes the form of sixty chapters covering the lifeworld of the Soviet Union – its values, practices, routines, styles, manners, institutions and biographies – and such topics as bazaars, medals, tattoos, borders, parades, queues, telephones, and so on. For Schlögel, pursuing the 'unachievable ideal' of *histoire totale*, 'The totality grows out of the details'.[80]

Another set of recent studies have been interested less in extending this tradition and more in reflecting on its popularization, especially via mass photography and film projects. Annebella Pollen describes these projects in *Mass Photography*.[81] They include: A Day in the Life of Australia (1981), One Day for Life (1987), Heart of Britain (1996), Dawn of the 21st Century – The Millennium Photo Project (2000), One Digital Day (2003), A Minute in the Life (2007), A Moment in Time (2009), Picturing the Seven Billion (2011), World Wide Moment (2011), One Day on Earth (2011), Life in a Day (2011) and A Day in the World (2012). Pollen herself is most interested in One Day for Life. People were asked to submit photos taken on 14 August 1987. They paid a fee of £1, which went to Search 88 Cancer Trust. A selection of the photos were published in a book. All of them were archived in the Mass Observation Archive. Daniel Ashton has studied *Life in a Day*, a crowdsourced documentary produced in collaboration with YouTube, and *Britain in a Day*, the sequel produced in collaboration with the BBC.[82] Again, there is a link to Mass Observation, claimed as inspiration by the producers. Between them, Pollen and Ashton note the concerns of these projects and their producers: the opportunities provided by new technologies; the amateur, the participatory, the democratic, the crowd (-sourced); the diversity of the crowd; the national self-portrait or family album; global connectedness and community; and the creation of archives, time capsules and chronicles for future generations. Not all such concerns are straightforwardly compatible. Indeed, Pollen and Ashton reflect critically on these projects, their intentions and outcomes.

I include these reflections in the next section, a more critical discussion of everyday life studies, but let me complete the present section by summarizing the strengths or opportunities presented by this tradition and its repertoire. A cross-sectional approach (especially focused on just one day), the techniques of Surrealism (especially montage and juxtaposition), quotation (especially from ordinary people speaking or writing from multiple perspectives) and non-hierarchical structures (especially the encyclopedic form) together allow for and encourage numerous achievements. Events can be described in ways that bring them to life, make them graphic and vivid, capture their feel and meaning and put the reader there. Multiple constituents of events can be included in descriptions – sites, acts, thoughts, feelings, sights, sounds, smells, textures, memories, fantasies – making up full and democratic accounts. The usually overlooked or taken-for-granted can be included – the familiar, habitual, routine – and made visible, strange, marvellous, shocking, open to critique and reform (or revolution). Multiple voices and perspectives can be included – speaking in their own terms, allowed to be unique – making for democratic, participatory accounts that decentre the author and their assumptions and prejudices. An alternative, unofficial, street-level view of events can be provided – what Alexievich terms 'missing history'[83] – that punctures the official rhetoric of politicians and journalists (and academics). A record or archive of that missing history can be provided for historians and future generations. A view of society as complex, diverse and eccentric can be presented that undercuts myths of 'the people'. A view of society as contradictory, paradoxical and ambiguous can be presented that encourages modesty and care in societal engagement. A creative, inventive form of theorizing can be facilitated, where new encounters and vibrations lead to the questioning of existing categories and hierarchies, and the making of novel connections, ideas and research questions.

Crude, naïve empiricism?

If these are the strengths of the everyday life studies repertoire, then it also has weaknesses, which have been in the background so far, but need discussing (as a prelude to discussion of this book's strengths and weaknesses). Indeed, many such weaknesses correspond to the strengths listed above. The experience of an event, especially an event like a pandemic, could never be fully captured in writing. Similarly, the excess of everyday life could never be fully registered. An event or place, as Perec found, could never be fully exhausted.[84] Exclusions will always remain. Also, the fewer exclusions remain, the more likely the description will be long and unwieldy. This approximates James Hinton's assessment of the original *May the Twelfth*, which in turn aligns with some assessments at the time (especially that of Harrisson): it was 'huge and sprawling' and 'as likely to evoke boredom as emotional involvement'.[85] One assessment of the broader M-O project at the time came from Malinowski, who supported M-O (as we have seen), but worried about its ambition to observe everything; its 'crude empiricism'.[86] For Malinowski, the usually overlooked was usually overlooked for a reason. M-O should have been focused on phenomena 'relevant' to existing knowledge and 'practical' for analysis.

Another criticism is that attempts to collect data on the ordinary (e.g. an ordinary day) constitute interventions that risk making the ordinary *extra*ordinary. Was 12 May 2020 transformed by MO's scrutiny of it? Pollen found that mass photography projects like One Day for Life certainly transformed their objects.[87] Calls for photographs – of the normal, the natural, the everyday – transformed particular days into special events. On such days, people did what they imagined would make for a good photograph, would interest future historians, would be universally understandable (as a symbol of common culture and experience). So they performed humanist universality (e.g. love) or local specificity (e.g. tradition). They submitted photographs that didn't so much depict everyday life – flowing, ceaseless – as made sentimental, celebratory statements about 'ordinary life' in 'our small world'.

Another criticism of studies focused on just one day or short period (amenable to exhaustive description) is that such a focus overlooks the longer term in which both causation and subjectivity might be seen. Benjamin was criticized for this. Adorno and Horkheimer, his sponsors at the Institute for Social Research, thought his undialectical Marxism privileged superstructure over base.[88] They encouraged a rebalancing away from 'representation' and the 'poetic' or 'romantic' form towards historical materialism and Marx's analysis of capital.[89] The balance they encouraged was probably best achieved not by Benjamin, but – a few years later – by Henri Lefebvre. In Volume 1 of *Critique of Everyday Life*, he sought to describe bourgeois society *sociologically*: to describe what is done (the small, individual event), but also the tangle of reasons and causes surrounding what is done – the actor's biography, job, family, class, habits and opinions, and the state of the market (*the complex social event*).[90] In Volume 3, he describes everyday actions like eating, drinking, dressing and sleeping, but also their social context: the social relations in which they occur; the structures implicit and concealed in such acts; the mode of production realized in everyday actions.[91] In doing so, Lefebvre was keen to go beyond endorsing or ratifying everyday life – a risk he saw in cross-sectional studies concerned with simultaneous detail. He researched everyday life to illuminate the mode of production and, ultimately, to create a different everyday.

The criticism directed at Benjamin by Adorno and Horkheimer was later directed by the New Left at M-O and specifically Madge.[92] For Marxists like Raymond Williams, Stuart Hall and E. P. Thompson, when everyday life studies attempted exhaustive description it became 'naïve empiricism'. A different but related criticism has been

273

directed at horizontal approaches to writing collected by the contemporary MO. For Hinton, such writing is usually autobiographical. Read vertically, with a focus on, say, one person writing across the years – as opposed to many people writing on just one day – it illuminates the historical agency of ordinary people, who drive forward 'molecular historical processes' by struggling, making choices and constructing selves.[93]

Horizontal approaches, then, risk missing both causation and subjectivity. Against this criticism, on the other side of the balance, are placed strengths like inclusiveness – the way spatial or temporal constraints (the focus on just one place or moment) facilitate inclusion of multiple perspectives on that particular event. But this claim to inclusiveness is also questionable. Everyday life studies has been dominated by white, middle-class men who've located everyday life in the city, the street and public space – not least by exploiting their freedom to walk and observe 'others'.[94] The tradition has neglected private space, the domestic sphere, the home, social reproduction, gendered labour and much feminist scholarship on such topics.[95] It has rarely included the full range of perspectives on events.

But even if the full range of perspectives could be included, other difficulties would remain. Can ordinary people know and communicate their own everyday lives? Marxists tend to think not. For Marx, everyday life was not self-evident. Real material circumstances, such as the division of labour, are hidden by ideology. Everyday life consists of surface experience, available for scrutiny, but also underpinning structures, only available for scrutiny once revealed by (dialectical, historical materialist) analysis.[96] Such analysis, in the field of everyday life studies, is again best exemplified by Lefebvre. The key concept of Volume 1 of *Critique of Everyday Life* is alienation. The division of labour atomizes people. Economic objects – commodities, money, capital – conceal social relations. People therefore lack consciousness of their own lives. They see only illusions, appearances and mystifications. The critique of everyday life aims for transformation by revealing the reality beneath such illusions.

Ordinary people, in this view, are not Marxists able to see the reality of everyday life. For critics of M-O, which depended so heavily on mass observation – observation of the masses by the masses – ordinary people lack a different kind of training: they are not anthropologists (trained to see rituals, symbols and superstitions). This criticism has been made of the Mass Observers used as ethnographers by Harrisson in his Worktown project, including by Malinowski,[97] but also of those used more as autoethnographers by Madge in his National Panel.[98] While the ethnographers faced difficulties entering working-class cultures as outsiders, the autoethnographers faced difficulties exiting their own cultures to gain a more distant perspective. In this view, ordinary people are too close to their own lives to know and communicate them without need for additional analysis or interpretation by trained outsiders. Furthermore, there is another way in which ordinary people might be too close to their own lives or at least to recent events in their lives. Alexievich identified this while conducting oral history interviews over the twenty-year period following the Chernobyl disaster.[99] Initially, in the first few years, interviewees struggled to express themselves. They were trapped in the language of war: 'nuclear', 'explosion', 'heroes', 'refugees', 'monuments'. It was only over time that people found new idioms and concepts to capture this new experience; that people 'caught up with reality'. How long might it take for people to catch up with and find words appropriate to the Covid-19 pandemic?

Another limitation of the everyday life studies repertoire is that collecting the multiple perspectives of ordinary people at one particular time (or in one particular place) – assuming that was both possible and revealing – before arranging those perspectives non-hierarchically as a montage of quotations with little mediation, framing, interpretation or narrative structure, can produce a cacophony, an incoherent text, easily ignored for its lack of clear findings, argument and programme. This was Harrisson's response to the original *May the Twelfth*. His own ambitions for M-O were that it should not only present but also classify and analyse mass culture. According to Hinton, Harrisson 'hated the book' (edited by Jennings and Madge) and 'deplored the picture it painted of M-O's work'.[100] After publication, and after Jennings had left M-O, Harrisson moved forward with Madge on a rebalanced programme of work that weighed classification and analysis more heavily.[101] The methodological implications of this rebalancing included replacement of the day-surveys (on which *May the Twelfth* was based) with more focused directives on topics like consumption habits and preparations for war.

One justification for producing a cacophony, an incoherent text lacking framing and interpretation, might be that authors – especially white, middle-class, male authors – need decentring. However, this is not easily achieved. When surveying a day or exhausting a place, authors generally choose the day or place. When giving voice to ordinary people, authors generally choose the quotations. When arranging fragments in a montage, authors generally choose the order, which in turn sets up the juxtapositions. When using the encyclopedic form, authors generally choose the entries, imposing their own classification. The centrality of the author – alongside the archivist – endures by more subtle means too. Dorothy Sheridan and colleagues describe writers for the contemporary MO as 'correspondents'.[102] They enter a relationship with MO. Their writing emerges from an ongoing dialogue with MO, in which the archivists are never quite peripheral. Pollen makes a similar point.[103] MO directives address panellists imagined as particular people (historically conscious, civic-minded, often older, more often than not women). By return, panellists address their writing to an imagined audience (of future historians and curious citizens). Just collecting perspectives on everyday life requires intersubjective negotiation, even before the author proceeds to compose such perspectives. At the point of composition, authors – alongside organizers, sponsors, judges and editors (in the case of mass photography and film projects) – become even more central. Pollen's study of One Day for Life demonstrates how the books, films and exhibitions produced from such projects tend to reflect the preferences and prejudices of those leading them. She concludes:[104]

> For all their democratic promise and ideals of self-representation, mass-participation projects are mediated by the interests of the organisers and funders and all are, inevitably, shaped by their project's brief. The resulting material is always solicited, produced, and performed for a particular purpose rather than

offering a direct interception of lived experience; they are never ordinary in any sense of the term.

Regarding *Life in a Day* and *Britain in a Day*, Ashton reaches a similar conclusion.[105] These montages of crowdsourced videos were shaped by the submission guidance provided by the producers. This guidance emphasized particular themes and norms (community, inclusion, the personal). In the resultant films, a diversity of contributors did not translate into a diversity of contributions.

A pretty full account

Where does all this discussion of strengths and weaknesses leave the present book? What are its strengths and weaknesses as an account of the Covid-19 pandemic? It does not fully capture the experience of everyday life in the pandemic, even just in the UK. No single book could – especially when based on a sample of just one collection (10 per cent of MO's 12th May diaries), and edited to fit a publisher's word limit (from a much longer original draft). However, like Gumbrecht's attempt to capture the worlds of 1926, it is worth experimenting. It is worth seeing how far it is possible to go in such an exercise.[106] And the account provided in this book is pretty full. It covers experiences of people from all age groups, genders, regions of the UK and occupational classifications. And it covers the activities, events and rituals of everyday life in the pandemic (from birdsong to working from home); sites or stages (from shops to Zoom); roles or subject positions (from furloughed workers to shielding 'vulnerable' or 'high-risk' individuals); frames (from luck to 'the new normal') and moods (from anxiety to hope).

By focusing on just one day (12 May 2020), the book trades the advantages of a cross-sectional, horizontal view – detailed description and inclusion of multiple perspectives – for other things: coverage of other days in the pandemic; coverage of days in the pandemic when a day-survey had not transformed the day from ordinary to extraordinary and coverage of the longer term in which might be seen causation and subjectivity. By focusing on just diaries collected by MO, the book is not formally representative of the UK population and no doubt misses some voices and perspectives (e.g. people unlikely to volunteer for a social history project), but it does include some voices and perspectives often missed by everyday life studies (e.g. those of women and teenagers). Furthermore, while the sample of diarists may not be fully representative from a social science perspective, the book does take seriously *representation* (from an arts and humanities perspective). This is important. The sampling, statistical, input problem of representativeness – the problem of the social constitution of the MO dataset and whether it can be generalized from – is only one problem confronting a study like this. An equally significant problem is the aesthetic, literary, output problem of representation: the problem of how to select and compose from the MO dataset to construct an account of the pandemic that does justice to the general and particular, and the clear and ambiguous – in both the archive and society as a whole. The book takes this problem seriously, inspired by – and having learned from – experimental, non-linear writing on previous pandemics (the introductory chapter) and everyday life (this chapter).

The core of the book – the main work – is made up of quotations with little in the way of interpretation and analysis. This provides only a surface view of pandemic experience. It leaves interpretation and analysis to others. However, the interpretative and analytical work done by MO diarists themselves should not be overlooked or dismissed. The quotations included in this book are already interpretations. In this respect, they are similar to writing for MO more generally. Such writing has often been reflexive.[107] Correspondents generally scrutinize the task they are given; acknowledge their own vantage points; position themselves as particular cases; contextualize their experiences; and reflect on tensions, contradictions and uncertainties in their lives (and the societies in which they live). The summary paragraphs at the top of each entry in this book should not be forgotten either. By providing these, I am attempting to balance two things: the principle of giving voice to ordinary people (letting them speak in their own terms and letting them be unique) and the desire of many potential readers for at least some coherence and some listening guide (to the otherwise intentional cacophony).

On the question of authorship and my own centrality, assumptions and prejudices, the book is very much a product of MO's relationship with its diarists, the archivists' organization of the 12 May 2020 day-survey and my own editorial choices. For example, I selected extracts from within the diaries and arranged them in entries developed from my initial reading of the material. Nevertheless, certain devices did allow me to decentre myself in the book. The entries are arranged alphabetically, so juxtapositions between entries are set up automatically and without my authorship. Similarly, within entries quotations are arranged numerically (by the code given to each diarist by MO). Overall, I think the book sets up many encounters, connections and vibrations, and suggests many ideas and questions (some of which I signpost in the introductory chapter). The book, I think, largely avoids humanistic cliché and instead depicts society as complex, diverse and eccentric; impossible to mythologize as 'the people'; demanding a modest and careful engagement with others. These are the book's politics. They are a different politics to, say, the politics of Harrisson, who disliked the original *May the Twelfth* or Lefebvre, who modelled a different everyday life studies. The final section discusses and contextualizes the book's politics.

Science of the people, by the people, for the people

My aim in writing this book was to produce a humanizing, democratic account of the Covid-19 pandemic as it was experienced in the UK. It was to produce something different from those accounts provided by the health and social sciences – based on statistics, focused on the immediate concerns of governments and other agencies seeking to govern the pandemic and criticized by Richard Horton, editor-in-chief of *The Lancet*, for 'biologising' and 'dehumanising' the pandemic; for raising mathematical summaries over the meanings of the disease and the biographies of those who lived and died with it.[108] My aim in writing this book was also to produce something different from certain accounts provided by the arts and humanities. The pandemic was a 'diarological moment',[109] with diaries and similar writing collected by numerous research projects and archives. Such large, qualitative datasets, however, pose methodological challenges for researchers. How to analyse the material? And how to present it? Many researchers have analysed a small proportion of these datasets and presented the material, or *re*presented it, alongside their own interpretations (as illustrations of their own expert interpretations). I wanted to include more of MO's Covid-19 collections in this book and to present the writing of diarists with less mediation from my own interpretations. This would make not only a humanizing account of the pandemic, at least compared to those accounts from the health and social sciences, but also a democratic account – with more people able to speak in their own voices. The idea for the book was both to provide such an account of the pandemic and to model such an account – humanizing, democratic – for use by other researchers interested in other events. The model I have in mind is captured by the title of this final section: a science of the people (describing the everyday lives of ordinary people), by the people (involving such people as observers and writers), for the people (involving ordinary people as readers of such writing).

This particular science – with 'science' used loosely in the same way it was used by the surrealists ('science of the everyday')[110] or the original M-O ('science of ourselves')[111] – was pioneered by the original M-O, at least in its early phase when Madge and Jennings were still involved. The original M-O was a political project that responded to the context of 1930s Britain. This context included: the recent advent of near universal suffrage; the rise of the Labour Party; the emergence of mass media (the popular press, cinema, radio); the recent economic depression; the growing threat of war; and concerns about how mass democracy would succeed.[112] For Nick Hubble, it included a view of modern life as depoliticized.[113] Representative democracy was thought to have transformed a debating public into a mass electorate. There were concerns that a great distance had opened up between political leaders and an apathetic people. Such people might be susceptible to propaganda (a threat) but also to interventions in everyday life (an opportunity – disruption of the symbolic order to promote a revolutionary mass consciousness).

How did M-O respond? It sought to close the gap between political leaders and the masses. It collected the voices of the people and sought to publish them to two different audiences for two different purposes.[114] Harrisson, the reformer, focused on a potential audience of political leaders. He would help them to understand the masses and so to rule more effectively. Madge, the revolutionary, focused on a potential audience of ordinary people. He would help the masses to understand themselves – their situation and potential.

The politics of the original M-O is perhaps best articulated in *Britain*.[115] Madge and Harrisson identified the problem as follows:[116]

There are two kinds of focus on society. One is the ordinary focus of the ordinary man or woman which centres round the home and family, work and wages. The other is the political focus, which centres round government policy and diplomacy. What happens in this political sphere obviously affects the sphere of home and work; equally obviously, political developments are affected by the reactions of ordinary people. But between the two there is a gulf – of understanding, of information, and of interest. This gulf is the biggest problem of our highly organised civilisation.

Britain was meant to be a democracy. So the people were meant to know about events, and their leaders were meant to know about the people (and what they thought of events). However, this did not appear to be happening. The newspapers and politicians were not providing the masses with facts or a voice. M-O would therefore have to perform this function: gathering facts about everyday life and publishing them to both elites and the people. Such a function was becoming increasingly important as the masses responded to successive crises – the abdication crisis of 1936 and the war crisis of 1938 – with uncertainty, anxiety, fear and a susceptibility to rumour and panic.

Britain contains analysis of the war crisis, but also cultural phenomena like the Lambeth Walk (a popular dance), on which Madge and Harrisson wrote:[117]

> What people feel about the war danger is an obviously serious subject, but it is less obvious why the popularity of a dance is of anything more than a frivolous interest. But if we can get at the reason for the fashion, and see it in its setting, it may help us to understand the way in which the mass is tending. We may learn something about the future of democracy if we take a closer look at the Lambeth Walk.

Madge and Harrisson appear to have found this dance interesting because it accommodated both mass participation and individual expression. Highmore has developed this point.[118] The Lambeth Walk was 'ritualistic without being hypnotic'. It was 'a practice that unites without unifying'. In this view, the dance contained the potential for a response to Fascism. Indeed, this was the broader politics of M-O, as Highmore sees it: to search out and highlight images of society as unified (meeting the desire for unity), but unified less through sameness and more through difference and creativity. One such image was found in the Lambeth Walk. Another was found in, or constructed from, the day-survey of 12 May 1937. The book based on that day-survey, *May the Twelfth*, emphasized both commonality ('everyone experienced the same day, the same coronation') and diversity.[119] It depicted society as 'a totality of fragments'.[120] This was the politics of the original *May the Twelfth*. It is also the politics of the present book.

I've referred to this politics as science of the people, by the people, for the people. Similar phrases have been used by other scholars of MO. David Pocock wrote:[121] 'The founders of the Mass-Observation "movement", as it was called, all shared a belief that whether the observation was *of* the masses or *by* the masses (it was in fact a combination of both) it was certainly *for* the masses.' M-O asked people to observe themselves and each other. Such observations were then published back to the masses. The idea was 'to feed into the public mind the truth about contemporary Britain'. Publications like *May the Twelfth* 'were somehow to work in the collective mind like the insights of the psychoanalyst, dissolving repressions, disentangling complexities [. . .] extending consciousness'.[122] Jeremy MacClancy described a central aim of M-O as 'the production of ethnography of the people by the people for the people'.[123] This would involve 'working with a mass of observers' to collect observations and then publishing those observations 'to all observers, so that their environment might be understood, and thus constantly transformed. By gaining knowledge people would emancipate themselves'.[124] Hubble also referred to 'observation of the masses by the masses for the masses'. Again, the phrase was used to capture two moves in the political education of British citizens: observation of the masses by the masses and publication of observations to the masses.

M-O aimed to raise consciousness in 1930s Britain. It invited people to participate in its science of the everyday and to constitute themselves as a public of Mass Observers.[125] It sought to construct a civil society and public sphere where superstition would be a focus of observation and conscious reflection.[126] To achieve all this, M-O mobilized ordinary people in two ways: as observers and writers (of reports), and as readers (of observations in books like *May the Twelfth*). There is disagreement regarding the success or failure of this latter mode of mobilization. Some researchers have noted the large size of M-O's National Panel during the late 1930s (over 2,000 panellists) and the way M-O fed results and examples back to panellists via its regular bulletin (*Us*) and other publications; and have argued that M-O was a popular social movement that contributed to the emergence of a new cadre of the intellectually and scientifically engaged, provided this cadre with models for self-observation and facilitated the routinization of social research during and after the Second World War – the mundane embedding of social research in everyday life, including the normalization of mass surveillance and opinion polling as a collective habit.[127] Others, though, have noted how publications like *May the Twelfth* were expensive and did not sell well.[128] Such publications were also infrequent as M-O struggled to process all the reports received from Mass Observers, not least after the organization began losing editors to the war effort.[129]

The mobilization of ordinary people as readers may not have been entirely successful, but it does appear to be one characteristic of the original M-O distinguishing it from the contemporary MO. The Mass Observation Archive and its ongoing research projects are focused primarily on mobilizing participants as writers. The Mass Observation Project, for example, is commonly viewed as a life history project and archive of autobiographical writing. Correspondents are encouraged and enabled to 'write themselves' and, by doing so, to 'write Britain'.[130] The writing submitted is rarely published back to participants or more widely, at least in relatively unmediated form, and at least in publications aimed beyond a relatively narrow readership of academics and students. Indeed, with only a few exceptions,[131] the contemporary MO has been more successful in publishing material collected during the 1930s and 1940s than material collected over the last four decades.[132]

The present book publishes material collected in 2020. In doing so, it seeks to revive the politics of the original M-O: to mobilize people as both writers and readers. And it seeks to revive the politics of the original *May the Twelfth*: to provide readers with a street-level view of events; a contrast to the official record; fragments of description and experience that put readers there (in the event); and a montage of juxtapositions that portray society as complex, diverse and eccentric. Today's context is different from the 1930s, of course, but there are similarities too. Myths and superstitions are being mobilized and amplified by old and new media. There is anxiety related to recent economic crises and the threat of war. There are concerns about democratic functioning and especially the gap between politicians and the people. There is the rise of populism, exploiting this gap and mobilising myths of 'the people'. There is even the return of Fascism to power in Europe. All this means that, just like in the 1930s, there is a need today for depictions of society as unified, but unified through difference and creativity. This need exists despite new forms of mass observation, including public opinion polls and social media. While public opinion polls are representative (in the statistical sense) and good at summarizing society, they are less good at *presenting* society (as a collection of unique voices). And while social media platforms allow people to speak for themselves, they don't seem to encourage or facilitate the frankness, thoughtfulness and reflexivity we see in writing for MO. There remains a need today for MO's writing projects and publication of that writing as widely as possible.

This book, then, is really two books. It is a book about the Covid-19 pandemic. It seeks to remember the pandemic – its novelty, strangeness, difficulty and painfulness – and to preserve stories about everyday life in the pandemic for future generations. It is an experiment in narrating the pandemic that seeks to provide a humanizing account (covering biographies, meanings, feelings, compromises, moral ambiguities, paradoxes, contradictions) and a democratic account (in which ordinary people get to speak in their own voices from multiple perspectives). It is composed to set up encounters, connections and vibrations; to illuminate and to shock; to suggest new ideas and questions; to make the world bigger; and so to encourage a certain orientation to the world: uncertain, modest, caring. In these ways, the book is also a contribution to a larger project. It tries to model a revived science of the people, by the people, for the people. It is certainly a call for research of this kind – focused on the ordinary, participatory, publicly engaged – built around a repoliticized MO for these repoliticized times.

Diarist 924 (female, 30s, Scotland, midwife)

Today was a bit of a rubbish day.
Maybe tomorrow will be better.

Diarist 1209 (female, 70s, North East England, retired doctor)

This is the spring of lock-down due to Covid-19, though I expect it will extend through summer and into autumn and winter. At present it is tolerable as the days are long and sunny. Heaven help us when it's dark, cold and gloomy.

Diarist 2205 (male, 70s, North West England, retired teacher)

Night all! And – as many say at the moment – Stay Safe!

Diarist 2721 (female, 40s, North West England, clinician)

I tell a friend about this diary and suddenly get paranoid when she says her day isn't interesting enough… is mine?

Diarist 2750 (female, 40s, South East England, heritage collections manager)

It is 9pm now [. . .] I feel like I haven't contributed much to the world today, other than keeping my family safe, but maybe recording and writing this is contribution enough.

Diarist 2957 (female, 50s, North West England, careers consultant)

Whatever happens in the year ahead, I just hope (and pray, sometimes) that we will keep safe. That we can stay positive. That I'll be able to write another diary entry, for May 2021.

NOTES

Introduction

1. On the sequence of events in late 2019 and early 2020, the UK's response and its consequences, see British Academy No Date, Farrar 2021, Freedman 2020, Horton 2021 and House of Commons Health and Social Care and Science and Technology Select Committees 2021. On public support for and compliance with lockdown and associated regulations and guidance, see Drury et al. 2021, Fancourt et al. 2020, and Reicher and Drury 2021.

2. Horton 2021: xvi.

3. Horton 2021: 153.

4. Hubble 2010, Jeffery 1978.

5. For more on the human science of the contemporary Mass Observation, see Clarke and Barnett 2023.

6. Jennings and Madge 1937/1987.

7. Buzard 1997, Hinton 2013.

8. Marcus 2001.

9. Pocock 1987: 419.

10. Highmore 2002a: 92.

11. Highmore 2023.

12. Highmore 2002a.

13. Brophy-Harmer 2023.

14. Madge and Harrisson 1937: 44.

15. Kushner 2004.

16. Brophy-Harmer 2023.

17. On the responses of different countries, see also Boin et al. 2021 and Capano et al. 2020.

18. Pollen 2023.

19. Cvetkovich 2003.

20. Langhamer 2016. On MO as an archive of feelings, see also Cook 2017.

21. Williams 1977.

22. Schlögel 2023.

23. Schlögel 2023: 6.

24. Spinney 2018: 4–5.

25. Krastev 2020: 5.

26. Wall 2003: xx–xxi; see also Defoe 1722/2003.

Notes

27. Burgess 1966/2003: 275.
28. Burgess 1966/2003: 272.
29. Camus 1947/2020: 20.
30. Camus 1947/2020: 91.
31. Camus 1947/2020: 87.
32. Judt 2020.
33. Grover 1987.
34. See Williams 1976.
35. Erni and Striphas 2021: 216.
36. On seeing and writing 'flatly', see Perec 1974/2008.
37. On Walter Benjamin's 'illuminations', understood in this way, see Tiedemann 1988/2002.
38. Highmore 2023.
39. Gumbrecht 1997.
40. Perec 1978/2008.
41. On the constituent parts of this myth of national disunity, especially panic buying and lockdown fatigue, see Drury et al. 2021 and Reicher and Drury 2021.
42. Hennessy 2022.
43. On 'COVID-19, the multiplier', see Erni and Striphas 2021.

Conclusion

1. Highmore 2002a, 2002b.
2. Highmore 2002a: 22.
3. Highmore 2002b: 19.
4. Highmore 2002b: 20.
5. Joyce 1922/1993, Woolf 1925/1992.
6. Johnson 1993: xxiv.
7. Levin, cited in Johnson 1993: ix.
8. Enright 2022.
9. Enright 2022: no page number.
10. Showalter 1992.
11. Showalter 1992.
12. Showalter 1992: xix.
13. Showalter 1992: xxi.
14. Showalter 1992: xxx.
15. Highmore 2002a.
16. Highmore 2002a: 46.
17. Highmore 2002a: 51.
18. Jennings and Madge 1937/1987.

19. Pocock 1987: 419.
20. Marcus 2001.
21. Madge and Harrisson 1938/2009.
22. Madge and Harrisson 1938/2009.
23. Harrisson et al. 1937.
24. Madge and Harrisson 1938/2009.
25. Highmore 2002a.
26. Hinton 2013.
27. Sheridan et al. 2000.
28. Hubble 2010.
29. Highmore 2023.
30. Jardine 2018.
31. Jennings 1985/2012.
32. Jennings 2012.
33. Jennings 1985/2012: xiii.
34. Jennings 1985/2012: xv.
35. Cottrell-Boyce 2012.
36. Benjamin 1929/2021: 266.
37. Benjamin 1929/2021: 267.
38. Arendt 1955/2015.
39. Eiland and McLaughlin 2002: xii.
40. Highmore 2002a.
41. Highmore 2002a.
42. Arendt 1955/2015.
43. Highmore 2002a: 71.
44. Arendt 1955/2015.
45. Tiedemann 1988/2002.
46. Benjamin, cited in Tiedemann 1988/2002: 931.
47. Benjamin 1926/2021.
48. Benjamin 1982/2002.
49. Eiland and McLaughlin 2002.
50. Arendt 1955/2015: 51.
51. Arendt 1955/2015: 51.
52. Eiland and McLaughlin 2002: xi.
53. Benjamin, cited in Arendt 1955/2015: 43.
54. Terkel 1970/2004.
55. Alexievich 1997/2016: 24.
56. In the 1960s, Perec worked as a research assistant for Lefebvre.
57. Perec 1973/2020: 31.

Notes

58. Perec 1973/2020: 32.
59. Perec 1974/2008.
60. Perec 1978/2008.
61. Perec 1975/2010.
62. Perec 1975/2010: 3.
63. Sturrock 2008.
64. Perec 1974/2008.
65. Phillips 2018.
66. Lowenthal 2010.
67. Perec 1974/2008: 92.
68. Barthes 1977/2002.
69. Gumbrecht 1997.
70. Gumbrecht 1997: 475.
71. Gumbrecht 1997: 435.
72. Gumbrecht 1997: ix.
73. Pile and Thrift 2002.
74. Pile and Thrift 2002: xix.
75. Featherstone and Venn 2006.
76. Matless 2015.
77. Berlant and Stewart 2019.
78. McFarlane 2021.
79. Schlögel 2023: 3.
80. Schlögel 2023: 2.
81. Pollen 2020.
82. Ashton 2015.
83. Alexievich 1997/2016.
84. Perec 1975/2010.
85. Hinton 2013: 67.
86. Malinowski 1938/2009.
87. Pollen 2020.
88. Arendt 1955/2015.
89. Tiedemann 1988/2002.
90. Trebitsch 2014.
91. Lefebvre 1981/2014.
92. Campsie 2016.
93. Hinton 2010.
94. Highmore 2002b.
95. Hall 2020.
96. Highmore 2002b.

97. Malinowski 1938/2009.

98. Buzard 1997.

99. Alexievich 1997/2016.

100. Hinton 2013: 68–74.

101. Madge and Harrisson 1938/2009.

102. Sheridan et al. 2000.

103. Pollen 2014.

104. Pollen 2020: 211.

105. Ashton 2015, 2017.

106. Gumbrecht 1997.

107. Kramer 2014, Wilson-Kovaks 2014.

108. Horton 2021.

109. Murray et al. 2020.

110. Highmore 2002a.

111. Madge and Harrisson 1939/2009.

112. Ashplant 2021.

113. Hubble 2010.

114. Hinton 2013.

115. Madge and Harrisson 1939/2009.

116. Madge and Harrisson 1939/2009: 25.

117. Madge and Harrisson 1939/2009: 140.

118. Highmore 2002a: 109.

119. Highmore 2002a: 92.

120. Highmore 2002a: 92.

121. Pocock 1987: 416.

122. Pocock 1987: 416.

123. MacClancy 1995: 495.

124. MacClancy 1995: 499.

125. Highmore 2023.

126. Highmore 2023.

127. Harrison 2014, Savage 2010.

128. Hinton 2013, Pocock 1987.

129. Highmore 2002a.

130. Sheridan et al. 2000.

131. The most notable exception is probably 'Observing the 80s', a collaboration between MO and the British Library, funded by Jisc (see https://blogs.sussex.ac.uk/observingthe80s/).

132. See, for example, Calder and Sheridan 1984, Garfield 2005, Sheridan 2009.

REFERENCES

Alexievich, S. (1997/2016), *Chernobyl Prayer: A Chronicle of the Future*, London: Penguin.

Arendt, H. (1955/2015), 'Introduction: Walter Benjamin: 1892–1940', in W. Benjamin, *Illuminations*, 7–60, London: The Bodley Head.

Ashplant, T. G. (2021), 'Mass Observation (1937–2017) and Life Writing: An Introduction', *The European Journal of Life Writing*, X: MO1–MO15.

Ashton, D. (2015), 'Producing Participatory Media: (Crowd)sourcing Content in *Britain/Life in a Day*', *Making Media Participatory*, 154: 101–11.

Ashton, D. (2017), 'Digital Stories, Participatory Practices, and *Life/Britain in a Day*: Framing Creativity and Debating Diversity', in S Malik, C Chapain, and R Comunian (eds), *Community Filmmaking: Diversity, Innovation, Policy, and Practice*, 26–44, London: Routledge.

Barthes, R. (1977/2002), *A Lover's Discourse: Fragments*, London: Vintage.

Benjamin, W. (1926/2021), *One-Way Street*, London: Verso.

Benjamin, W. (1929/2021), 'Surrealism: The Last Snapshot of the European Intelligentsia', in W. Benjamin and NLB (ed.), *One-Way Street*, 261–79, London: Verso.

Benjamin, W. (1982/2002), *The Arcades Project*, Cambridge, MA: The Belknap Press.

Berlant, L. and K. Stewart (2019), *The Hundreds*, Durham: Duke University Press.

Boin, L., A. McConnell, and P. t'Hart (2021), *Governing the Pandemic: The Politics of Navigating a Mega-Crisis*, Basingstoke: Palgrave Macmillan.

British Academy (n.d.), *The COVID Decade: Understanding the Long-Term Societal Impacts of COVID-19*, London: British Academy.

Brophy-Harmer, K. (2023), 'An "Anthropology of Whites": Race, Diversity, and Mass Observation', *Mass Observation Online* (Essays), https://www.massobservation.amdigital.co.uk.

Burgess, A. (1966/2003), 'Introduction to the 1966 Edition', in D. Defoe, *A Journal of the Plague Year*, 264–75, London: Penguin.

Buzard, J. (1997), 'Mass-Observation, Modernism, and Auto-Ethnography', *Modernism/Modernity*, 4 (3): 93–117.

Calder, A. and D. Sheridan (1984), *Speak for Yourself: A Mass-Observation Anthology*, London: Jonathan Cape.

Campsie, A. (2016), 'Mass-Observation, Left Intellectuals, and the Politics of Everyday Life', *English Historical Review*, CXXXI (548): 92–121.

Camus, A. (1947/2020), *The Plague*, London: Penguin.

Capano, G., M. Howlett, D. S. L. Jarvis, M. Ramesh, and N. Goyal (2020) 'Mobilising Policy (In)capacity to Fight COVID-19: Understanding Variations in State Responses', *Policy and Society*, 39 (3): 285–308.

Clarke, N. and C. Barnett (2023), 'Archiving the COVID-19 Pandemic in Mass Observation and Middletown', *History of the Human Sciences*, 36 (2): 3–25.

Cook, M. (2017), '"Archives of Feeling": The AIDS Crisis in Britain, 1987', *History Workshop Journal*, 83: 51–78.

Cottrell-Boyce, F. (2012), 'Forward', in H. Jennings, M.-L. Jennings, and C. Madge (eds), *Pandæmonium, 1660–1886: The Coming of the Machine As Seen by Contemporary Observers*, vii–xii, London: Icon.

Cvetkovich, A. (2003), *An Archive of Feelings: Trauma, Sexuality, and Lesbian Public Cultures*, Durham: Duke University Press.

Defoe, D. (1722/2003), *A Journal of the Plague Year*, London: Penguin.

Drury, J., H. Carter, E. Ntontis, and S. T. Guven (2021), 'Public Behaviour in Response to the COVID-19 Pandemic: Understanding the Role of Group Processes', *BJPsych Open*, 7 (1): E11.

Eiland, H. and K. McLaughlin (2002), 'Translators' Forward', in W. Benjamin and R. Tiedemann (eds), *The Arcades Project*, ix–xiv, Cambridge, MA: The Belknap Press.

Enright, A. (2022), 'My Mother Considered it a Dirty Text, but This Profoundly Democratic Book has Liberated Female Irish Authors', *The Guardian*, 29 January.

Erni, J. N. and T. Striphas (2021), 'Introduction: COVID-19, the Multiplier', *Cultural Studies*, 35 (2–3): 211–37.

Fancourt, D., A. Steptoe, and L. Wright (2020), 'The Cummings Effect: Politics, Trust, and Behaviours During the COVID-19 Pandemic', *The Lancet*, 396: 464–5.

Farrar, J. (2021), *Spike: The Virus vs the People*, London: Profile.

Featherstone, M. and C. Venn (2006), 'Problematising Global Knowledge and the New Encyclopedia Project', *Theory, Culture, and Society*, 23 (2–3): 1–20.

Freedman, L. (2020), 'Strategy for a Pandemic: The UK and COVID-19', *Survival*, 62 (3): 25–76.

Garfield, S. (2005), *Our Hidden Lives: The Remarkable Diaries of Post-War Britain*, London: Ebury Press.

Geertz, C. (1993), *The Interpretation of Cultures: Selected Essays*, London: HarperCollins.

Grover, J. Z. (1987), 'AIDS: Keywords', *October*, 43: 17–30.

Gumbrecht, H. U. (1997), *In 1926: Living at the Edge of Time*, Cambridge, MA: Harvard University Press.

Hall, S. M. (2020), 'Revisiting Geographies of Social Reproduction: Everyday Life, the Endotic, and the Infra-Ordinary', *Area*, 52: 812–19.

Harrison, R. (2014), 'Observing, Collecting, and Governing "Ourselves" and "Others": Mass-Observation's Fieldwork *Agencements*', *History and Anthropology*, 25 (2): 227–45.

Harrisson, T., H. Jennings, and C. Madge (1937), 'Anthropology at Home', *New Statesman and Nation*, 30 (January): 155.

Hennessy, P. (2022), *A Duty of Care: Britain Before and After Corona*, London: Allen Lane.

Highmore, B. (2002a), *Everyday Life and Cultural Theory: An Introduction*, London: Routledge.

Highmore, B. (2002b), *The Everyday Life Reader*, London: Routledge.

Highmore, B. (2023), '"The Observation by Everyone of Everyone": The Project of Mass-Observation in 1937', in J. J. Purcell (ed.), *Mass-Observation: Text, Context, and Analysis of the Pioneering Pamphlet and Movement*, 7–28, London: Bloomsbury.

Hinton, J. (2010), *Nine Wartime Lives: Mass-Observation and the Making of the Modern Self*, Oxford: Oxford University Press.

Hinton, J. (2013), *The Mass Observers: A History, 1937–1949*, Oxford: Oxford University Press.

Horton, R. (2021), *The COVID-19 Catastrophe*, 2nd edn, Cambridge: Polity.

House of Commons Health and Social Care, and Science and Technology Committees (2021), *Coronavirus: Lessons Learned to Date*, London: House of Commons.

Hubble, N. (2010), *Mass Observation and Everyday Life: Culture, History, Theory*, Basingstoke: Palgrave Macmillan.

Jardine, B. (2018), 'Mass-Observation, Surrealist Sociology, and the Bathos of Paperwork', *History of the Human Sciences*, 31 (5): 52–79.

Jeffery, T. (1978), *Mass Observation: A Short History*, Birmingham: University of Birmingham Centre for Contemporary Cultural Studies.

References

Jennings, H. (1985/2012), *Pandæmonium, 1660–1886: The Coming of the Machine As Seen by Contemporary Observers*, London: Icon.

Jennings, H. and C. Madge (1937/1987), *May the Twelfth: Mass-Observation Day-Surveys 1937*, London: Faber and Faber.

Jennings, M.-L. (2012), 'Humphrey Jennings and This Book', in H. Jennings, M.-L. Jennings, and C. Madge (eds), *Pandæmonium, 1660–1886: The Coming of the Machine As Seen by Contemporary Observers*, xx–xxviii, London: Icon.

Johnson, J. (1993), 'Introduction', in J. Joyce, *Ulysses*, ix–xxxvii, Oxford: Oxford University Press.

Joyce, J. (1922/1993), *Ulysses*, Oxford: Oxford University Press.

Judt, T. (2020), 'Afterword', in A. Camus, *The Plague*, 243–53, London: Penguin.

Kramer, A.-M. (2014), 'The Observers and the Observed: The "Dual Vision" of the Mass Observation Project', *Sociological Research Online*, 19 (3): 226–36.

Krastev, I. (2020), *Is It Tomorrow Yet? Paradoxes of the Pandemic*, London: Allen Lane.

Kushner, T. (2004), *We Europeans? Mass-Observation, 'Race', and British Identity in the Twentieth Century*, Aldershot: Ashgate.

Langhamer, C. (2016), 'An Archive of Feeling? Mass Observation and the Mid-century Moment', *Insights*, 9 (4): 1–15.

Lefebvre, H. (1981/2014), *Critique of Everyday Life: The One-Volume Edition*, London: Verso.

Lowenthal, M. (2010), 'Translator's Afterword', in G. Perec, *An Attempt at Exhausting a Place in Paris*, 49–54, Cambridge, MA: Wakefield Press.

MacClancy, J. (1995), 'The Meeting, in Mass-Observation, of British Surrealism and Popular Anthropology', *The Journal of the Royal Anthropological Institute*, 1 (3): 495–512.

Madge, C. and T. Harrisson (1937), *Mass-Observation*, London: Frederick Muller.

Madge, C. and T. Harrisson (1938/2009), *First Year's Work, 1937–1938*, London: Faber and Faber.

Madge, C. and T. Harrisson (1939/2009), *Britain*, London: Faber and Faber.

Malinowski, B. (1938/2009), 'A Nation-Wide Intelligence Service', in C. Madge and T. Harrisson (eds), *First Year's Work, 1937–1938*, 81–121, London: Faber and Faber.

Marcus, L. (2001), 'Introduction: The Project of Mass-Observation', *New Formations*, 44: 5–20.

Matless, D. (2015), *The Regional Book*, Axminster: Uniformbooks.

McFarlane, C. (2021), *Fragments of the City: Making and Remaking Urban Worlds*, Oakland: University of California Press.

Murray, P., K. Munro, S. Taylor, and R. Moffitt (2020), 'Note to Self: A Pandemic is a Great Time to Keep a Diary, Plus 4 Tips for Success', *The Conversation*, 30 August.

Perec, G. (1973/2020), 'Approaches to What?', in G. Perec, *Brief Notes on the Art and Manner of Arranging One's Books*, 30–3, London: Penguin.

Perec, G. (1974/2008), *Species of Spaces and Other Pieces*, London: Penguin.

Perec, G. (1975/2010), *An Attempt at Exhausting a Place in Paris*, Cambridge, MA: Wakefield Press.

Perec, G. (1978/2008), *Life: A User's Manual*, London: Vintage.

Phillips, R. (2018), 'George Perec's Experimental Fieldwork; Perecquian Fieldwork', *Social and Cultural Geography*, 19 (2): 171–91.

Pile, S. and N. Thrift (2002), *City A-Z*, London: Routledge.

Pocock, D. (1987), 'Afterword', in H. Jennings and C. Madge (eds), *May the Twelfth: Mass-Observation Day-Surveys 1937*, 415–23, London: Faber and Faber.

Pollen, A. (2014), 'Shared Ownership and Mutual Imaginaries: Researching Research in Mass Observation', *Sociological Research Online*, 19 (3): 214–25.

Pollen, A. (2020), *Mass Photography: Collective Histories of Everyday Life*, London: Routledge.

Pollen, A. (2023), '"There is Nothing Less Spectacular Than a Pestilence": Picturing the Pandemic in Mass Observation's COVID-19 Collections', *History of the Human Sciences*, 36 (2): 71–104.

Reicher, S. and J. Drury (2021), 'Pandemic Fatigue? How Adherence to COVID-19 Regulations has been Misrepresented and Why it Matters', *BMJ*, 372: n137.

Savage, M. (2010), *Identities and Social Change in Britain Since 1940: The Politics of Method*, Oxford: Oxford University Press.

Schlögel, K. (2023), *The Soviet Century: Archaeology of a Lost World*, Princeton: Princeton University Press.

Sheridan, D. (2009), *Wartime Women: A Mass Observation Anthology*, London: Weidenfeld and Nicolson.

Sheridan, D., B. Street, and D. Bloome (2000), *Writing Ourselves: Mass-Observation and Literary Practices*, Cresskill: Hampton Press.

Showalter, E. (1992), 'Introduction', in V. Woolf, *Mrs Dalloway*, xi–xlix, London, Penguin.

Spinney, L. (2018), *Pale Rider: The Spanish Flu of 2018 and How it Changed the World*, London: Vintage.

Sturrock, J. (2008), 'Introduction', in G. Perec and J. Sturrock (ed.), *Species of Spaces and Other Pieces*, ix–xvii, London: Penguin.

Terkel, S. (1970/2004), *Working: People Talk About What They Do All Day and How They Feel About What They Do*, New York: The New Press.

Tiedemann, R. (1988/2002), 'Dialectics at a Standstill', in W. Benjamin and R. Tiedemann (ed.), *The Arcades Project*, 929–45, Cambridge, MA: Harvard University Press.

Trebitsch, M. (2014), 'Preface', in H. Lefebvre, *Critique of Everyday Life: The One-Volume Edition*, 5–24, London: Verso.

Wall, C. (2003), 'Introduction', in D. Defoe, *A Journal of the Plague Year*, xvii–xxxiii, London: Penguin.

Williams, R. (1976), *Keywords: A Vocabulary of Culture and Society*, London: Croom Helm.

Williams, R. (1977), *Marxism and Literature*, Oxford: Oxford University Press.

Wilson-Kovaks, D. (2014), '"Clearly Necessary", "Wonderful", and "Engrossing"? Mass Observation Correspondents Discuss Forensic Technologies', *Sociological Research Online*, 19 (3): 161–76.

Woolf, V. (1925/1992), *Mrs Dalloway*, London: Penguin.

GENERAL INDEX

INDEX OF DIARISTS